Human Behavior, Learning, and the Developing Brain

TYPICAL DEVELOPMENT

EDITED BY

Donna Coch
Kurt W. Fischer
Geraldine Dawson

THE GUILFORD PRESS
New York   London

In memory of
Patricia S. Goldman-Rakic, a pioneer

For those who provided inspiration and support
—D. C.

To my children—
Seth, Johanna, Lukas, and Kara
—K. W. F.

To Blake, Colin, and Ellie

© 2007 The Guilford Press
A Division of Guilford Publications, Inc.
72 Spring Street, New York, NY 10012
www.guilford.com

Paperback edition 2010

Printed in the United States of America

This book is printed on acid-free paper.

Last digit is print number: 9 8 7 6 5 4 3 2

Library of Congress Cataloging-in-Publication Data

Human behavior, learning, and the developing brain. Typical development / edited by Donna Coch, Kurt W. Fischer, Geraldine Dawson.
   p. ; cm.
Includes bibliographical references and index.
ISBN 978-1-59385-136-1 (hardcover : alk. paper)
ISBN 978-1-60623-968-1 (paperback : alk. paper)
   1. Cognitive neuroscience.   I. Coch, Donna.   II. Fischer, Kurt W.   III. Dawson, Geraldine.   IV. Title: Typical development.
   [DNLM: 1. Behavior—physiology. 2. Adolescent. 3. Brain—growth & development. 4. Child. 5. Infant. 6. Learning—physiology.
7. Psychophysiology. WS 105 H918 2007]
   RJ506.D47H863   2007
   618.92′89142—dc22

                                                        2007004332

About the Editors

Donna Coch, EdD, is Assistant Professor in the Department of Education at Dartmouth College. She earned a doctoral degree from the Harvard University Graduate School of Education and conducted postdoctoral research at the University of Oregon. Using a noninvasive brain wave recording technique, Dr. Coch's research focuses on what happens in the brain as children learn how to read, particularly in terms of phonological and orthographic processing. A goal of both her research and teaching is to make meaningful connections between the fields of developmental cognitive neuroscience and education.

Kurt W. Fischer, PhD, is Charles Bigelow Professor of Education and Human Development at the Harvard University Graduate School of Education and founder and director of the program in Mind, Brain, and Education. He studies cognitive and emotional development from birth through adulthood, combining analysis of the commonalities across people with the diversity of pathways of learning and development. Dr. Fischer's studies concern students' learning and problem solving, brain development, concepts of self in relationships, cultural contributions to social-cognitive development, reading skills, emotions, and child abuse. One product of Dr. Fischer's research is a single scale for measuring learning, teaching, and curriculum across domains, which is being used to assess and coordinate key aspects of pedagogy and assessment in schools. He is the author of several books as well as over 200 scientific articles. Leading an international movement to connect biology and cognitive science to education, Dr.

Fischer is founding president of the International Mind, Brain, and Education Society and the new journal *Mind, Brain, and Education.*

Geraldine Dawson, PhD, is Professor of Psychology at the University of Washington, where she is also Director of the Autism Center. She has had an active career as a scientist and clinician specializing in autism and the effects of experience on early brain development, and is internationally recognized for her pioneering research on early diagnosis and brain function in autism and early biological risk factors for psychopathology. Dr. Dawson has published over 125 scientific articles and chapters on these topics, and edited or authored a number of books, including *Autism: Nature, Diagnosis, and Treatment* (1989), *Human Behavior and the Developing Brain* (1994), and *A Parent's Guide to Asperger Syndrome and High-Functioning Autism: How to Meet the Challenges and Help Your Child Thrive* (2002), all published by The Guilford Press. She has been the recipient of continuous research funding from the National Institutes of Health for her studies on autism and child psychopathology.

Contributors

Denise R. Adkins, PhD, Department of Psychology, Shippensburg University, Shippensburg, Pennsylvania. Her research focuses on individual differences in the development of attention, working memory, and inhibitory control during middle childhood.

Martha Ann Bell, PhD, Department of Psychology, Virginia Polytechnic Institute and State University, Blacksburg, Virginia. Her research focuses on individual differences in frontal lobe development during infancy and childhood, with an emphasis on electrophysiology and cognition.

Gal Ben-Yehudah, PhD, Departments of Psychology and Neuroscience, Learning Research and Development Center, University of Pittsburgh, Pittsburgh, Pennsylvania. Her research focuses on the neural correlates of reading and working memory and the relationships between these cognitive functions. Dr. Ben-Yehudah is interested in applying findings from her research to advance literacy and learning.

James R. Booth, PhD, Department of Communication Sciences and Disorders, Northwestern University, and Department of Radiology, Evanston Northwestern Healthcare, Evanston, Illinois. His research focuses on the neural bases of learning and development, with a particular focus on reading, language, attention, and inhibition.

James P. Byrnes, PhD, Department of Psychological Studies in Education, College of Education, Temple University, Philadelphia, Pennsylvania. His research focuses on the development of decision-making skills and on explaining individual, gender, and ethnic differences in achievement.

Julie A. Fiez, PhD, Departments of Psychology and Neuroscience, Learning Research and Development Center, University of Pittsburgh, Pittsburgh, Pennsylvania. Her research focuses on the neural basis of language processing and reading, as well as the neural basis of reward and motivation.

Kurt W. Fischer, PhD (See "About the Editors.")

Jay N. Giedd, MD, Brain Imaging Unit, Child Psychiatry Branch, National Institute of Mental Health, Bethesda, Maryland. His research focuses on the relationship among genes, brain, and behavior in healthy development and in neuropsychiatric disorders of childhood onset.

Mary Helen Immordino-Yang, EdD, Brain and Creativity Institute and Rossier School of Education, University of Southern California, Los Angeles, California. Her research interests focus on the intersection of neuroscience and education, especially on the developmental and neurological relations among cognition, emotion, and language, and on the neurological bases of social emotions.

Mark H. Johnson, PhD, Centre for Brain and Cognitive Development, School of Psychology, Birkbeck, University of London, London, England. His research focuses on brain and cognitive development in human infants and other species.

Jerome Kagan, PhD, Department of Psychology, Harvard University, Cambridge, Massachusetts. His research focuses on human temperament.

Rhoshel K. Lenroot, MD, Brain Imaging Unit, Child Psychiatry Branch, National Institute of Mental Health, Bethesda, Maryland. Her research focuses on the relationship among genes, brain, and behavior in healthy development and in neuropsychiatric disorders of childhood onset.

Debra L. Mills, PhD, Department of Psychology, Emory University, Atlanta, Georgia. She uses the event-related potential technique to study how the organization of the brain changes during the course of language development, including the role of experience in setting up cerebral specializations for different aspects of language processing in typical and atypical populations.

Seth D. Pollak, PhD, Department of Psychology, Psychiatry, and Pediatrics and Waisman Center for Human Development, University of Wisconsin at Madison, Madison, Wisconsin. His research focuses on the biological mechanisms underlying children's emotional development and risk for psychopathology, with special emphasis on the effects of early adversity and biobehavioral plasticity.

Sidney J. Segalowitz, PhD, Department of Psychology, Brock University, Ontario, Canada. His research focuses on the control of attention and working memory across development and the maturation of the prefrontal cortex as indexed by the electroencephalogram and event-related potentials.

Elizabeth A. Sheehan, MA, doctoral candidate in the Department of Psychology, Emory University, Atlanta, Georgia. Her research focuses on language development and understanding how children increase their communicative competence through their interactions with others.

Nancy Snidman, PhD, Department of Psychology, Harvard University, Cambridge, Massachusetts and Judge Baker Children's Center, Boston, Massachusetts. Her research focuses on human temperament.

Linda Patia Spear, PhD, Department of Psychology and Center for Developmental Psychobiology, Binghamton University, Binghamton, New York. Her areas of research include adolescent sensitivity to ethanol; the neurobiology of risk taking; and the contribution of adolescent-relevant motivational strategies, alcohol/drug use, and peer affiliations to risk taking, impulsivity, and other problem behaviors of adolescents.

Sara Jane Webb, PhD, Department of Psychiatry and Behavioral Sciences, Center on Human Development and Disability, and UW Autism Center, University of Washington, Seattle, Washington. She uses multiple neuroimaging and behavioral methods to examine the development of information processing and memory in individuals with autism spectrum disorders and typical development, focusing on the neurobiological bases of social perception and motivation, visual feature binding, and cortical connectivity.

Alison B. Wismer Fries, MS, doctoral candidate in clinical psychology, University of Wisconsin at Madison, Madison, Wisconsin. Her research focuses on understanding the mechanisms through which early adverse experiences of maltreatment influence later social and emotional development in children, as well as increase risk for psychopathology.

Christy D. Wolfe, PhD, Department of Psychology, University of Louisville, Louisville, Kentucky. Her research focuses on individual differences in the development of working memory and inhibitory control during early childhood.

Preface

Just over a decade ago, in one of the first books to gather together chapters on brain–behavior connections in human development, it was noted that "a new era ha[d] emerged from the wedding of two fields of inquiry, developmental psychology and developmental neurobiology" (Dawson & Fischer, 1994, p. xiii). In the years since this new era first emerged, there has been a veritable explosion of innovative research and findings in a newborn field encompassing developmental, cognitive, social, and emotional neuroscience research in context. In this volume, we selectively highlight some of the central research and theory shaping this interdisciplinary field that is focused on the connections among brain science, cognitive science, and behavioral science in human development and learning.

Investigators in this new field have the common goal of scientifically exploring the development of brain–behavior relations in both typically- and atypically-developing populations (see also the companion volume, *Human Behavior, Learning, and the Developing Brain: Atypical Development*). Here, we focus on human functional brain development from infancy through adolescence, as indexed by both cross-sectional and longitudinal measures of change. Furthermore, development is investigated at multiple levels of analysis, including the neurophysiological, behavioral, sociocultural, and contextual—from molecules of neurotransmitters at the synaptic gap to complex learned behaviors, such as reading a printed word in a classroom environment. Indeed, one hallmark of this new approach to a scientific understanding of the development of the whole child in context is the integration of multiple sources of information at many different levels, yielded from varied research methods ranging from the traditional (e.g., child interviews and standardized tests) to the innovative (e.g., functional magnetic resonance imaging and diffusion tensor imaging with children and adolescents).

Although translations between and across these levels of analysis are often not transparent, many investigators in this new field are concerned with the practical application of research findings to developmental, educational contexts; thus, the terms *mind, brain, and education, educational neuroscience,* and *brain science and education* have been used to describe a new, interdisciplinary science of learning. One goal of this volume is to highlight the potential connections between neuroscientific research on cognitive, social, and emotional development and education and intervention programs, particularly in terms of the future for this emerging discipline. Although the words *translation* and *application* are often used to describe a potentially fruitful cross-disciplinary connection, in many cases the direct translation and application of scientific findings into the classroom may await future advances. Presently, the endeavor to build a multifaceted understanding of human development and learning may serve researchers, educators, and policymakers more indirectly through building a shared, usable, foundational knowledge base, as represented in this book.

PLAN OF THE BOOK

The chapters in this book are organized into three sections. The first section provides a framework for understanding the new science of mind, brain, and education in terms of history, method, and theory. The second section focuses on the developing brain and behavior in infancy and toddlerhood, and the third section focuses on the developing brain and behavior in school-age children and adolescents.

History, Method, and Theory

Sidney J. Segalowitz opens with a chapter offering both a historical and a contemporary perspective on the relation between the fields of neuroscience and developmental psychology. He traces some of the reasons for developmental psychology's historical difficulty in embracing the issues of brain development and explains why this situation is now changing and why we can expect a more productive blending of the two fields. Provocatively, he uses the central Piagetian concept of constructivism as an illustration of the possibility of fruitful integration between brain and developmental sciences. Segalowitz claims that in order to have a brain that is involved in its own construction, experience must influence the maturational path of the human brain across a lifetime, and some subset of these influences must be accessible to mental manipulation by the individual by means of conscious choices. He shows that contemporary developmental neuroscience has yielded data that are consistent with the notion that the human brain is indeed involved in its own construction, demonstrating the interdisciplinary blending that is characteristic of a new science of learning and development.

The chapter that follows directly addresses the potential relevance of neuroscientific findings to educational practice and policy. In this chapter, James P. Byrnes takes a measured approach and cautions that evidence from neuroscience research is only one piece of the learning and development puzzle. Byrnes argues that neuroscience may be particularly helpful in understanding learning and development in terms of componential analysis and illustrates this point by reviewing findings from the fields of learning and memory, attention, and math skills. He closes his chapter with an interesting and worrisome review of how neuroscience findings have been "translated" into the educational world in the past, a convincing argument for improving scientific and neuroscience literacy for both educators and policymakers and for increasing educational literacy for researchers.

In the next chapter, Rhoshel K. Lenroot and Jay N. Giedd present magnetic resonance imaging (MRI) data from an ongoing cross-sectional and longitudinal study designed to chart anatomical trajectories of brain development. These impressive data, based on over 3,500 scans from 1,800 participants, clearly illustrate the heterochronicity of gray matter development—different brain regions develop at different rates and times—and more linear, less variable progressive development of white matter from age 4 to age 25. These data also show consistent gender differences, but simultaneously highlight the vast individual variability in typical brain development across the childhood and adolescent years. Although the central data are purely structural, Lenroot and Giedd do offer some provocative speculation regarding possible connections to functional brain development.

In the next chapter, Mary Helen Immordino-Yang and Kurt W. Fischer make the connections between behavior and brain development even more explicit while focusing on the complementary roles of the two cerebral hemispheres in development and learning. In a tripartite chapter, the authors first outline the dynamic skills theory of cyclical growth in brain and behavior development, reviewing evidence for discontinuities in development that mark reorganizations in neural and behavioral systems and noting a recurrent global right-to-left hemispheric cycle of development. Next, they review evidence for a similar right-to-left hemispheric shift in the specific domain of learning music. Finally, they present data from two hemispherectomized boys that further highlight the roles of the cerebral hemispheres and the complexities of developmental research. In the authors' view, this theory and these findings serve as a starting point for the creation of more complex studies of learning and development that take into account, among other factors, the cyclical nature of these processes; the organizing influences of the environment, experience, emotion, and cultural support; and the roles of the cerebral hemispheres and other brain regions.

The Developing Brain and Behavior in Infancy and Toddlerhood

To open the next section, Mark H. Johnson highlights the challenge of relating brain and behavioral development, framing three different theoretical approaches: maturational, skill learning, and interactive specialization. In the context of the development of the social brain in infancy, he reviews behavioral and neuroimaging evidence from face perception, eye gaze, and the perception of action and biological motion that is, for the most part, consistent with the interactive specialization approach. In this view, functional brain development involves the organization of patterns of interactions among cortical regions, with an outcome of increasing specialization over time. It appears that experience with the environment in terms of early social interactions during infancy is a critical factor in the eventual development of specialized processing for salient social information.

In the next chapter, Sara Jane Webb reviews a large body of literature on memory development, drawing on adult, nonhuman primate, lesion, and infant and child behavioral and electrophysiological (event-related potential) data. She notes the critical role of memory in many aspects of human development and focuses on behavioral and neuroimaging studies of novelty preference, familiarity, and recognition memory, charting the early developmental time courses for these different aspects of the memory system. She highlights studies of brain–behavior relations and convincingly argues that the systems involved in remembering in the infant may not be the same systems involved in remembering in the adult.

In Chapter 7, Debra L. Mills and Elizabeth A. Sheehan take a close look at how the brain becomes specialized for processing language across developmental time. The chapter reviews a series of event-related potential studies with infants and adults designed to investigate how brain activity in response to linguistic stimuli might be associated with chronological age, linguistic experience, and proficiency. The authors present electrophysiological data indicating that lateralization of brain activity to spoken words changes during development and discuss the functional significance of these observed changes, using data from monolingual and bilingual infants, children, and adults to build their arguments. In addition, the authors discuss the possible roles of both language-specific and domain-general processes in the development of vocabulary. Finally, they comment on the potentially powerful role of educational experience in the development of language skills and related neurocognitive networks.

In the chapter on temperament and biology that follows, Jerome Kagan and Nancy Snidman provide an overview of their longitudinal work, tracing potential biological and behavioral markers of human temperamental categories. In addition, they provide a fascinating array of evidence corroborating the theoretically central role of the amygdala in the temperamental types of high-reactive and low-reactive. Moreover, they repeatedly emphasize the value of multiple sources of evidence and the complex interaction of biology and environment in both behavior and brain development related to temperament, echoing central themes in the new science of learning and development.

Martha Ann Bell, Christy D. Wolfe, and Denise R. Adkins close this section with a chapter integrating current knowledge about working memory and inhibitory control in relation to language and temperament by focusing on frontal lobe development during infancy and early childhood. In infants, these authors report that performance on a looking working memory task is related to electroencephalogram (EEG) recordings and individual differences in temperament. In early childhood, they report connections between performance on other working memory/inhibitory control tasks (the day–night and yes–no tasks) and EEG recorded at medial frontal sites, aspects of temperament, and language comprehension ability. In the same children at 8 years old, performance on another working memory/inhibitory control task (Wisconsin Card Sort) is related to right frontal EEG activity and child-reported temperament. Longitudinally, Bell, Wolfe, and Adkins have found that infant and child measures of EEG and of temperament are correlated, whereas infant and child measures of working memory/inhibitory control skills are not; however, infant temperament appears to be a predictor of working memory/inhibitory control ability. This fascinating chapter begins to characterize the complexity of brain–behavior relations in the early development of working memory and inhibitory control skills.

The Developing Brain and Behavior in School-Age Children and Adolescents

The final section begins with a chapter on reading, a topic central to education and a topic for which there is a growing body of evidence linking brain and behavior. James R. Booth reviews the complexities of the developing language and reading system in the human brain, focusing on orthographic processing in the fusiform gyrus, phonological processing in the superior temporal region, semantic processing in the middle temporal gyrus, and syntactic processing in the inferior frontal gyrus. He also highlights the role of the inferior parietal cortex in developing automaticity in reading skills and the top-down influence of the prefrontal cortex; he illustrates that dynamic causal modeling, used to investigate the patterns of effective connectivity among brain regions, confirms the modulatory role of the inferior frontal gyrus. Discussing processes of elaboration and specialization and methods for determining effective connectivity, Booth outlines the developmental course of language and reading systems.

Next, Gal Ben-Yehudah and Julie A. Fiez provide a review of current knowledge about the development of verbal working memory, integrating information from theory, behavioral studies, and neuroimaging investigations. As they chart the developmental course of verbal working memory across the preschool and early elementary school years, both behaviorally and neurally, they begin to build a convincing argument for a specific connection among speech production, reading, and verbal working memory skills. It appears likely that the common thread is the development of fine-grained phonological representations. The authors conclude that some changes in verbal working memory may be due to structural maturation, but other changes may be due to literacy; that is, literacy may play an important role in developing verbal working memory skills.

In the next chapter, summarizing much of what is currently known about emotion processing and the developing brain, Alison D. Wismer Fries and Seth D. Pollak build a preliminary developmental model of emotion processing, including descriptions of the biological and environmental mechanisms involved in early sensory processing related to the perception of change, attention to emotionally relevant and salient information, integration with stored associations, and generation of a behavioral response. Consistent with the new, interdisciplinary approach to understanding human development, the model is informed by multiple sources of evidence, including behavioral, cognitive, and neuroimaging work with humans and animals. The authors note the preliminary nature of the model and the need for more research, particularly with regard to the complex interconnectivity of the neural systems involved in socioemotional processing and the complexity of emotional behavior in context across developmental time.

In the closing chapter, Linda Patia Spear deftly reviews a large and wide-ranging literature on adolescent development in humans and other species. She presents an evolutionary argument regarding many typical adolescent behaviors, including a changing focus for social behaviors; changing eating and sleeping habits; changes in cognition and reward sensitivity; and changing affect regulation, risk-taking, and novelty-seeking behaviors. At the same time, she offers a neurobiological explanation, discussing puberty, hormonal changes, and especially brain changes that characterize adolescence. She weaves together these strands to clearly illustrate the complexity of adolescent behavior and development, influenced not only by brain and biology, but also by evolution, experience, and environment. She closes with the provocative speculation that the normal processes of brain development during adolescence, usually considered in a negative light, may actually provide a "unique window of opportunity" during which education and enrichment experiences may have "ameliorative or protective influences on the maturing adolescent."

REFERENCE

Dawson, G. D., & Fischer, K. W. (Eds.). (1994). *Human behavior and the developing brain*. New York: Guilford Press.

Contents

PART III. The Developing Brain and Behavior in School-Age Children and Adolescents

PART I

HISTORY, METHOD, AND THEORY

The Role of Neuroscience in Historical and Contemporary Theories of Human Development

Sidney J. Segalowitz

For much of the last century, developmental psychology has had an ambivalent partnership with the neurosciences. Although these two disciplines coexist in the same university departments, the same textbooks, and even occasionally the same undergraduate courses, the tentative marriage has been one filled with sudden flirtations followed by the disillusionment of long-term incompatibility. Developmentalists who are not themselves physiologically oriented have accepted the notion that understanding the brain can have some clinical utility, that it can impress the general public (because the medical sciences are always headline-worthy topics), and that it has an ever-increasing place in textbooks claiming to be complete. However, there had been little in classic developmental theories that really owed anything *specifically* to an understanding of the brain and its developmental growth patterns. Brain mechanisms relating to behaviors might be used to bolster the arguments for some psychological constructs, but these mechanisms have often been treated as circumstantial evidence only. However, developmental neuroscience has progressed enough recently that we are now in an era when knowledge of brain–behavior relations can contribute to developmental psychology. The fields of developmental neuropsychology (clinical fields and developmental cognitive and affective studies of brain function, utilizing primarily behavioral measures) and developmental cognitive neuroscience (basic research, mostly with animals, involving cognitive or learning functions)—the disciplines that relate brain growth to behavior in a developmental context—can be usefully informative to developmental psychology and can drive developmental theory. Although much of this crossover is rooted in the study of interactions between genes and experience (e.g., Caspi et al., 2002), there is also a growing trend to relate macromorphological brain characteristics to psychological development—themes that are covered in detail elsewhere in this volume. However, it is with standard neuroscience advancements that we can see a major integration. Somewhat ironically, this integration includes Piaget's concept of constructivism, which captures the major historical controversies in developmental psychology and which he devised because he perceived such integration as not possible.

The field has been at this threshold before, and we may wonder what happened to the promising integration of developmental psychology and brain maturation that seemed ready to flourish in the 1920s and 1930s. This review presents some of the reasons for developmental psychology's historical difficulty in embracing the issue of brain maturation during the last century, why it is currently changing, and how we can look for a fruitful blending of the two fields in the future, the evidence for which comprises the rest of this volume.

WHAT IS A "NEUROPSYCHOLOGY OF DEVELOPMENT" AND HAVE WE ALWAYS HAD ONE?

Psychology in the modern era has always been based on the notion that the brain is the organ of the mind, and psychologists have often made reference to reputed neurological mechanisms. More recently, developmental neuroscience has flourished with advances in brain imaging technologies and now includes many findings about human brain development. Traditionally, however, developmental neuroscience dealt almost exclusively with nonhuman brain development, and indeed there were very few comprehensive data sets concerning human cortical development, with the exception of Conel's (1939–1967). This early but limited developmental neuroscience work could not directly relate brain development to behavioral development due to a lack of appropriate technology and paradigms, and therefore links between brain anatomy and human psychological development were based on whatever speculation seemed reasonable at the time.

Sometimes this linkage was naive in the extreme, and sometimes it was impressively insightful, but in all cases it rested primarily on conjecture.

For the purposes of this chapter, I define a "neuropsychology of development" as a specification of possible brain correlates of developmental constructs; this we could refer to as a "physiology of development." Physiological reductionist positions—such as Burbank's (1909) Lamarckian treatment of child development and de Crinis's (1932) histological explanation of development (the latter is described further below)—were very popular a century ago. But such anatomical and physiological description is neither necessary nor sufficient for developmental psychology, even if the facts involved are correct. Knowing that a given psychological characteristic leads to a specific outcome is complemented by knowing the brain correlates of the characteristic and the outcome, but this knowledge does not by itself advance developmental theory. This theoretical advancement can only be accomplished if there is information about those brain correlates that can be used to inform the developmental theory rather than just correlate with or corroborate that theory. Physiological correlates in themselves are fascinating, may be useful clinically, and are prerequisites to constructing theories that, in the end, will bring psychological and neurological development together. However, they are not a prerequisite to developmental theory. For example, although Freud was a neurologist by training, he did not insist that psychological development from id to ego to superego had to involve physical maturation of specific brain areas, although presumably he would have been delighted to be able to specify some. Whether he would think that current attempts really have furthered his approach (e.g., Solms, 2004) is an open question.

In discussing neuropsychological development, we cannot avoid discussing the notion of maturation—a concept that has bothered many developmental psychologists because it is often interpreted as having reductionist implications. In fact, Piaget struggled with this concept, invoking it to account for cognitive development (Piaget, 1930/1960) yet later clearly opposing simple reductionism (Piaget, 1947/1966). A contemporary text defines maturation as "a sequence of changes that are strongly influenced by genetic inheritance and that occur as individuals grow old" (Cole & Cole, 2001, p. 34). This definition reflects accurately how the word is used today in general and in the field of psychology specifically. However, it omits the somewhat subtler view of the interplay between nature and nurture proposed 70 years ago, which still emphasizes inborn influences on development but focuses also on the dynamic aspects, whereby "growth is a process so intricate and so sensitive that there must be powerful stabilizing factors, intrinsic rather than extrinsic, which preserve the balance of the total pattern and the direction of the growth trend. Maturation is . . . a name for this regulatory mechanism" (Gesell, 1933, p. 232). Although one must see biological factors in such regulatory mechanisms, this approach to maturation is actually more in line with very contemporary discoveries in developmental neuroscience, and in returning to this approach, a true blending of brain science and developmental science (of nature and nurture) is possible. Gesell further outlined both maturation and development in what appears to be a highly modern perspective:

> *Maturation* is a term which has recently come to the fore in the literature of child psychology. It is not a precise and altogether indispensable term, but it has come into usage as an offset to the extravagant claims which have been made for processes of conditioning and of habit formation. In spite of some inevitable vagueness, the concept of maturation may serve, at least for a period, as a useful aid both to experimental investigation and theoretical interpretation. . . .
>
> *Development is a process* in which the mutual fitness of organism and environment is brought to progressive realization. . . . It is unnecessary to draw an absolute distinction between physical and mental developments. "They" occur in close association and may be considered basically unitary. Both express themselves in changes of form and of patterning which may be investigated from a morphological standpoint. (1933, pp. 209–210)

Unfortunately, this same author, who was so influential in developmental psychology during the first half of the 20th century, turned to emphasizing a genetic view. Although he reiterated that "growth . . . [is] a physiological process of organization which is registered in the structural and functional unity of the individual . . . a unifying concept which resolves the dualism of heredity and environment" (Gesell, 1954, p. 358), all the compelling examples he provided concerned the stability of characteristics from birth to adulthood, implying a lack of possible change due to biological restrictions and constraints.

Consistent with this definition (but not with Gesell's emphasis), in this chapter *brain maturation* refers to the physical growth of the brain in terms of general processes (e.g., dendritic expansion, myelination) and in terms of regional development (e.g., subcortical centers, various regions of the cortex), whatever their apparent origin. These characteristics are now being related to the development of specific psychological systems (e.g., language, social behavior, perception mechanisms, and executive control functions).

Beyond the foundational definitional issues, the focus of this chapter is on "grand" theories of psychological development, with an eye to how some current trends are leading to a new, somewhat eclectic integration of psychology and developmental neurophysiology in a way that did not seem possible to developmentalists up until a few decades ago. The progress in just the last decade has greatly opened up possibilities. Many of the other chapters in this book are devoted to explaining the details of these current trends; the sheer number of them places us at a very exciting time in the development of our interdisciplinary field.

A BRIEF SYNOPSIS OF THE FIRST HALF-CENTURY (1895–1946)

Freud and Baldwin

We are now a decade past the centenary of the publication of two important books, each of which represents an attempt to integrate some aspects of brain physiology and function into central concepts in developmental psychology and psychology in general. Freud (1895/1966) sketched a quasi-cell-assembly model of the brain mechanisms corresponding to processes central to his psychodynamic approach, including the underpinnings of cathexis and identification (Pribram & Gill, 1976). This exercise was certainly ambitious, and it represented the common notions of the time that the nervous system acts to reduce stimulation and that development consists only of a quantitative increase in connectivity of (the recently discovered) synapses (Holt, 1965). There was little place in Freud's framework either for an overall inhibitory mechanism that would help focus attention on internal cognitive processes (Macmillan, 1992) or for qualitative changes in brain function as a result of maturation.

Baldwin (1894/1925) also speculated on the relationship between brain function and child development, with a keen appreciation for the complexity of the central nervous system and the near impossibility of ever really accounting for the current issues in consciousness within a brain model. Both Baldwin and Freud were acutely aware of the need for progress in neuroscience before they could speak about these issues with confidence—a recurrent theme with other major developmentalists who followed them.

Freud and Baldwin, and later Piaget, had a great interest in the phylogenesis of the brain but surprisingly little interest in its ontogenesis. This bias might have reflected the fact that biological science was just coming through two tremendous intellectual revolutions: (1) Darwin's (1859/1901) theory of evolution firmly removed the assumption that biological structures are permanently fixed for all time, and (2) the rediscovery of Gregor Mendel's notion of genetic material fixed at conception placed the possibility of fluidity in phylogenesis and not ontogenesis (see Moore, 1972). Thus, Baldwin argued that brain structures do not change with growth, but their functions recombine as the child develops new skills:

[A] psychology which holds that we have a "speech faculty," an original mental endowment which is incapable of further reduction, may appeal to the latest physiological research and find organic confirmation, at least as far as a
determination of its cerebral apparatus is concerned; but such support for the
position is wanting when we return to the brain of the infant. Not only do we
fail to find the series of centres into which the organic basis of speech has been
divided, but even those of them which we do find have not taken up the function, either alone or together, which they perform when speech is actually realized. In other words, the primary object of each of the various centres involved
is not speech, but some other simpler function; and speech arises by development from a union of these separate functions. (1894/1925, pp. 6–7)

It is interesting to note the basic similarity of this position to a contemporary one on hemispheric specialization (Witelson, 1977, 1987). What is
missing is a growth model of the brain, despite this position being completely compatible with one. It is curious how firmly all the main developmental theorists held to this notion of nondevelopmental macrostructure of
the brain while the histologists were discovering the ontogenesis of the
microstructure (e.g., Ramón y Cajal, 1894) as well as major macrostructure
changes (see Noback & Moss, 1956, for a review of this period).

Carmichael and Gesell

During the 1920s and 1930s, Carmichael (1926, 1927, 1928, 1946), Gesell
(1929), and their students began to write about how the physiological maturation of the brain must be held accountable for some of the development
of skills during childhood. Their basic animal work expressed an appreciation for maturation in the growth of motor function, but the question
remained as to whether this maturation process could be extrapolated to
mental functions. Gesell, in fact, sought what we would see as a modern
integration, recognizing the paucity of the nature–nurture division:

If we manage to envisage maturation as an active physiological process, we
overcome the rather stilted antithesis of the nature-versus-nurture problem.
Galton tells us that in his day the very term *heredity* was strange. With the
advent of Mendelism the term took on popularity and became oversimplified.
Individual unit characters of inheritance were too specifically identified with
discrete chromosome particles, and heredity came to be regarded too mechani-
cally as a fixed mode of transmission. Geneticists now emphasize the fact that
these particles are chemicals which interact with each other and with many
other factors to produce the organism. And if we but knew the biochemistry
and biophysics of the interactions we should be making much less earnest use
of such words as *heredity, environment,* and *maturation.* (1933, p. 209)

This very modern-sounding attitude nevertheless was held simultaneously with rigid views about fixed traits; maturation was seen as controlled by heredity. That is, environmental factors could modify development in minor ways but could not dictate the overall structural pattern of development (Gesell, 1933). Clearly ideas were in flux, as they are today (especially with respect to how experience can influence the activation patterns of genes; see Rutter, Moffit, & Caspi, 2006, for a review). However, although feeling confident that developmental psychology must embrace a conceptual integration of brain maturation with experience in some ways, Gesell did express concern about anyone's ability to document such integration:

> The role of maturation in the higher spheres of intellectual and moral life is, on the basis of present knowledge, difficult to determine. On theoretical grounds some may even question whether the concept of maturation can be applied to these higher and more rarefied fields of behavior accessible to introspection but not to photography. *Nevertheless, if there is a general physiology of growth which governs the entire development of the individual, we may well believe that maturation maintains a role in the higher orders of thought and feeling.* (1933, pp. 223–224; emphasis added)

Piaget

Whereas Gesell remained firmly committed to a neurodevelopmental approach, Piaget took an alternate route. He appreciated the theoretical implications and complexities of the phylogenesis of the brain, and also, as he indicated later, realized that he did not have enough information about brain development and brain function to be able to articulate the role of brain maturation in child development (Piaget & Inhelder, 1966/1969). He recognized that a truly developmental theory of neuropsychology would be needed, but he seemed to have no vision of how such a theory might look (as compared to McGraw, 1946 [see below], who had such a vision but did not have a developmental theory into which to place her observations). Piaget tried to apply the principles of biological functioning in phylogeny and ontogeny to philosophical constructs such as epistemology (MacNamara, 1976), while rejecting any further involvement of physiological constructs in mental development. He maintained that such constructs are inherently nondevelopmental and that they represent "vitalism, apriorism and Gestalt: habit deriving from intelligence, habit unrelated to intelligence and habit explained, like intelligence and perception, by structurings whose laws remain independent of development" (Piaget, 1947/1966, p. 88). Piaget's view of any attempt to introduce brain factors would necessarily include only fixed characteristics. One example of this perspective is the argument that the child's sense of speed is a basic construct inherent in the structure of the retina (Piaget, 1970).

His attempt to reconcile evolutionary biology with his notion of genetic epistemology (the ontogenetic "evolution" of mind) was truly valiant (Piaget, 1947/1966). However, it still resulted in no notion of brain development, save for the idea that experience leads to further neuronal connections—a position that he, like Baldwin before him, immediately recognized as nothing more than pure associationism. This position "is scarcely upheld any longer in its pure associationist form, except for some authors, *of predominantly physiological interests*, who think they can reduce intelligence to a system of 'conditioned' responses" (Piaget, 1947/ 1966, p. 16; emphasis added).

The Integration That Slipped Away

At this point, Myrtle McGraw (1946) presented an intriguing review of the issue of maturation in child development. She argued strongly for an integration of brain growth and experience, along the lines that Carmichael and Gesell had suggested before her, with her own data focusing again on motor development, as did the others'. However, she also knew that differential cortical maturation must be necessary for some type of understanding in developmental theory and quoted an intriguing paper by de Crinis (1932) on this issue. De Crinis had mapped out histologically those cortical areas (in humans) where dendritic growth matured earlier versus later, using a technique that he claimed would reflect functional maturation and not just physical growth. This research supported the earlier speculation, derived from the data on myelin growth, that functional development is first found in sensory and motor areas and last in what we now consider to be multimodal or tertiary areas of integrative functions (Segalowitz, 1992). What is interesting is that we would recognize this pattern as fitting not only the mapping sequence of primary sensorimotor cortex to unimodal association areas to heteromodal cortex (Mesulam, 1985; Segalowitz & Schmidt, 2003), but also our current conception of stages in cognitive development. Unfortunately, de Crinis interpreted his findings in an entirely reductionist framework—a sort of "histology of the mind" that Ramón y Cajal (1894) had suggested a generation earlier, in which experience was not seen as being able to influence brain development. At the time of McGraw's paper, developmental theory (at least in the United States) was perhaps too reductionistic to be able to provide a framework for recognizing the good fit between de Crinis's maturational map and a type of developmental theory separating habit from intelligence, as Piaget would have put it.

This slippage into determinism is perhaps one of the primary reasons for the difficulties in the marriage of neuroscience and developmental psychology alluded to earlier. By focusing on single factors in development, those factors are necessarily isolated in such a way that they always appear to account for growth and therefore are deemed "causes." This erroneous conclusion reflects the fundamental methodological problem of not appreciating a multivariate model and has led historically to many of the chronic debates in developmental psychology concerning determinism, including the intertwining of political issues with developmental psychology.

The Political Ramifications

Jumping ahead in time for a moment, we see that developmental psychologists in the 1960s and 1970s often sought a nondeterministic approach, requiring inclusion of complex interacting systems in their developmental models and rejecting single sources of variance. Perhaps one goal of embracing such a general systems theory approach was to reject the radical behaviorism and biological reductionism that had been historically prominent. Many developmentalists at this time sought to put a child's consciousness in some sort of control position. The hallmark of the social movements in Western societies during the 1960s, after all, was a respect for the individual over oppressive societal systems, leading in the United States to the Civil Rights Act and special social programs for groups that were considered disadvantaged by the wider society.

It is important to keep in mind that developmental and clinical psychology are branches of the discipline that have political ramifications because, unlike other subfields, they can have direct applications to people's lives and effects on government policy. In the 1970s, theoretical issues concerning intellectual growth and variation were debated in the public forum with considerable heat. A biologically reductionist position, touted by Jensen (1969), had serious immediate implications for social policy in the United States (with respect to funding for Head Start) and Britain (with respect to immigration policy). A ruggedly deterministic, behaviorist position would similarly imply that individuals not fitting into the system are not to be respected for their differences. Thus, the two extreme deterministic approaches could be seen to contribute to a politically conservative agenda of rejecting those who do not quite conform to societal expectations. In particular, suspicions concerning the political agenda of those supporting the debate on the role of genetics in intelligence aroused strong feelings within the developmentalist community (Montagu, 1975).

For some the solution in the 1960s to avoiding these twin extremes was to embrace the Piagetian constructivist alternative, in which a child is seen as the center of his or her own growth, with a careful path being drawn that emphasizes experience over environment and "constitutional" factors over physiology. Politically, such a position was less contentious; theoretically, it moved the field away from the nature–nurture extremes without, however, integrating the two sets of factors.

Summary

The result of this half-century of mismatch between those who wanted to integrate brain maturation into a theory of child development and those who had the epistemological constructs into which such development could be placed was an abandonment of the enterprise for the time. Freud, Baldwin, and Piaget would no doubt applaud the current activity in developmental neuropsychology, but they had to work without a reliance on a construct of brain maturation. Although their writings continued to respect such an eventual alliance, their followers were often nonbiologically oriented, being nonmedically oriented psychoanalysts, behavioral psychologists, educationalists, and social and cognitive anthropologists. The genius of these theorists is shown in their ability to have gotten so far in their models of behavior and development with only analogies of biological constructs and no direct biological bases, despite their own predilections for such an approach. Gesell, despite his initial inclinations to form such an integration, was not able to marshal the evidence necessary for it. The next quarter-century saw a flourishing of such purely cognitive-behavioral work. Since then, however, we have begun to see a return to the integration so longed for by Freud, Baldwin, Carmichael, Gesell, and Piaget.

FREUD AND PIAGET IN TODAY'S NEUROPSYCHOLOGICAL CLIMATE

Before moving on to more contemporary issues, it is an interesting exercise to speculate on how Freud and Piaget might have taken advantage of today's notion of brain ontogeny, in which growth and experience are seen to complement each other in maturation (Greenough, Black, & Wallace, 1987).

Freud could have sought brain changes corresponding to the expansion of the id to ego to superego. The discovery of such brain changes would have obviated many of the processes in his theory if it could be shown that the development of the ego and superego depends on physiological maturation, perhaps in the sequence mentioned earlier, of primary sensorimotor cortex first, then unimodal association areas, and finally heteromodal cortex (Mesulam, 1985; Segalowitz & Schmidt, 2003). Whereas the details of psychological development could still be determined by life's traumas, the speed of ego and superego growth (faster in some people, slower in others) could then be attributed to other (physiological) factors. This perspective would have relieved psychodynamic theory from having to explain so much, and even from having to account for the developmental sequence at all. It may even have loosened the connection, so difficult for Freud's contemporaries, between psychosexual development in the phallic stage and the growth of the superego—a connection that led to what are seen today as astonishing claims about gender differences in superego strength.

Similarly, Piaget had to account for both change from stage to stage and the sequence of skill development. As he formulated it, the motivating energy for development is the conflict between the principle of organization (a tendency to make sense of experience) and a recalcitrant environment, producing adaptation and decentration (the push to adapt one's mental constructs to more sophisticated levels of understanding). A truly biological framework, however, would center on the development of the neural networks underpinning the skills at each stage. For example, the notion that babies develop the intellectual structures of object permanence simply from experience does not free us from having to explain what drives the timetable (if anything) and why other species seem to have other timetables. Physiological networks that are capable of performing the behaviors seen in object permanence tasks would presumably have a timetable of development that is partly dependent on physiological factors and partly on experiential factors. Diamond and Goldman-Rakic (1989) and Goldman-Rakic (1987) have tried to show that the basis for types of behavior reflecting object permanence is dependent on networks involving the dorsolateral prefrontal cortex (DLPFC; see Diamond, Werker, & Lalonde, 1994). Presumably, factors contributing to the functional development of tissue— such as dendritic elaboration, myelination, and maturation of other critical brain areas that feed information to and from the DLPFC—might account for the timetable of object permanence in a way that reduces the need to rely on the traditional sequence of sensorimotor structures as the sole cause (Jordan, 1972; Segalowitz, 1979; Segalowitz & Hiscock, 2002). A similar argument can be made, of course, for later development of formal operations. For example, evoked potential measures that are regulated by the dorsolateral prefrontal area successfully differentiate 12-year-old adolescents from adults, and those measures are related specifically to standard psychometric measures of executive control functions, but not to simpler, domain-specific cognitive functions (Segalowitz, Unsal, & Dywan, 1992; also, cf. Segalowitz & Davies, 2004; Thatcher, 1994).

In a similar vein, Scheibel (1990) suggests that his data on the pattern of early versus later dendritic growth in Broca's area in the left hemisphere reflect the later development of language (i.e., after infancy). If Piaget were alive to view these data, it seems reasonable that he would now want to consider the factor of physiological maturation rate when accounting for the timing of language. In an argument with a similar structure, Tucker (1992) provided numerous possible relations between socioemotional development and supportive brain structures. None of these physiological models denies a role for experience, because brain structure must reflect experience and learning in some way. However, such models also suggest that the structure of development must depend on brain physiology and maturation to some extent.

Although we can only speculate on what Piaget's and Freud's personal reactions would be to the kinds of suggestions being made here, they may have been extremely pleased to incorporate neural maturation models of a nonreductionist sort.

INCORPORATING THE CONSTRUCT OF BRAIN DEVELOPMENT INTO DEVELOPMENTAL THEORY

Similar to the earlier theorists discussed above, most schools of developmental psychology that flourished over the subsequent years ignored a link with brain maturation not only implicitly but also explicitly, and have supported this inattention with particular sorts of arguments. For example, although one may argue that the brain matures to some extent during the psychologically impressionable early years, these maturational changes are limited in two ways: (1) They are universal and of a general sort, so that whereas one individual may generally be more mature than another, there are no specific interactions in brain development that could account for interesting variations among children as they grow; and (2) such changes are so gradual and so small, compared to the dramatic environmental changes children encounter in early childhood, that there is little to suggest that most of the variance involved in growth could be attributable to the maturation of the brain, even including dramatic developmental milestones such as the acquisition of language. Thus, Skinner (1957) could confidently discuss language acquisition as just another learned behavior; Dollard and Miller (1950) could deal with socialization, including the metacognitive structures for mature social behavior, as simply a product of a reinforcement schedule; and Piaget (1970), of course, could describe how a child constructs higher and higher levels of cognition through assimilation and accommodation. In all these cases, the focus was on universal aspects of development—on how the broad strokes of development are the same across children—whereas individual differences are primarily nuisance factors. But the dramatic increase in interest in individual differences in development (e.g., Anastasi, 1958; Maccoby, 1966), aided greatly by physiological approaches, started to supersede these theoretical frameworks.

The status that individual differences have in growth and behavior rests on the constructs that theorists permit. If a theorist focuses on universals and does not permit any constructs that reflect differences among people, then the strength of that theory in accounting for individual differences is necessarily weak. However, in the approaches already considered, we find a variety of constructs for variability. For example, Gesell's maturational approach permits differences in the rate of growth (Gesell & Amatruda, 1941). This monolithic variable cannot account for qualitative differences among children, such as how some become more verbal, some more shy, or some more athletic. Yet, to the extent that there are general developmental structures, one could at least support a developmental psychology that includes differing rates of global maturation.

Similarly, Piaget's approach acknowledges differential rates of maturation, whether during the earlier sensorimotor period or the later operational periods. His approach, also resting on universal stages, could naturally incorporate an individual growth rate construct. However, the real engine of cognitive development for him is exposure to cognitive conflict (disequilibrium), with individual differences in the rate of growth resulting from differing experiential backgrounds simply perturbing the rate (Piaget, 1972). From a neuropsychological approach, this perspective leads to an interesting debate as to whether the Piagetian constructivist approach has subtly captured the results of some interaction between brain growth and experience (Segalowitz & Hiscock, 2002) or has, rather, described the forces *driving* those changes (Keating, 1990). I return to these ideas below.

Behaviorist theory has its own constructs for dealing with individual variation: differences in reinforcement schedules and differential stimulus–stimulus pairing. This is not the place to explore the adequacy of these notions, but one does wonder about the exceptional cases in which early talent develops in the absence of social support or even normal intellectual functioning, such as cases of children who have a level of linguistic sophistication completely at odds with their general intellectual level (Bellugi, Lichtenberger, Mills, Galaburda, & Korenberg, 1999; Obler & Fein, 1988).

A neuropsychological approach is partly compatible with all of these traditional developmental theories, with the proviso that we recognize the mind–brain isomorphism. Any mental differences must be reflected in some way by variation in brain structure and activity. Psychological development involves brain changes, just as differences across people must involve variations in brain structure and function (Bunge, 1980).

The Past 40 Years:
Lenneberg's *Biological Foundations of Language*

We can trace much of the current interest among developmental psychologists in the maturation of the brain to Eric Lenneberg's book *Biological Foundations of Language*, published in 1967. Hemispheric specialization had already aroused general interest with the popular work of the California group investigating commissurotomy patients (e.g., Gazzaniga, 1970; Sperry, 1968). Lenneberg's breakthrough involved a melding of developmental issues with brain maturation in a way that was accessible to developmental psychologists and educationalists. He proposed that the hitherto unending debate over why there seems to be a critical period for second-language (and presumably first-language) acquisition was missing a critical variable. The issue for him was not whether learning styles of children differ at various ages, but whether the left hemisphere of the brain is still adaptable enough to acquire language in adulthood and whether adaptability decreases as brain tissue becomes specialized for cognitive functions. Within 10 years of the publication of his seminal book there was a rush of activity concerning the role of brain lateralization in children's mental growth, much of it showing that some basic assumptions in Lenneberg's model were wrong, despite their widespread acceptance at the time (Kinsbourne & Hiscock, 1977; Segalowitz & Berge, 1995; Segalowitz & Gruber, 1977). However, the lasting effect of *Biological Foundations of Language* was an appreciation that there is a biological context for human mental functions, even complex ones.

Lenneberg's (1967) description of the biological basis for language was readable, it was addressed to psychologists, and it was promising as a model for a new developmental framework that was inaccessible from traditional, behaviorally oriented approaches. In historical terms, although many other influences were certainly at play simultaneously, *Biological Foundations of Language* was a critical catalyst that eventually broke through some very powerful, even political, forces in developmental psychology that resisted the incorporation of any brain construct.

An irony here is that appreciating that the brain has specific mechanisms for language (or for any other mental function) does not necessarily lead to any alteration of our conception of that mental function, except to confirm its existence. That is, our notion of how that function is structured need not change solely because of its having a biological correlate (James, 1892). Historically, however, this new approach did lead to two new appreciations. First, we expect some individual differences in mental function to take particular forms and not others, solely because of biological differences among people. Second, the brain may be seen to provide constraints on development that purely behavioral models cannot predict. The first factor concerning individual differences is historically the stronger in drawing developmental psychologists to neurophysiology, but it is the second issue that keeps them there.

Individual Differences and Mental Growth

As has been argued elsewhere (Bourgeois, 2001; Segalowitz, 1987), we must come to grips with the notion that everyone's brain does not appear to be organized in the same way. This statement sounds like a truism of a trivial sort, and some of the implications are indeed trivial. However, once we accept the notion of individual variation in, for example, cerebral specialization for language, it is not a long leap to try to conclude that some of these differences are responsible for individual differences in language or cognitive functioning. For example, Semrud-Clikeman, Hynd, Novey, and Eliopoulos (1990) provided evidence that individual differences in reading skill are related to specific anatomical brain asymmetries in children.

That individual differences in mental functioning must be at least partly due to differences in brain structure and chemistry is a concept that was appreciated by Gesell 70 years ago. However, the technologies required to document such effects within a principled, causative framework have been slow in coming. The advent of functional magnetic resonance imaging (fMRI) technologies within the last 15 years or so may mark another critical historical shift in the quest for brain–behavior connections. But it is important to sound a note of caution regarding the power of such new technologies: It is very possible that we will go too far in expecting to find large biological differences for every large difference in psychological function—something that, of course, need not be the case. For some developmentalists, the field has already gone too far in this direction.

In the past 60 years, brain growth has been invoked to account for many aspects of the child's mental development. After Sperry's dramatic findings regarding commissurotomy patients were reported and Lenneberg's book appeared in the 1960s, hemispheric specialization was in vogue as an explanatory construct for very many aspects of children's (and adults') mental attributes—in some cases beyond what the data could support. It was as if some in the community of developmentalists were eager to embrace any brain construct, even one that appeared to have only a single dimension. At the same time the dramatic developmental sequence of myelin growth was first reported (Yakovlev & Lecours, 1967), and this finding also inspired single-dimensional explanations (Konner, 1991). A few more complex models that dealt with both laterality and other regional maturational schemes were also introduced during this time period (e.g., Best, 1988). However, for much of the 1960s and 1970s, there appeared to be a return to the dichotomous thinking that had concerned Gesell in the 1930s.

Accounting for Change: Gradual or Epigenetic?

The 1960s, 1970s, and 1980s saw a return to single-factor models of development in other ways. In particular, the behavior geneticists started to have much more influence in developmental theory as they founded the twin-study paradigm that would yield intrinsically fascinating data (Burt, 1966; Eysenck, 1971; Jensen, 1969). The inherent limitations of heritability coefficients were not well known and the arguments perhaps were too complex or not yet well enough articulated to break through the consciousness of the general public (Rutter et al., 2006; Segalowitz, 1999; Wahlsten, 1990).

In addition, although Piaget's approach gained enormous popularity in North America during this period, the so-called neo-Piagetians were finding that his structuralist approach succumbed to many challenges, raising the possibility that simpler models might suffice (Case, 1991; Fischer, 1980; Gelman, 1978). Not only did the particulars of Piaget's epistemological model receive challenges, but also his whole constructivist model began to look as if it might have weak foundations. For example, if the development of representational thought did not depend on sensorimotor operations (Jordan, 1972; Segalowitz, 1979), in what sense was the child's reality self-constructed? If the development of language depended on simple maturation of tissue of the left hemisphere, then perhaps Piaget's description of how language comes to reflect concepts was just that—a vivid description but not an explanation.

A constructivist perspective such as Piaget's emphasizes the general reasoning skills underlying concrete problem solving. For example, a child's performance on problems of the Tower of Hanoi sort (i.e., moving a size-ordered set of rings from one post to another post, one at a time, without ever placing a larger one on a smaller one) can improve somewhat because of very specific facts learned about the task at hand, but most would agree that improvements in the development of general problem-solving strategies and in working memory capacity are more important factors (Shallice, 1988; see Karmiloff-Smith, 1994, for an argument against the domain-free cognitive model). Was such gradual improvement during the childhood years due to improved strategies for remembering, such as the clustering of information or development of mnemonic strategies for self-cueing (Brown, Bransford, Ferrara, & Campione, 1983; Gelman, 1978), or due to brain maturation? Circumstantial evidence for the brain hypothesis started to accrue during the 1980s (Diamond, 1990; Goldman-Rakic, 1987; Howard & Polich, 1985) with a great emphasis (that still continues) on the physical maturation of the frontal lobes (Happeney, Zelazo, & Stuss, 2004; Segalowitz & Rose-Krasnor, 1992). Indeed, we are potentially at the threshold of another "grand theory" in developmental psychology, in which the fundamental constructs are neuropsychological functions associated primarily with the frontal lobes, rather than purely behavioral or psychological constructs.

In all of this debate about brain maturation, about the growth of cognitive strategies (that themselves may rely on neural growth), and about the extent to which genes play a predictive role in individual differences in both of these, the primary Piagetian theme of how children invent their own reality and character got lost. However, developmental neuroscience is once again bringing us back to this view, fleshing out, in concrete ways, the details of this perspective.

A CLOSER LOOK: CONSTRUCTIVISM
AND DEVELOPMENTAL NEUROSCIENCE

The contemporary link between neuroscience and constructivism is probably not obvious, considering that neuroscience has traditionally been associated with a reductionist–determinist view of development. As outlined earlier, this deterministic aspect should make neuroscience the last place to consider support for the concept of *constructivism*—that is, the notion that a person can influence his or her own psychological growth. However, some aspects of neuroscience have radically changed in the last decade, and it has become increasingly clear that, in some very important ways, the neuroscience approach is far from traditional determinism. In fact, developmental neuroscience may now provide the best evidence in developmental psychology in favor of the notion of constructivism.

The new view is that biological systems certainly provide structure, but that this structure is tailored for flexibility, that brain growth is the basis for individuality, and even that there are genes for adaptability. The notion that the brain is a fixed entity from birth is wrong; rather, it is a dynamically growing organ in which we can see the evidence for the self-constructivist principle in child development. As long as we accept that mental structures are stored in the brain, the constructivist principle requires that one's actions and thoughts must influence the neural networks related to them.

Building Blocks of Constructivism

What would one need in order to have a brain that is involved in its own construction? First, experience must influence the maturational path of the brain; second, the period of this influence must cover the entire developmental period of the brain (essentially, lifelong); and third, at least some subset of these influences must be accessible to mental manipulation by the individual by means of conscious choices. Without this last component, the individual has no influence over the growth of the system, and therefore it is not constructivist. (In describing a constructivist versus selectionist model of cortical maturation, Quartz & Sejnowski, 1997, present much of the neuroscientific detail for the first two points but omit the last essential psychological component.)

The first principle—the notion that the brain's experience influences its own structure—is now well established empirically (besides being a logical necessity for learning to occur). Early work beginning in the 1960s established that dendritic spread and synaptic growth vary as a function of stimulating experience, that being deprived of such experience can dramatically reduce this growth, and that continued stimulation helps ward off the reductions expected with aging in rats (Diamond, 1988). Similar behavioral findings in children had already been documented with respect to the effect of poorly staffed orphanage experiences (Dennis, 1960). In a more positive vein, behavioral activity has been shown to directly influence cortical representation in humans, especially within the modality being experienced (Draganski et al., 2004; Elbert, Pantev, Wienbruch, Rockstroh, & Taub, 1995). For example, in language acquisition, a second language learned fluently after childhood has a different neural base than one learned as a young child (Kim, Relkin, Lee, & Hirsch, 1997). The behavioral influence can also transcend the modality: Having the early experience of learning a second language has implications for executive functions not normally associated with language per se (Bialystok et al., 2005; Bialystok, Craik, Klein, & Viswanathan, 2004).

The second component of lifelong development involves relatively recent discoveries. The connectivity of the brain is a constantly dynamic process, made especially so by the early proliferation of connections that later need to be pruned. Moreover, reports indicate that there is continual birth of new neurons in the hippocampus, a key structure for memory and learning, and that the fate of these new neurons is affected by both experiences and stressors, whether considered psychological or physical (Gould

& Tanapat, 1999). The pattern of growth of dendrites and synapses generally, and hippocampal neurons specifically, extends well past childhood, and therefore there is plenty of time for the brain to be affected by experience, whether generated by the individual whose brain we are considering or by others (Nithianantharajah & Hannan, 2006).

We now know that large individual differences in the particulars of neural networks can arise from differential experiences. Even mild stressors influence dendritic growth in the medial frontal cortex, an area critical for the development and functioning of emotional self-regulation, socialization, and self-monitoring of behavior, in general (Brown, Henning, & Wellman, 2005; Cook & Wellman, 2004). At least some of this stress-induced reduction in medial frontal connections is reversible (Radley et al., 2005), thus opening up another major role for environmental influences. Similarly, maternal behavior regulates some activation patterns of genes that, in themselves, have important influences on brain growth (Meaney & Szyf, 2005; Rutter et al., 2006). Thus, the continual growth and loss of neural connections are influenced by specific experiences of the individual related to voluntary behavior and to environmental factors beyond the individual's control.

The third component has an obvious psychological corollary: For experience to influence the growth of skills and brain structures, one preferably should be mentally active and interactive with experience. Practicing a task that requires one to identify the visual orientation of objects improves coding in the primary visual cortex, even in adult brains (Schoups, Vogels, Qian, & Orban, 2001), and the early experience of violinists affects the somatosensory representation of the fingers in proportion to the degree of use (Elbert et al., 1995). Thus, voluntary overt activity has measurable long-term effects on brain structure. These effects have even been demonstrated, without such obvious task-oriented activity, in perceptual–motor learning tasks. For example, a classic study with kittens showed that an active kitten that explores the environment develops normal spatial vision, whereas one yoked to passively experience the same perceptions as the active one does not (Held & Hein, 1963). Anecdotally and experientially, we all know that children's spontaneous engagement in a learning activity increases the likelihood of success. In other words, attention and engagement are major catalysts for learning.

Attention as a catalyst for learning works at the neurological level by the basic principle of top-down control, whereby attending to a certain aspect of one's experience over others increases the neural activations associated with the experience. For example, although experiencing a visual input certainly activates the visual cortex, covertly attending to one side of visual space (while maintaining a straight-ahead gaze) increases the cortical activation within the visual cortex of the hemisphere to which the more-attended input arrives (Worden, Foxe, Wang, & Simpson, 2000). Similarly, when a visual display containing both moving and stationary dots is presented to someone, the visual-movement region of the cortex (area MT/V5) increases or decreases in activation depending on which set of dots is attended (O'Craven, Rosen, Kwong, Triesman, & Savoy, 1997; see also Hopfinger, Buonocore, & Mangun, 2000; Macaluso, Frith, & Driver, 2000). In the same way, attending to a vibratory stimulus increases activation in the somatosensory cortex (Meyer et al., 1995). More dramatically, *imagining* movements affects the networking in the motor cortex (Caldara et al., 2004; Halpern, Zatorre, Bouffard, & Johnson, 2004; Lotze et al., 1999). Thus, just thinking about an activity activates tissue and fine-tunes the primary cortex at the most basic level—not only at the level of associative cortex, which is involved with the abstract level of planning.

This top-down effect is, of course, critical for learning what one wants to learn and may be linked to the basic reward system. When dopaminergic neurons in a region critical for processing unexpected stimuli and rewards (the ventral tegmental area) are stimulated following an auditory stimulus, the cortical representation of that sound is increased and the representation of nearby sound frequencies is reduced (Bao, Chan, & Merzenich, 2001). The overall effect of the top down system is to increase neuronal activation in certain areas by voluntarily shifting attention; as indicated above, increased activation can lead to increased connectivity in the tissue involved. It appears that increased attention synchronizes neural firing, and the more challenging the task, the greater the increase in synchronized firing (Steinmetz et al., 2000). Therefore, simply attending to particular input—that is, being interested in a certain way—ultimately has a role in shaping the growth of the cortex.

Given these three constructivist principles of growth and functioning, the child's decision to focus on one aspect of available multimodal experience over another shapes the brain to have the capacity to better or more efficiently process that aspect. This is a positive feedback loop that is highly adaptive in a complex environment. Brain circuits keep changing physically by growing and losing connections, and the functioning of the brain alters the degree to which regions become activated, thereby feeding back on the growth pattern. In this way, early propensities and interests could lead to later talents. The system is built to take advantage of the experiences available, so that expertise is efficiently developed to interact with the world.

As many developmental psychologists have noted, Piaget among them, the play behavior of the child is serious business indeed, being the method for the self-construction of the hardware with which the world will be challenged and engaged. Thus, children's mental engagement furthers the healthy maturation of the specific function being engaged in, at both the behavioral and neural levels simultaneously. Contemporary developmental neuroscience is thus supplying the concrete details of, and therefore the basic justification for, a fundamental constructivist tenet of child development. We are in the midst of an important historical period in developmental theory: For the first time, epigenetic change in cognitive structures can be attributed to maturation of specific cortical structures; this finding provides us with a truly maturational construct that accounts for the timing of certain cognitive developments and perhaps for their existence. We are starting to see a way to return to the integration for which Baldwin and Gesell hoped, an integration that was simply outside the grasp of their time—but an integration whose time may finally have come.

ACKNOWLEDGMENTS

I would like to thank the editors for their insightful comments on earlier drafts of this chapter.

REFERENCES

Anastasi, A. (1958). *Differential psychology: Individual and group differences in behavior* (3rd ed.). Oxford, UK: Macmillan.

Baldwin, J. M. (1925). *Mental development in the child and the race.* New York: Macmillan. (Original work published 1894)

Bao, S., Chan, V. T., & Merzenich, M. M. (2001). Cortical remodelling induced by activity of ventral tegmental dopamine neurons. *Nature, 412,* 79–83.

Bellugi, U., Lichtenberger, L., Mills, D., Galaburda, A., & Korenberg, J. R. (1999). Bridging cognition, the brain and molecular genetics: Evidence from Williams syndrome. *Trends in Neurosciences, 22*(5), 197–207.

Best, C. T. (1988). The emergence of cerebral asymmetries in early human development: A literature review and a neuroembryological model. In D. L. Molfese & S. J. Segalowitz (Eds.), *Brain lateralization in children: Developmental implications* (pp. 5–34). New York: Guilford Press.

Bialystok, E., Craik, F. I., Grady, C., Chau, W., Ishii, R., Gunji, A., et al. (2005). Effect of bilingualism on cognitive control in the Simon task: Evidence from MEG. *NeuroImage, 24*(1), 40–49.

Bialystok, E., Craik, F. I., Klein, R., & Viswanathan, M. (2004). Bilingualism, aging, and cognitive control: Evidence from the Simon task. *Psychology and Aging, 19*(2), 290–303.

Bourgeois, J. P. (2001). Synaptogenesis in the neocortex of the newborn: The ultimate frontier for individuation? In C. A. Nelson & M. Luciana (Eds.), *Handbook of developmental cognitive neuroscience* (pp. 23–34). Cambridge, MA: MIT Press.

Brown, A., Bransford, J. D., Ferrara, R. A., & Campione, J. C. (1983). Learning, remembering, and understanding. In J. H. Flavell & E. M. Markman (Vol. Eds.), *Handbook of child psychology: Vol. 3. Cognitive development* (4th ed., pp. 77–166). New York: Wiley.

Brown, S. M., Henning, S., & Wellman, C. L. (2005). Mild, short-term stress alters dendritic morphology in rat medial prefrontal cortex. *Cerebral Cortex, 15*(11), 1714–1722.

Bunge, M. (1980). *The mind–brain problem.* Oxford, UK: Pergamon Press.

Burbank, L. (1909). *The training of the human plant.* New York: Century.

Burt, C. (1966). The genetic determination of differences in intelligence: A study of monozygotic twins reared together and apart. *British Journal of Psychology, 57*, 137–153.

Caldara, R., Deiber, M. P., Andrey, C., Michel, C. M., Thut, G., & Hauert, C. A. (2004). Actual and mental motor preparation and execution: A spatio-temporal ERP study. *Experimental Brain Research, 159*(3), 389–399.

Carmichael, L. (1926). The development of behavior in vertebrates experimentally removed from the influence of external stimulation. *Psychological Review, 33*, 51–58.

Carmichael, L. (1927). A further study of the development of behavior in vertebrates experimentally removed from the influence of external stimulation. *Psychological Review, 34*, 34–47.

Carmichael, L. (1928). A further experimental study of the development of behavior. *Psychological Review, 35*, 253–260.

Carmichael, L. (1946). The onset and early development of behavior. In L. Carmichael (Ed.), *Manual of child psychology* (pp. 43–166). New York: Wiley.

Case, R. (1991). *The mind's staircase: Exploring the conceptual underpinnings of children's thought and knowledge.* Hillsdale, NJ: Erlbaum.

Caspi, A., McClay, J., Moffitt, T. E., Mill, J., Martin, J., Craig, I. W., et al. (2002). Role of genotype in the cycle of violence in maltreated children. *Science, 297*, 851–854.

Cole, M., & Cole, S. R. (2001). *The development of children* (3rd ed.). New York: Worth.

Conel, J. L. (1939–1967). *The postnatal development of the human cerebral cortex.* Cambridge, MA: Harvard University Press.

Cook, S. C., & Wellman, C. L. (2004). Chronic stress alters dendritic morphology in rat medial prefrontal cortex. *Journal of Neurobiology, 60*(2), 236–248.

Darwin, C. (1901). *The origin of species by means of natural selection.* New York: Collier. (Original work published 1859)

de Crinis, M. (1932). Die Entwicklung der Grosshirnrinde nach der Geburt in ihren Beziehungen zur intellektuellen Ausreifung dese Kindes [The development of the cerebral cortex after birth and its relation to the intellectual maturity of the child]. *Wiener Klinische Wochenschrift, 45*, 1161–1165.

Dennis, W. (1960). Causes of retardation among institutional children: Iran. *Journal of Genetic Psychology, 96*, 47–59.

Diamond, A. (1990). Introduction. In A. Diamond (Ed.), The development and neural bases of higher cognitive functions. *Annals of the New York Academy of Sciences, 608,* viii–lvi.

Diamond, A., & Goldman-Rakic, P. S. (1989). Comparison of human infants and rhesus monkeys on Piaget's AB task: Evidence for dependence on dorsolateral prefrontal cortex. *Experimental Brain Research, 74,* 24–40.

Diamond, A., Werker, J. F., & Lalonde, C. (1994). Toward understanding commonalities in the development of object search, detour navigation, categorization, and speech perception. In G. Dawson & K. W. Fischer (Eds.), *Human behavior and the developing brain* (pp. 380–426). New York: Guilford Press.

Diamond, M. C. (1988). *Enriching heredity: The impact of the environment on the anatomy of the brain.* New York: Free Press.

Dollard, J., & Miller, N. (1950). *Personality and psychotherapy: An analysis in terms of learning, thinking, and culture.* New York: McGraw-Hill.

Draganski, B., Gaser, C., Busch, V., Schuierer, G., Bogdahn, U., & May, A. (2004). Neuroplasticity: Changes in grey matter induced by training. *Nature, 427,* 311–312.

Elbert, T., Pantev, C., Wienbruch, C., Rockstroh, B., & Taub, E. (1995). Increased cortical representation of the fingers of the left hand in string players. *Science, 270,* 305–307.

Eysenck, H. J. (1971). *The IQ argument: Race, intelligence, and education.* New York: Library Press.

Fischer, K. W. (1980). A theory of cognitive development: The control and construction of hierarchies of skills. *Psychological Review, 87,* 477–531.

Freud, S. (1966). Project for a scientific psychology. In J. Strachey (Ed. & Trans.), *The standard edition of the complete psychological works of Sigmund Freud* (Vol. 1, pp. 294–397). London: Hogarth Press. (Original work published 1895)

Gazzaniga, M. S. (1970). *The bisected brain.* New York: Appleton-Century-Crofts.

Gelman, R. (1978). Cognitive development. *Annual Review of Psychology, 29,* 297–332.

Gesell, A. (1929). Maturation and infant behavior pattern. *Psychological Review, 26,* 307–319.

Gesell, A. (1933). Maturation and the patterning of behavior. In C. Murchison (Ed.), *A handbook of child psychology* (2nd ed., pp. 209–235). New York: Russell & Russell.

Gesell, A. (1954). The ontogenesis of infant behavior. In L. Carmichael (Ed.), *Manual of child psychology* (2nd ed., pp. 335–373). New York: Wiley.

Gesell, A., & Amatruda, C. S. (1941). *Developmental diagnosis.* New York: Harper & Row.

Goldman-Rakic, P. S. (1987). Circuitry of the prefrontal cortex and the regulation of behavior by representational knowledge. In F. Plum & V. Mountcastle (Eds.), *Handbook of physiology: Section I. The nervous system. Vol. 5. Higher functions of the brain* (pp. 373–417). Bethesda, MD: American Physiological Society.

Gould, E., & Tanapat, P. (1999). Stress and hippocampal neurogenesis. *Biological Psychiatry, 46*(11), 1472–1479.

Greenough, W. T., Black, J. E., & Wallace, C. S. (1987). Experience and brain development. *Child Development, 58,* 539–559.

Halpern, A. R., Zatorre, R. J., Bouffard, M., & Johnson, J. A. (2004). Behavioral and neural correlates of perceived and imagined musical timbre. *Neuropsychologia, 42*(9), 1281–1292.

Happaney, K., Zelazo, P. D., & Stuss, D. T. (2004). Development of orbitofrontal function: Current themes and future directions. *Brain and Cognition, 55*(1), 1–10.

Held, R., & Hein, A. (1963). Movement-produced stimulation in the development of visually guided behavior. *Journal of Comparative and Physiological Psychology, 56*(5), 872–876.

Holt, R. R. (1965). A review of some of Freud's biological assumptions and their influence on his theories. In N. S. Greenfield & W. C. Lewis (Eds.), *Psychoanalysis and current biological thought* (pp. 93–124). Madison: University of Wisconsin Press.

Hopfinger, J. B., Buonocore, M. H., & Mangun, G. R. (2000). The neural mechanisms of top-down attentional control. *Nature Neuroscience, 3*(3), 284–291.

Howard, L., & Polich, J. (1985). P300 latency and memory span development. *Developmental Psychology, 21,* 283–289.

James, W. (1892). *Psychology: Briefer course.* London: Macmillan.

Jensen, A. (1969). How much can we boost IQ and scholastic achievement? *Harvard Educational Review, 39,* 1–123.

Jordan, N. (1972). Is there an Achilles' heel in Piaget's theorizing? *Human Development, 15,* 379–382.

Karmiloff-Smith, A. (1994). Précis of beyond modularity: A developmental perspective on cognitive science. *Behavioral and Brain Sciences, 17*(4), 693–745.

Keating, D. P. (1990). Developmental processes in the socialization of cognitive structures. In *Development and learning: Proceedings of a symposium in honour of Wolfgang Edelstein on his 60th birthday* (pp. 37–72). Berlin: Max-Planck-Institut fur Bildungsforschung.

Kim, K. H., Relkin, N. R., Lee, K. M., & Hirsch, J. (1997). Distinct cortical areas associated with native and second languages. *Nature, 388,* 171–174.

Kinsbourne, M., & Hiscock, M. (1977). Does cerebral dominance develop? In S. J. Segalowitz & F. A. Gruber (Eds.), *Language development and neurological theory* (pp. 171–191). New York: Academic Press.

Konner, M. (1991). Universals of behavioral development in relation to brain myelination. In K. R. Gibson & A. C. Peterson (Eds.), *Brain maturation and cognitive development: Comparative and cross-cultural perspectives* (pp. 181–223). London: de Gruyter.

Lenneberg, E. H. (1967). *Biological foundations of language.* New York: Wiley.

Lotze, M., Montoya, P., Erb, M., Hulsmann, E., Flor, H., Klose, U., et al. (1999). Activation of cortical and cerebellar motor areas during executed and imagined hand movements: An fMRI study. *Journal of Cognitive Neuroscience, 11*(5), 491–501.

Macaluso, E., Frith, C. D., & Driver, J. (2000). Modulation of human visual cortex by crossmodal spatial attention. *Science, 289,* 1206–1208.

Maccoby, E. E. (1966). *The development of sex differences*. Palo Alto, CA: Stanford University Press.

Macmillan, M. (1992). Inhibition and the control of behavior: From Gall to Freud via Phineas Gage and the frontal lobes. *Brain and Cognition, 19*, 72–104.

MacNamara, J. (1976). Stomachs assimilate and accommodate, don't they? *Canadian Psychological Review, 17*, 167–173.

McGraw, M. B. (1946). Maturation of behavior. In L. Carmichael (Ed.), *Manual of child psychology* (pp. 332–369). New York: Wiley.

Meaney, M. J., & Szyf, M. (2005). Environmental programming of stress responses through DNA methylation: Life at the interface between a dynamic environment and a fixed genome. *Dialogues in Clinical Neuroscience, 7*(2), 103–123.

Mesulam, M.-M. (1985). Patterns in behavioral neuroanatomy: Association areas, the limbic system, and hemispheric specialization. In M.-M. Mesulam (Ed.), *Principles of behavioral neurology* (pp. 1–70). Philadelphia: Davis.

Meyer, E., Ferguson, S. S. G., Zatorre, R. J., Alivisatos, B., Marrett, S., Evans, A. C., et al. (1995). Attention modulates somatosensory cerebral blood flow response to vicrotactile stimulation as measured by positron emission tomography. *Annals of Neurology, 29*, 440–443.

Montagu, A. (Ed.). (1975). *Race and IQ*. London: Oxford University Press.

Moore, J. M. (1972). *Heredity and development* (2nd ed.). New York: Oxford University Press.

Nithianantharajah, J., & Hannan, A. (2006). Enriched environments, experience-dependent plasticity and disorders of the nervous system. *Natures Reviews: Neuroscience, 7*, 697–709.

Noback, C. R., & Moss, M. L. (1956). Differential growth of the human brain. *Journal of Comparative Neurology, 105*, 539–551.

Obler, L. K., & Fein, D. (Eds.). (1988). *The exceptional brain: Neuropsychology of talent and special abilities*. New York: Guilford Press.

O'Craven, K. M., Rosen, B. R., Kwong, K. K., Triesman, A., & Savoy, R. L. (1997). Voluntary attention modulates fMRI activity in human MT-MST. *Neuron, 18*, 591–598.

Piaget, J. (1960). *The child's conception of physical causality*. Totowa, NJ: Littlefield, Adams. (Original work published 1930)

Piaget, J. (1966). *The psychology of intelligence*. Totowa, NJ: Littlefield, Adams. (Original work published 1947)

Piaget, J. (1954). Language and thought from the genetic point of view. *Acta Psychologica, 10*, 51–60.

Piaget, J. (1970). *Genetic epistemology*. New York: Columbia University Press.

Piaget, J. (1972). Intellectual evolution from adolescence to adulthood. *Human Development, 15*, 1–12.

Piaget, J., & Inhelder, B. (1969). *The psychology of the child*. New York: Basic Books. (Original work published 1966)

Pribram, K. H., & Gill, M. M. (1976). *Freud's Project reassessed*. London: Hutchison.

Quartz, S., & Sejnowski, T. J. (1997). The neural basis of cognitive development: A constructivist manifesto. *Behavioral and Brain Sciences, 20*(4), 537–596.

Radley, J. J., Rocher, A. B., Janssen, W. G., Hof, P. R., McEwen, B. S., & Morrison, J. H. (2005). Reversibility of apical dendritic retraction in the rat medial prefrontal cortex following repeated stress. *Experimental Neurology, 196*(1), 199–203.

Ramón y Cajal, S. (1894). *La fine structure des centre nerveux* [The fine structure of the central nerves]. Croonian Lecture, March 8, 1894. *Royal Society of London Proceedings, 55*, 444–468.

Rapoport, J. L. (1991). Basal ganglia dysfunction as a proposed cause of obsessive compulsive disorder. In B. J. Carroll & J. E. Barrett (Eds.), *Psychopathology and the brain* (pp. 77–95). New York: Raven Press.

Rutter, M., Moffitt, T. E., & Caspi, A. (2006). Gene–environment interplay and psychopathology: Multiple varieties but real effects. *Journal of Child Psychology and Psychiatry, 47*, 226–261.

Scheibel, A. B. (1990). Dendritic correlates of higher cognitive function. In A. B. Scheibel & A. F. Wechsler (Eds.), *Neurobiology of higher cognitive function* (pp. 239–270). New York: Guilford Press.

Schoups, A., Vogels, R., Qian, N., & Orban, G. (2001). Practising orientation identification improves orientation coding in V1 neurons. *Nature, 412*, 549–553.

Segalowitz, S. J. (1979). Piaget's Achilles' heel: A safe soft spot? *Human Development, 23*, 137–140.

Segalowitz, S. J. (1987). Individual differences in hemispheric specialization: Sources and measurement. In A. Glass (Ed.), *Individual differences in hemispheric specialization* (pp. 17–29). New York: Plenum Press.

Segalowitz, S. J. (1992, May). *The developmental neurobiology of Max de Crinis: Neuropsychology catches up 60 years later*. Paper presented at the third annual meeting of TENNET, Universite du Quebec, Montreal.

Segalowitz, S. J. (1999). Why twin studies don't really tell us much about human heritability. *Behavioral and Brain Sciences, 22*, 904–905.

Segalowitz, S. J., & Berge, B. E. (1995). Functional asymmetries in infancy and early childhood: A review of electrophysiological studies and their implications. In R. Davidson & K. Hugdahl (Eds.), *Brain asymmetry* (pp. 579–616). Cambridge, MA: MIT Press.

Segalowitz, S. J., & Davies, P. L. (2004). Charting the maturation of the frontal lobe: An electrophysiological strategy. *Brain and Cognition, 55*, 116–133.

Segalowitz, S. J., & Gruber, F. A. (Eds.). (1977). *Language development and neurological theory*. New York: Academic Press.

Segalowitz, S. J., & Hiscock, M. (2002). The neuropsychology of normal development: Developmental neuroscience and a new constructivism. In S. J. Segalowitz & I. Rapin (Vol. Eds.), *Handbook of neuropsychology: Vol. 8. Child neuropsychology* (pp. 7–28). Amsterdam: Elsevier.

Segalowitz, S. J., & Rose-Krasnor, L. (Eds.). (1992). The role of frontal lobe maturation in cognitive and social development [Special issue]. *Brain and Cognition, 20*, 1–213.

Segalowitz, S. J., & Schmidt, L. A. (2003). Developmental psychology and the neurosciences. In J. Valsiner & K. J. Connolly (Eds.), *Handbook of developmental psychology* (pp. 48–71). London: Sage.

Segalowitz, S. J., Unsal, A., & Dywan, J. (1992). Cleverness and wisdom in 12-year-olds: Electrophysiological evidence for late maturation of the frontal lobe. *Developmental Neuropsychology, 8,* 279–298.

Semrud-Clikeman, M., Hynd, G., Novey, E., & Eliopoulos, E. (1990). Relationships between brain morphology and neurolinguistic measures in children with dyslexia, ADD/H, and normal controls. *Journal of Clinical and Experimental Neuropsychology, 12,* 97.

Shallice, T. (1988). *From neuropsychology to mental structure.* Cambridge, UK: Cambridge University Press.

Skinner, B. F. (1957). *Verbal behavior.* New York: Appleton-Century-Crofts.

Solms, M. (2004). Freud returns. *Scientific American, 290*(5), 82–88.

Sperry, R. W. (1968). Hemispheric deconnection and unity of conscious awareness. *American Psychologist, 23,* 723–733.

Steinmetz, P. N., Roy, A., Fitzgerald, P. J., Hsiao, S. S., Johnson, K. O., & Niebur, E. (2000). Attention modulates synchronized neuronal firing in primate somatosensory cortex. *Nature, 404,* 187–190.

Thatcher, R. W. (1994). Cyclic cortical reorganization: Origins of human cognitive development. In G. Dawson & K. W. Fischer (Eds.), *Human behavior and the developing brain* (pp. 232–266). New York: Guilford Press.

Tucker, D. M. (1992). Developing emotions and cortical networks. In M. R. Gunnar & C. A. Nelson (Eds.), *Developmental behavioral neuroscience* (pp. 75–128). Hillsdale, NJ: Erlbaum.

Wahlsten, D. (1990). Insensitivity of the analysis of variance to heredity-environment interaction. *Behavioral and Brain Sciences, 13*(1), 109–161.

Witelson, S. F. (1977). Early hemispheric specialization and interhemispheric plasticity: An empirical and theoretical review. In S. J. Segalowitz & F. A Gruber (Eds.), *Language development and neurological theory* (pp. 213–289). New York: Academic Press.

Witelson, S. F. (1987). Neurobiological aspects of language in children. *Child Development, 58,* 653–688.

Worden, M. S., Foxe, J. J., Wang, N., & Simpson, G. V. (2000). Anticipatory biasing of visuospatial attention indexed by retinotopically specific alpha-band electroenephalography increases over occipital cortex. *Journal of Neuroscience, 20,* RC63.

Yakovlev, P. I., & Lecours, A.-R. (1967). The myelogenetic cycles of regional maturation in the brain. In A. Minkowski (Ed.), *Regional development of the brain in early life* (pp. 3–70). Oxford, UK: Blackwell.

CHAPTER 2

Some Ways in Which Neuroscientific Research Can Be Relevant to Education

James P. Byrnes

Over the past 10 years, many educators and government officials have become enamored with the idea that it is possible to "teach to the brain" (Bruer, 1997; Byrnes, 2001b). Correspondingly, there has been quite a demand for professional development workshops, curricula, videos, and books that attempt to explain the educational implications of brain research to teachers. My goal in writing this chapter is twofold. First, I briefly unpack the claim that brain research should guide instructional decision making. Then, I consider the possible educational implications of certain kinds of neuroscientific findings in more detail.

What do educators and curriculum developers mean when they say that it is possible to "teach to the brain"? My reading of educator-oriented literature is that instruction can be more or less compatible with basic cortical and subcortical processes (e.g., Jensen, 2000). By *compatible*, I mean that information is presented in a manner that is consistent with the way the brain normally processes information. Compatibility, in turn, is argued to be a compelling basis for instructional decision making. That is, one should choose more compatible approaches over less compatible approaches because the former will produce more knowledge growth and skill development than the latter. For example, advocates of brain-based education sometimes argue that reading instruction should be grounded in phonics, because studies using fMRI methods (e.g., Pugh et al., 1997) have shown that phonological processing areas of the brain are active when skilled readers read. Any approach that does not emphasize phonics (e.g., extreme versions of the whole-language approach) is argued to be inconsistent with what we know about the brain (and therefore should be avoided).

Although the logic of making instructional decisions on the basis of research is well founded, the degree to which the education community has embraced this logic is a rather new development. It would appear that the motivation for grounding instructional decisions in neuroscientific evidence is that findings revealed through neuroscientific methods seem to be more credible and definitive than evidence provided through other means (e.g., traditional psychological experiments). Hypothetically, then, if psychological experiments suggest that children should be taught using Approach X, whereas neuroscientific work implicates Approach Y, Approach Y should be selected.

Although I am in complete agreement with the suggestion that one should base instructional decisions on issues of compatibility and credible experimental evidence, there is an important intermediary link between instruction and outcomes that is missing from the brain-based account described above. Rather than argue that instruction should be compatible with the basic operations of the brain, I argue instead that instruction should be compatible with the basic operations of the *mind* (see Byrnes, 2001a). Given that the mind (or cognition) is produced by a brain (Kosslyn & Koenig, 1994), however, it is probably not a good idea to remain agnostic about the value of certain kinds of neurological findings. Doing so would be analogous to a physicist ignoring the role of physical entities (e.g., wires) when studying emergent properties of these entities (e.g., the electromagnetic waves that are produced when an electric current runs through wires).

I align myself with scholars who argue that the primary role for neuroscientific research is to provide additional insight into the best ways to "carve up" a psychological skill or process (e.g., reading) into its components (e.g., Kosslyn & Koenig, 1994). A detailed and accurate componential analysis of a skill is a crucial aspect of knowing how to improve it. To understand this premise by way of an analogy, consider how the first step in producing effective medicines (e.g., anticholesterol drugs) is to understand the component operations of individual organs or systems (e.g., the liver). When scientists have a detailed understanding of the chain of events that occurs within a biological process (e.g., how the liver produces cholesterol), they can then figure out how to interfere with, or enhance, this process chemically. I have argued that psychologists who have interests in education should behave analogously; that is, they should endeavor to understand the chain of mental events that occurs within psychological processes such as reading and figure out ways to enhance this process (Byrnes, 2001a).

In my view, neuroscientific research is potentially relevant to education to the extent that it helps refine our understanding of (1) psychological events that take place in learning contexts (e.g., reading, mathematical thinking, learning and memory, attention) or (2) brain development (because anatomical changes in the brain could eventually be part of the explanation of the emergence of new skills over time; see below). But I underscore the word *potentially* in the prior sentence because we still have to make sure that the neuroscientific findings in question are credible and consistently observed in distinct laboratories. Poorly conducted neuroscientific research is no more informative or credible than poorly conducted psychological research. Similarly, isolated or nonreplicated findings in neuroscience are no more informative than isolated or nonreplicated findings in psychology. There are many isolated psychological findings that have been overturned once meta-analyses of multiple studies revealed that these findings were due to sample fluctuations (e.g., gender differences in math skills prior to adolescence).

In what follows, I provide a brief summary of neuroscientific findings that have the potential to provide refined insight into either brain development or psychological events that take place in learning contexts (see also other chapters in this volume). After discussing various relevant studies, I conclude by first characterizing our current level of understanding of these matters. Then I provide examples of how some researchers, educators, or policymakers have overinterpreted neuroscientific findings. Finally, I make suggestions for future research.

SOME FINDINGS THAT MAY HAVE RELEVANCE TO EDUCATION

For expository purposes, I have organized relevant findings with respect to whether they pertain to brain development, learning, memory, attention, or math skills. Each area of research is briefly discussed in turn. A more comprehensive treatment of these and other topics appears in Byrnes (2001b). Although neuroscientific research on reading and phonological processing is also clearly relevant to educators, I do not review this work here because it is discussed more fully in other chapters in the present volume (e.g., see Booth, Chapter 10, this volume).

Brain Development

The research on brain development is potentially relevant to education for several reasons. First, it is reasonable to assume that there is a neural basis to human abilities such as (a) forming and storing representations of experiences, (b) carrying out various cognitive operations (e.g., computing math answers, parsing sentences), and (c) planning and executing various physical skills (e.g., walking across the room, writing a note to a friend, shooting a foul shot, driving a stick-shift car). The only alternative to this neural-basis assumption is a radical kind of mind–brain dualism that is contradicted by a variety of findings in neuropsychology (see Byrnes, 2001b; Temple, 2000; or Warrington & McCarthy, 1989, for reviews). For example, numerous studies have shown that people lose the ability to retrieve specific items of information (e.g., addition facts) or perform specific tasks (e.g., move their right arms) when specific areas of the brain are injured. Second, it is also reasonable to assume that when a normal adult brain carries out specific, routine cognitive tasks (e.g., storing mental representations), it does so via neural architectures or assemblies that are configured in such a way that these tasks are performed in a relatively rapid, efficient, and reliable way. Prior to adulthood, however, these architectures may not be so configured. As a result, children may perform the same tasks more slowly, less efficiently, and less reliably (i.e., make more errors).

The differences between the adult versions of the neural assemblies and those of children (that could affect speed, efficiency, and reliability) could pertain to such things as the number and types of cells in these assemblies, the patterns of connectivity among cells, and the degree of myelination of connecting fibers (see also Lenroot & Giedd, Chapter 3, this volume). As the adult version of the assembly is slowly constructed during development, changes in structure could partly explain the following common developmental progression: from (a) phase 1—not being able to perform a task at all (e.g., walk, talk, hold items in working memory); to (b) phase 2—performing it in a relatively slow, inefficient, and error-prone way; to (c) phase 3—performing it in a relatively fast, efficient, and nearly errorless fashion.

If precise kinds of anatomical and performance changes could be identified and correlated in such ways, the findings would be informative to educators. Minimally, the results could help explain why children at particular ages perform more poorly on certain academic tasks than children at older ages. Given the arguments above, developmental differences may derive from the fact that the neural assemblies that are active when a skill is executed could have the wrong number or wrong mixture of specific cell types (i.e., too few or too many pyramidal and stellate cells), or be connected to the wrong number of other cells (i.e., too few or too many connections), or contain too few myelinated fibers.

However, it is important to be clear about the kinds of inferences that can be drawn from the foregoing analysis. Although one could partly explain children's poor performance by appealing to the fact that their neural assemblies may not be configured optimally (once relevant, well-done studies confirm this fact), such an account would provide little insight into how teachers could solve this problem. Gaining the latter kind of insight requires that we provide teachers with additional information about *developmental mechanisms* that explain how earlier states of brain development get transformed into later states of brain development (e.g., how a neural assembly that has too many cells, too many synapses, or too few myelinated fibers becomes transformed into one that has a more optimal number of cells, synapses, and myelinated fibers). If teachers are told that the primary developmental mechanism involved is the expression of regulatory genes that operate according to a particular timetable, it would be reasonable for teachers to assume that they should wait until children's genes have crafted sufficiently developed assemblies before asking children to engage in particular kinds of tasks. This stance is, of course, the traditional *readiness* view of instruction. In contrast, if teachers are told that the primary mechanism involved is experience in the domain of interest, the correct inference is to ask children to immediately engage in domain-relevant tasks (i.e., not wait) in order to make use of the sculpting effects of experience.

To illustrate the latter possibility, several contemporary theories suggest that children acquire segmented phonological representations of spoken words not because of endogenous (i.e., experience-independent) brain maturation per se, but in response to the acquisition of a large number of words (Metsala & Walley, 1998). In particular, the claim is that each time children acquire a new word that shares phonological components with already known words (e.g., the child has *cat* in her vocabulary and learns a new word, *rat*), the representations of the known word become segmented (e.g., *cat* is segmented into *cuh* + *-at*, or its onset and rime). These original and segmented representations would, of course, be reflected or grounded in specific patterns of connectivity in neural assemblies. Similarly, the segmentation processes would have some sort of neurological analog (e.g., synaptic reorganizations). Such an account could explain why neurologically intact, low-income second graders who lack phonemic awareness skills can acquire these skills relatively quickly in intervention studies (Vellutino et al., 1996) and why their truly disabled peers do not respond to training as readily. The fact that the former children are 2–3 years beyond the age when middle-class children demonstrate such phonological processing skills implies that a maturational account of their lack of phonemic awareness is not as plausible as one that suggests that these children were not exposed to a sufficient quantity of vocabulary words during their preschool years (Hart & Risley, 1995).

It should also be noted that in order for a maturational explanation of cognitive development to be even minimally plausible, it has to be consistent at least with findings regarding the timetables for the seven major processes of brain development: proliferation, migration, differentiation, growth, synaptogenesis, regressive processes (cell death and axonal pruning), and myelination (Byrnes, 2001b; Nelson & Luciana, 2001). Each of these processes has either a relatively fixed or relatively open timetable. Those with fixed timetables (i.e., proliferation, migration, differentiation, and growth) start and largely stop at specific ages. Those with open timetables start early and continue well into adulthood (i.e., synaptogenesis, regressive processes, and myelination). Whereas maturational accounts that appeal to processes with open timetables have the potential to be plausible at any age, those accounts that appeal to processes with fixed timetables can sometimes be implausible if the age of emergence of the skill to be explained (e.g., age 7) is later than the end of the timetable for the process in question (e.g., proliferation, which ends at the seventh prenatal month for most brain regions).

Said another way, maturational accounts that attempt to explain the emergence of a cognitive skill after age 6 (when the brain is 90% of its adult volume) will generally have to appeal primarily to processes such as synaptogenesis, regressive processes, and myelination. MRI studies suggest that there are significant reductions in gray matter (in the frontal and parietal regions mainly) and significant increases in white matter between ages 6 and 20 (Giedd, 2004; see also Lenroot & Giedd, Chapter 3, this volume). The loss of gray matter is thought to show that an initial overproduction of brain cells and synapses is progressively pruned down to a more optimal number (Durston et al., 2001). The increase in white matter, in contrast, demonstrates the progressive myelination of connecting fibers. From childhood to adolescence, myelination of cortical fibers proceeds from the back of the head (occipital lobe) to the front (frontal lobe). Given that the frontal region is involved in abilities such as working memory, executive function skills, and inhibition, one would predict that these abilities would continue to develop during adolescence (Giedd, 2004). In the corpus callosum, in contrast, myelination of connecting fibers between the hemispheres proceeds from the anterior (frontal) portions to the posterior regions. This latter change would mean that during adolescence, regions of the temporal and parietal lobes become more capable of communicating and working together to process language, math, and spatial problems more quickly. In addition, improvements in long-term memory would be expected (see the learning and memory and math sections below).

This is not to say, of course, that synaptogenesis and myelination are the only possible maturational processes that could, in principle, be responsible for cognitive development after infancy. Other candidates include growth of new neurons (e.g., in the hippocampus); growth and recession of dendrites; growth of glial cells (which recently have been found to play a role in neural functioning); and neural network reorganization, as indicated by coherence changes (Angulo, Kozlov, Charpak, & Audinat, 2004; Barry et al., 2004; Bell & Fox, 1994; Gould, Tanapat, Rydel, & Hastings, 2000; Quartz & Sejnowski, 1997). But the general logic of argumentation remains the same in that the maturational account has to appeal to the latter kinds of processes and consider the possible consequences of these changes.

Learning and Memory

To understand the developmental neuroscience of learning and memory, it is helpful to consider several established findings in the traditional psychological literature on these processes. The first pertains to the role of repetition in learning. With the exception of so-called "flashbulb" memories, in which traumatic events are seemingly seared into one's memory in a single episode, the storage of all other experiences normally requires multiple exposures (Anderson, 1990). The second relevant finding pertains to the distinction between recognition and recall. When we *recognize* something (e.g., a face), a stimulus cue in the environment (i.e., an actual face) matches the representation that we are trying to retrieve from long-term memory (i.e., our mental representation of that face). When we *recall* something, in contrast, the cue (e.g., a person's name) is merely associated with the object in question (e.g., the person's face) and the representation of this object in our minds. Children and adults nearly always perform better on recognition tasks than they do on recall tasks (Schneider & Bjorklund, 1998). The third pertains to the distinctions among (a) the learning of facts (declarative memory), (b) the learning of habits or skills (procedural or skill learning), (c) our ability to remember events in which we participated (episodic memory), and (d) the ability to hold verbal or spatial information temporarily in our conscious awareness (i.e., verbal and spatial working memory; see Ben-Yehudah & Fiez, Chapter 11, this volume). Psychological studies have shown that these aspects of memory are dissociable. For example, students may be better at executing math computations than they are at recalling math facts. Also, people may remember participating in an event (e.g., attending a course) but not recall any facts learned during that event.

Through a combination of studies that utilized methodologies such as surgically ablating sections of animal brains, assessing the impairments of adults with brain injuries, and using functional magnetic resonance imaging (fMRI) to determine areas of the brain that are active during memory tasks, researchers have revealed a neuroscientific basis for all of these psychological phenomena (Squire & Schacter, 2002). In the case of repetition, for example, there is the adage that frequently appears in the neuroscience literature: "Neurons that fire together, wire together" (e.g., Staley, 2004). That is, neurons that are (1) in close proximity to each other and (2) repeatedly active at the same time tend to form synapses with each other. Clusters of neurons will fire simultaneously, however, only when they share input fibers from afferent pathways (e.g., from the eyes and ears) or from other regions of the brain that send stimulation to these neurons at the same time (Johnson, 1997). Over time, correlated activity can cause the strengthening of particular synaptic connections within an assembly as well as the pruning of other connections. Either way, the psychological term *learning* can be said to correspond to the neuroscientific term *synaptic reorganization* (Squire, 1991). Correlated activity promotes a noticeable anatomical change in synapses that enables a rapid and efficient pattern of "communication" among the neurons in an assembly (Goodman & Tessier-LaVigne, 1997). The formation of stable synapses and elimination of synapses, however, is a relatively conservative process that normally takes time and multiple repetitions.

Further insights into the neuroscience of learning come from studies of amnesia. In certain adults who experience anterograde amnesia, there is an impairment in the ability to acquire new information (Broadbent, Clark, Zola, & Squire, 2002; Kopelman & Stanhope, 2002; Shimamura, 2002). These patients, as a rule, sustain damage to key structures in the medial temporal lobe (i.e., hippocampus, entorhinal cortex, parahippocampal gyrus, and perirhinal cortex). According to *relational binding theory* (Shimamura, 2002), these structures participate in the creation of new memories in the following way. First, the hippocampal complex acts to bind co-activated cortical representations through projections that extend from areas of cortical activity to the hippocampus. This binding or mediation through the hippocampus increases the likelihood that these representations will be reactivated at a later time. Each time the pairs or sets of representations are reactivated, they slowly establish cortical–cortical connections with themselves. The binding through the hippocampus is needed because the cortical–cortical connections take a longer time to establish than the cortical–hippocampal projections. Eventually, however, the cortical–cortical connections become established. At that point, the cortical–hippocampal connections that supported the consolidation process are no longer necessary for retrieval; however, they can still contribute to the retrieval process.

In addition to playing a role in learning, the medial temporal lobe also plays a role in two other distinctions discussed above: recognition memory and episodic memory. In the case of recognition memory, unimodal and polymodal association areas in the frontal, temporal, and parietal lobes send projections to the perirhinal and parahippocampal cortices in the medial temporal lobe. The latter structures send projections to the entorhinal cortex, which in turn sends projections to the hippocampus (Broadbent et al., 2002). All of these projections between the aforementioned structures are reciprocal, so communication is bidirectional. To create new representations that can be used to recognize something (e.g., a face, a name, a song), the hippocampus plays a key role in the binding or consolidation process, as described above. The unimodal and polymodal association areas, in contrast, serve as storage areas for the representations themselves. It is generally the case that representations of a particular type (e.g., visual) are stored near the primary areas of the cortex involved in the initial processing of that kind of information (e.g., visual processing). In essence, then, if a lesion occurs in the hippocampal complex, the affected person will have trouble creating new representations (e.g., the face of a new acquaintance) but may still be able to recognize entities using already-established representations (e.g., the face of a spouse). In contrast, if the lesion occurs in the unimodal or polymodal association areas of the cortex, the representations themselves may be lost.

In the case of episodic or autobiographical memory, the left hippocampus, in conjunction with areas in the medial frontal lobe, seems to be important (Maguire, 2001). These areas are active in the brains of healthy adults when they are asked to remember if particular events happened to them recently or some time ago. Relatedly, damage to the left hippocampus often results in a diminished ability to remember personal experiences.

Studies of brain-injured adults also show that whereas amnesiacs have trouble creating new declarative memories, they do not seem to have trouble learning new habits or skills (Shimamura, 2002). In contrast, patients with basal ganglia disorders (e.g., Huntington's disease or Parkinson's disease) have trouble with motor skill learning but not with the recognition component of declarative memory (Knowlton, 2002). The subcortical basal ganglia, which include structures such as the striatum (caudate and putamen), are intimately connected to nearly all frontal regions (including motor cortices) as well as the thalamus and amygdala. The connections to the frontal regions can perhaps explain why Huntington's and Parkinson's patients have been found to have impairments in declarative memory as well. For example, their deficit in recall ability is disproportionate to their recognition ability. Moreover, they show less clustering during recall (suggesting a lower rate of strategy use) and impaired implicit association learning (see Knowlton, 2002, for a review).

Studies using fMRI generally support the distinction between verbal and spatial working memory as well. For example, when adults are asked to perform tasks that are thought to involve verbal working memory, areas of the left parietal and left frontal lobes are particularly active (Byrnes, 2001b). In contrast, when the same individuals are asked to perform tasks that are thought to involve spatial working memory, areas of the right parietal and right frontal lobes are active.

Given all of these findings related to the neuroscience of memory, it would be reasonable to assume that children would demonstrate increased memory skills as their brains develop. In fact, there are clear increases in children's ability to recall experiences and imitate actions over the first 2 years of life (Bauer, 2004). In addition, there are monotonic increases in working memory skills and strategic behavior from age 6 to adulthood (Schneider & Bjorklund, 1998; Swanson, 1999). These changes are clearly consistent with what has been learned about brain development in children (as briefly reviewed above, in the section on brain development), but many more studies are needed to confirm tight linkages between specific brain changes and children's abilities to learn and remember. Although there is a correlation between brain changes and memory increases, no causative relationship has yet been established in neuroscientific studies of children. The latter connection will only be known when we understand how it is that certain brain changes can induce skill enhancement or representational change.

Attention

All major theories of cognitive development assume, quite reasonably, that children cannot acquire meaningful amounts of declarative, conceptual, or procedural knowledge if they are not paying attention during instructional activities (Byrnes, 2001b). Thus, psychological research on attention is clearly relevant to education, but the question for the present chapter is whether *neuroscientific* research on attention is relevant to education. As suggested earlier, issues of relevance emerge from componential analyses of intellectual capacities.

Researchers have subdivided the cognitive process of attention into aspects such as arousal, engagement (and disengagement), selective attention (i.e., filtering, inhibition of distraction), and sustained attention (also known as vigilance). This componential analysis, in turn, has served as a guide for neuroscientific researchers who are interested in discovering the anatomical basis of these aspects of attention (Byrnes, 2001b; Posner & Raichle, 1994; Sarter, Givens, & Bruno, 2001). Decomposed in this way, it is relatively straightforward to make connections to the classroom. For example, numerous studies have shown that learning is optimized when arousal levels are moderate (as opposed to when students are sleepy or overaroused), when attention is engaged or focused on the task at hand, when students selectively attend to instructional information (as opposed to being distracted by events inside or outside the classroom), and when students maintain attention over time in anticipation of classroom events.

The results of studies with individuals with brain injuries, neuroimaging techniques, and animal models have been fairly consistent with respect to the brain regions that are most active when attention is engaged. Specifically, regions of the frontal lobes (especially in the right hemisphere and anterior cingulate) seem to form an anterior system that is involved in the detection of stimuli, executive control of attention, and maintenance of attention over time (Lawrence, Ross, Hoffmann, Garavan, & Stein, 2003; Sarter et al., 2001). Bilateral regions of the parietal lobes comprise the second, posterior half of the sustained attention system that works in conjunction with the anterior half. In addition, subcortical regions serve to mediate the level of arousal and activation in the anterior and posterior cortical regions, but there is some disagreement as to which subcortical regions provide these mediating functions (cf. Lawrence et al., 2003; Posner & Raichle, 1994; Sarter et al., 2001). Whatever the specific subcortical region turns out to be, it is relatively clear that the subcortical and cortical areas work together to provide arousal and sustained attention in classroom and other settings.

One other area of research that has the potential to provide additional insights into the role of attention in classroom contexts is that pertaining to attention-deficit/hyperactivity disorder (ADHD). Given the estimated prevalence of ADHD of 5% of children (Durston et al., 2003), it is likely that teachers will often have at least one child in their classrooms who has problems with hyperactivity/impulsiveness or inattentiveness (or both). Although it has been speculated that the orbitofrontal area may be underdeveloped in children with ADHD (Barkley, 1997), recent fMRI studies suggest that there is underactivation of a frontal–striatal network that corresponds to an inability to inhibit responses (Durston et al., 2003). At present, similar fMRI studies have not been conducted with children with ADHD who primarily have a problem with inattentiveness and underarousal rather than impulsivity. Moreover, whereas there are correlations between achievements in attention and brain development, imaging studies of children lag far behind those conducted with adults (Posner, 2001). When more studies of children are conducted, we will be in a better position to determine whether brain changes seem to precede or accompany attention changes.

Math Skills

Contemporary psychological and educational perspectives on mathematical thinking emphasize the ability to solve problems in a consistent, efficient, and effective manner (Byrnes, 2001a). In the educational and developmental literature (e.g., Bisanz, Sherman, Rasmussen, & Ho, 2005; Byrnes, 2001a), mathematical competence is said to involve five component aspects: (1) declarative knowledge, or an extensive storehouse of math facts (e.g., that $15^2 = 225$); (2) procedural knowledge, or an extensive storehouse of goal-directed processes such as computational algorithms, strategies, and heuristics (e.g., the least common denominator method for adding fractions); (3) conceptual knowledge, or an extensive network of concepts (e.g., ordinality, cardinality) that help problem solvers understand the meaning of facts and procedures (e.g., why one must invert and multiply when dividing fractions); (4) estimation skills; and (5) the ability to graphically depict and model mathematical relationships and outcomes.

In principle, neuroscientists who want to understand the anatomical basis of mathematical competence could use the aforementioned psychological framework as a guide. For example, researchers could attempt to discover brain regions that seem to participate in mathematical processes such as the retrieval of math facts, estimation of approximate answers to questions, comparison of the relative size of two numerical amounts, and construction of strategies for solving a math problem.

However, most of the neuroscientific work on math skills has not been guided by this multifaceted model of mathematical competence. Instead, many studies have been oriented toward documenting and systematizing various deficits of adults with brain injuries who lose specific, lower-level math skills (Byrnes, 2001b). Depending on the location of injury, deficits have been observed in the ability to recognize numerical symbols, provide the names of numerical symbols, retrieve mathematical facts, perform arithmetic operations (e.g., addition, subtraction, multiplication), and compare the relative size of two numerical quantities (Dehaene & Cohen, 1997; McClosky, Aliminosa, & Sokol, 1991). In addition, various double dissociations have been observed in terms of mathematical operations (e.g., a person can perform addition but not multiplication) and symbolic codes (e.g., a person can perform a task when numbers are presented as words, such as *three*, but not as Arabic symbols, such as *3*). In most of these cases (i.e., ~66%), the majority of lesions occurred in the left hemisphere.

In addition to neuropsychological research with brain-injured adults, a handful of neuroimaging studies of math skills have been conducted since the mid-1990s, although the results have not always been consistent. The results of two fMRI studies were, however, reasonably convergent. In one, Rickard and colleagues (2000) gave eight adult participants three tasks: single-digit multiplication problems ($2 \times 6 = 12$; true or false?), numerical magnitude problems (Which is larger: 14 or 81?), and a perceptual–motor control task. Three main brain areas were found to be active for the multiplication problems. First, there was a clear level of activation in the left parietal lobe for all eight subjects and also homologous activation in the right parietal lobe (but to a lesser extent). Second, there was bilateral activation in the fusiform and lingual gyri of the temporooccipital lobe. Third, there was activation located near Broca's area of the left frontal lobe and also in areas anterior and superior to Broca's area (Brodmann's areas 9 and 10).

In the second study that used fMRI technology, Schmithorst and Brown (2004) scanned 15 adults as they mentally added or subtracted fractions. Once again, there was bilateral activation in the inferior parietal lobes. In addition, activation was evident in the left perisylvian area and in inferior portions of the occipitotemporal area. The authors interpreted these findings as being supportive of Dehaene's triple code model of math skills that was originally proposed to account for performance of adults with brain injuries (Dehaene & Cohen, 1997). The triple code model proposes that math knowledge is represented in three kinds of codes: a visual Arabic code that is localized in the left and right inferior occipital–temporal areas, an analogical quantity or magnitude code that is localized in the left and right inferior parietal areas, and a verbal code that is localized in the left perisylvian area. The visual Arabic code, which subserves multidigit operations, is utilized during the identification of strings of digits and also during judgments of parity (e.g., knowing that numbers that end in 2 are even). The magnitude code, in contrast, is assumed to correspond to distributions of activation on an oriented number line. This code subserves the ability to evaluate proximity (e.g., that 18 is close to 20 on a number line) and ordinal relations (e.g., that 20 is a larger amount than 18). The verbal code represents numbers via a parsed sequence of words. It is involved when an individual retrieves rote memories of arithmetical facts.

Collectively, these results are of interest for several reasons. First, one of the best predictors of a child's ability to learn mathematics is his or her understanding of ordinality (Byrnes & Wasik, 1991; Case & Okamoto, 1996). In order for a maturational account of mathematical development to be minimally plausible, then, it would need to focus at least on anatomical changes in the inferior parietal lobes of both hemispheres and the caudal section of the corpus callosum, which contains fibers that connect homologous sections of the left and right parietal areas. For example, as children show increased mastery of ordinality over the course of childhood, are there indications that these sections of the parietal lobes and corpus callosum are maturing (e.g., increased myelination)? The second interesting aspect of the findings is that many of the focal regions are localized in the left hemisphere rather than the right. Such findings call into question proposals that suggest that math skills are predominately localized in the right hemisphere (see below). A related problem for such proposals is that areas that are active during math tasks (e.g., the inferior parietal lobes) are not the same areas that are active when people are engaged in spatial reasoning tasks (e.g., Barnes et al., 2000; Vanrie, Béatse, Wagemans, Sunaert, & Van Hecke, 2002). Such results undermine claims that spatial skills and math skills are intimately linked at an anatomical level. The third aspect of the results worth noting is that there is still a great deal to be discovered in the neuroscience of math. Few studies have been conducted (compared to reading or memory) and none has focused on problem solving per se. When such studies are conducted, it is likely that areas such as the frontal lobes will be found to play a more prominent role than has been noted to date.

CONCLUSIONS AND IMPLICATIONS

The goal of the present chapter was to describe the ways in which neuroscientific research is, or could be, relevant to education. I have argued that the issue of relevance chiefly pertains to whether or not a given body of research provides increased insight into cognitive development and the normal operations of the mind (Byrnes, 2001b). Just as physicians are more likely to make sound treatment decisions when they truly understand the internal processes of the body, I argue that educators are more likely to make sound instructional decisions when they truly understand the internal processes of the mind and the factors that promote learning and cognitive development (Byrnes, 2001a). Neuroscientific evidence is simply one of several forms of evidence that helps us determine which of several competing psychological models of the mind is closer to the truth. There is nothing inherent in neuroscientific evidence that makes it any more compelling or convincing than other forms of evidence (e.g., the results of traditional psychological experiments). But when psychological research and neuroscientific research both point to the same conclusion (e.g., that working memory should be decomposed into verbal and spatial components), this collective, dove-tailing evidence is certainly hard to dismiss and clearly informative.

In this chapter, I have reviewed neuroscientific studies related to brain development, memory and learning, attention, and mathematical thinking. In each case, I have included work that either clarifies the nature of these capacities or helps us form maturation-based conjectures about why skills might emerge or change at particular ages (if we were so inclined). Given the central premise of this chapter, then, these studies are clearly relevant to education. On the other hand, there is certainly a need for researchers to conduct a number of additional psychological and neuroscientific studies to further clarify the nature of school-related competencies and provide insight into the ways in which brain development could promote changes in competence. At present, all models of intellectual skills and maturation–cognition links are works in progress. In addition, there are a number of inconsistencies in the literature that need to be resolved. As such, it is not yet possible to say that particular models of some process (e.g., reading, mathematical thinking) are completely accurate and unlikely to be revised. Uncertainty about particular models, in turn, suggests that instructional decisions based on these models are more tenuous than many in the education community, the media, and curriculum sales would have us believe.

In addition to being at odds with such groups regarding certainty about models, readers familiar with the teacher-oriented literature on brain-based education will also find my conclusions to be somewhat at odds with the conclusions drawn in that literature. For example, the latter literature includes claims such as the following: (1) that music training improves mathematical and spatial ability, (2) that children need to be taught foreign languages before age 5 (when their brains are still alleged to be receptive to learning languages readily), (3) that neuroscientific research supports direct instruction in phonics, (4) that classrooms that promote divergent thinking will foster the creation of additional synaptic connections, and so on.

As I have argued in more detail elsewhere (Byrnes, 2001b), each of these claims is either a nonsequitur or based on a misreading of the neuroscientific literature. In the case of music training, for example, three problems can be identified. First, although it is true that certain kinds of music, math, and spatial skills are localized in the right parietal lobe, other kinds are localized in the left parietal, left temporal, and left frontal lobes. Thus, it is a mischaracterization to say that music, math, and spatial skills are all "right-brain activities." Second, brain regions responsible for reading music, interpreting music-related hand movements (e.g., recognizing a chord played by someone else), and controlling right-hand movements during playing are all localized in the left hemisphere for right-handers

(Hasegawa et al., 2004; Hickok, Buchsbaum, Humphries, & Muftuler, 2003; Meister et al., 2004). Thus, if anything, music training should enhance alleged *left*-brain activities, not right-brain activities. Third, there is no reason to think that simply using a brain region for one activity (e.g., music) would increase one's competence in other skills or activities that also apparently use that region (e.g., spatial ability). Competence usually involves knowledge and strategies. The cortex is highly specialized with respect to the locations in which different kinds of knowledge are stored. As such, representations of songs would not be stored in the same region in which representations of math facts are stored. It is also unlikely that regions specialized to process music would also be used to process math problems.

With respect to the claim that children must learn foreign languages before age 5, several problems can again be identified. This claim is based on two lines of evidence. One is the finding that young children's brains seem to metabolize considerably more glucose than the brains of older children and adults (according to their resting PET scans). Whereas some argue that this finding reflects the fact that young children have more synaptic connections than older individuals (e.g., Chugani, Phelps, & Mazziotta, 2002), it could also reflect many other possibilities. One, for example, is the fact that children are "universal novices." Studies have shown that individuals who are highly skilled in some domain (e.g., experts) tend to have lower levels of brain activation than novices in domain-relevant regions of the brain. The second finding that seemed to support the claim that children are especially receptive to learning languages before age 5 was an oft-cited finding (i.e., Johnson & Newport, 1991) that the later one learns a language, the less competence in the second language one demonstrates (grammatically and phonologically). However, these findings have recently been overturned in a series of experiments (see Birdsong, 1999). Thus, it would appear that adults do not seem to have a harder time learning a second language than young children.

As for the linkage between neuroscientific research on reading and instruction, it does not follow that one should teach phonics in a particular way (using a specific curriculum package) simply because neuroscientific research implicates phonological processing as being a key component of reading competence. Any program that is designed to enhance phonological processing and the alphabetic principle is compatible with what we have learned from both neuroscientific and psychological research.

Finally, some advocates of brain-based education have tried to link particular instructional methods to particular patterns of synapse generation. As noted above, for example, it has been argued that divergent thinking promotes the development of new synapses that fan out across the brain. Although it is true that "learning is in the synapses," there are two major kinds of synaptic reorganization that could underlie new learning or skill enhancement: the creation of new synapses and the pruning of existing synapses. It does not follow that there is a parallelism between instructional type and one or the other of these two possibilities. Divergent thinking could promote the pruning of synaptic connections, for example.

In sum, then, there are useful implications that can be drawn from neuroscientific research, but there are also unwarranted implications that have been drawn. In my view, the ability to tell the difference between warranted and unwarranted inferences is another reason why educators should become familiar with neuroscientific research. They will not only acquire more accurate models of the mind, they will also avoid falling prey to certain misguided claims that are unfortunately rampant in teacher-oriented literature and in the media.

REFERENCES

Anderson, J. R. (1990). *Cognitive psychology and its implications* (3rd ed.). New York: Freeman.

Angulo, M. C., Kozlov, A. S., Charpak, S., & Audinat, E. (2004). Glutamate released from glial cells synchronizes neuronal activity in the hippocampus. *Journal of Neuroscience, 24,* 6920–6927.

Barkley, R. A. (1997). Behavioral inhibition, sustained attention, and executive functions: Constructing a unifying theory of ADHD. *Psychological Review, 121,* 65–94.

Barnes, J., Howard, R. J., Senior, C., Brammer, M., Bullmore, E. T., Simmons, A., et al. (2000). Cortical activity during rotational and linear transformations. *Neuropsychologia, 38,* 1148–1156.

Barry, R. J., Clarke, A. R., McCarthy, R., Selikowitz, M., Johnstone, S. J., & Rushby, J. A. (2004). Age and gender effects in EEG coherence: I. Developmental trends in normal children. *Clinical Neurophysiology, 115,* 2252–2258.

Bauer, P. J. (2004). Getting explicit memory off the ground: Steps toward construction of a neuro-developmental account of changes in the first two years of life. *Developmental Review, 24,* 347–373.

Bell, M. A., & Fox, N. A. (1994). Brain development over the first year of life: Relations between electroencephalographic frequency and coherence and cognitive and affective behaviors. In G. Dawson & K. W. Fischer (Eds.), *Human behavior and the developing brain* (pp. 314–345). New York: Guilford Press.

Birdsong, D. (1999). *Second language acquisition and the Critical Period Hypothesis.* Mahwah, NJ: Erlbaum.

Bisanz, J., Sherman, J. L., Rasmussen, C., & Ho, E. (2005). Development of arithmetic skills and knowledge in preschool children. In J. I. D. Campbell (Ed.), *Handbook of mathematical psychology* (pp. 143–162). New York: Psychology Press.

Broadbent, N. J., Clark, R. E., Zola, S., & Squire, L. J. (2002). The medial temporal lobe and memory. In L. R. Squire & D. L. Schacter (Eds.), *Neuropsychology of memory* (3rd ed., pp. 3–23). New York: Guilford Press.

Bruer, J. T. (1997). Education and the brain: A bridge too far. *Educational Leadership, 56,* 14–18.

Byrnes, J. P. (2001a). *Cognitive development and learning in instructional contexts* (2nd ed.). Needham Heights, MA: Allyn & Bacon.

Byrnes, J. P. (2001b). *Minds, brains, and learning: Understanding the psychological and educational relevance of neuroscientific research.* New York: Guilford Press.

Byrnes, J. P., & Wasik, B. A. (1991). Role of conceptual knowledge in mathematical procedural learning. *Developmental Psychology, 27,* 777–786.

Case, R., & Okamoto, Y. (1996). The role of central conceptual structures in the development of children's thought. *Monographs of the Society for Research in Child Development, 61,* v–265.

Chugani, H. T., Phelps, M. E., & Mazziotta, J. C. (2002). Positron emission tomography study of human brain functional development. In M. H. Johnson, Y. Munakata, & R. O. Gilmore (Eds.), *Brain development and cognition: A reader* (2nd ed., pp. 101–116). Oxford, UK: Blackwell.

Dehaene, S., & Cohen, L. (1997). Cerebral pathways for calculation: Double dissociation between rote verbal and quantitative knowledge of arithmetic. *Cortex, 33,* 219–250.

Durston, S., Hilleke, E. H., Casey, B. J., Giedd, J. N., Buitlaar, J. K., & Van England, H. (2001). Anatomical MRI of the developing human brain: What have we learned? *Journal of the American Academy of Child and Adolescent Psychiatry, 40,* 1012–1020.

Durston, S., Tottenham, N. T., Thomas, K. M., Davidson, M. C., Eigsti, I., Yang, Y., et al. (2003). Differential patterns of striatal activation in young children with and without ADHD. *Biological Psychology, 53,* 871–878.

Giedd, J. N. (2004). Structural magnetic resonance imaging of the adolescent brain. *Annals of the New York Academy of Science, 1021,* 77–85.

Goodman, C. S., & Tessier-LaVigne, M. (1997). Molecular mechanisms of axon guidance and target recognition. In W. M. Cowan, T. M. Jessell, & L. S. Zipursky (Eds.), *Molecular and cellular approaches to neural development* (pp. 108–137). New York: Oxford University Press.

Gould, E., Tanapat, P., Rydel, T., & Hastings, N. (2000). Regulation of hippocampal neurogenesis in adulthood. *Biological Psychiatry, 48,* 715–720.

Hart, B., & Risley, T. R. (1995). *Meaningful differences in the everyday experience of young American children.* Baltimore: Brookes.

Hasegawa, T., Matsuki, K., Ueno, T., Maeda, Y., Matsue, Y., Konishi, Y., et al. (2004). Learned audio-visual cross-modal associations in observed piano playing activate the left planum temporale: An fMRI study. *Cognitive Brain Research, 20,* 510–518.

Hickok, G., Buchsbaum, B., Humphries, C., & Muftuler, T. (2003). Auditory–motor interaction revealed by fMRI: Speech, music, and working memory in Area SPt. *Journal of Cognitive Neuroscience, 15,* 673–682.

Jensen, E. (2000). *Teaching with the brain in mind.* Alexandria, VA: Association for Supervision and Curriculum Development.

Johnson, J. S., & Newport, E. L. (1991). Critical period effects on universal properties of language: The status of subjacency in the acquisition of a second language. *Cognition, 39,* 215–258.

Johnson, M. H. (1997). *Brain development and cognition: A reader.* Cambridge, MA: Blackwell.

Knowlton, B. J. (2002). The role of the basal ganglia in learning and memory. In L. R. Squire & D. L. Schacter (Eds.), *Neuropsychology of memory* (3rd ed., pp. 143–153). New York: Guilford Press.

Kopelman, M. D., & Stanhope, N. (2002). Anterograde and retrograde amnesia following frontal lobe, temporal lobe, or diencephalic lesions. In L. R. Squire & D. L. Schacter (Eds.), *Neuropsychology of memory* (3rd ed., pp. 47–60). New York: Guilford Press.

Kosslyn, S. M., & Koenig, O. (1994). *Wet mind: The new cognitive neuroscience.* New York: Free Press.

Lawrence, N. S., Ross, T. J., Hoffmann, R., Garavan, H., & Stein, E. A. (2003). Multiple neuronal networks mediate sustained attention. *Journal of Cognitive Neuroscience, 15,* 1028–1038.

Maguire, E. A. (2001). Neuroimaging studies of autobiographical event memory. *Philosophical Transactions of the Royal Society of London, B, 356,* 1441–1451.

McClosky, M., Aliminosa, D., & Sokol, S. M. (1991). Facts, rules, and procedures in normal calculation: Evidence from multiple single-patient studies of impaired arithmetic fact retrieval. *Brain and Cognition, 17,* 154–203.

Meister, I. G., Krings, T., Foltys, H., Boroojerdi, B., Müller, M., Töpper, R., et al. (2004). Playing piano in the mind: An fMRI study on music imagery and performance in pianists. *Cognitive Brain Research, 19,* 219–228.

Metsala, J. L., & Walley, A. C. (1998). Spoken vocabulary growth and the segmental restructuring of lexical representations: Precursors to phonemic awareness and early reading ability. In J. L. Metsala & L. C. Ehri (Eds.), *Word recognition in beginning literacy* (pp. 89–120). Mahwah, NJ: Erlbaum.

Nelson, C. A., & Luciana, M. (2001). *Handbook of developmental cognitive neuroscience.* Cambridge, MA: MIT press.

Posner, M. I. (2001). The developing human brain. *Developmental Science, 4,* 253–387.

Posner, M. I., & Raichle, M. E. (1994). *Images of mind.* New York: Scientific American Library.

Pugh, K. R., Shaywitz, B. A., Shaywitz, S. E., Shankweiler, D. P., Katz, L., Fletcher, J. M., et al. (1997). Predicting reading performance from neuroimaging profiles: The cerebral basis of phonological effects in printed word identification. *Journal of Experimental Psychology: Human Perception and Performance, 23,* 299–318.

Quartz, S., & Sejnowski, T. J. (1997). The neural basis of cognitive development: A constructivist manifesto. *Behavioral and Brain Sciences, 20,* 537–596.

Rickard, T. C., Romero, S. G., Basso, G., Wharton, C., Flitman, S., & Grafman, J.

(2000). The calculating brain: An fMRI study. *Neuropsychologia, 38,* 325–335.

Sarter, M., Givens, B., & Bruno, J. P. (2001). The cognitive neuroscience of sustained attention: Where top-down meets bottom-up. *Brain Research Reviews, 35,* 146–160.

Schmithorst, V. J., & Brown, R. D. (2004). Empirical validation of the triple-code model of numerical processing for complex math operations using functional MRI and group independent component analysis of mental addition and subtraction of fractions. *NeuroImage, 22,* 1414–1420.

Schneider, W., & Bjorklund, D. F. (1998). Memory. In W. Damon (Series Ed.), R. S. Siegler, & D. Kuhn (Volume Eds.), *Handbook of child psychology: Vol. 2. Cognition, perception, and language* (pp. 467–521). New York: Wiley.

Shimamura, A. P. (2002). Relational binding theory and the role of consolidation in memory retrieval. In L. R. Squire & D. L. Schacter (Eds.), *Neuropsychology of memory* (3rd ed., pp. 61–72). New York: Guilford Press.

Squire, L. R. (1991). *Memory and brain.* New York: Oxford University Press.

Squire, L. R., & Schacter, D. L. (2002). *Neuropsychology of memory* (3rd ed.). New York: Guilford Press.

Staley, K. (2004). Epileptic neurons go wireless. *Science, 305,* 482–483.

Swanson, H. L. (1999). What develops in working memory?: A life span perspective. *Developmental Psychology, 35,* 986–1000.

Temple, C. M. (2000). *Developmental cognitive neuropsychology.* Hove, UK: Taylor & Francis.

Vanrie, J., Béaste, E., Wagemans, J., Sunaert, S., & Van Hecke, P. (2002). Mental rotation versus invariant features in object perception from different viewpoints: An fMRI study. *Neuropsychologia, 40,* 917–930.

Vellutino, F. R., Scanlon, D. M., Sipay, E. R., Small, S. G., Pratt, A., Chen, R., et al. (1996). Cognitive profiles of difficult-to-remediate and readily remediated poor readers: Early intervention as a vehicle for distinguishing between cognitive and experiential deficits as basic causes of reading disability. *Journal of Educational Psychology, 88,* 601–638.

Warrington, R. A., & McCarthy, E. K. (1989). *Cognitive neuropsychology: A clinical introduction.* San Diego, CA: Academic Press.

CHAPTER 3

The Structural Development
of the Human Brain
as Measured Longitudinally
with Magnetic Resonance Imaging

Rhoshel K. Lenroot
Jay N. Giedd

Magnetic resonance imaging (MRI), with its lack of ionizing radiation, allows not only the safe scanning of healthy children and adolescents but also repeated acquisitions from the same people throughout the course of development. Such longitudinal data have proven indispensable in capturing the heterochronous and highly variable trajectories of anatomical brain development. The feasibility of longitudinal studies is supported by the relative stability of morphological measures from scans acquired at 2- to 4-week intervals (Giedd et al., 1995). This stability indicates that quantitative differences in longitudinal scans are reflections of genuine changes in brain structure and are not due to variability related to scan acquisition itself. The capacity for longitudinal pediatric brain imaging has expanded investigations that examine neuroanatomical differences between groups to include explorations of the journey, and not just the destination, of brain development.

There are many types of MRI, including functional, diffusion tensor, and magnetization transfer. The most common type of MRI performed clinically is usually referred to as "anatomical" or "structural" MRI and provides images similar to those seen in postmortem specimens. The smallest component of anatomical MRI output is termed a *voxel* (volume element). Each voxel is assigned a single value based on the average magnetic resonance characteristics present in the tissue of that voxel. Voxel sizes vary depending on the magnet strength, the time allowed for acquisition, and other factors, but for most structural MRI studies reported in the literature, voxel sizes are on the order of 1–2 milliliter (ml). Thus, each voxel may contain millions of neurons and hundreds of billions of synaptic connections (Pakkenberg & Gunderson, 1997). This reality has implications for the limitations of inferring functional and behavior capabilities from MR images.

One of the fundamental steps in analyzing MR images to describe, for example, differences related to brain development is to determine the type of tissue corresponding to each voxel. Brain regions such as the cortex and subcortical nuclei, which are composed primarily of neuronal cell bodies and glia, appear relatively dark on postmortem specimens and are commonly called "gray matter." "White matter" is the term for areas dominated by bundles of axons that extend between different regions of the brain; these bundles tend to appear lighter in color in postmortem specimens due to their myelin sheaths. Anatomical MR images are usually designed to optimize discrimination between gray matter, white matter, and the surrounding cerebrospinal fluid (CSF), because these three tissue types are used to define the boundaries of many brain structures. An additional complication in MRI scans in subjects up to about 2 years of age is that the myelin sheaths may not yet have formed around axons in all parts of the brain. Specialized MR images and analysis routines are necessary to take these regions of unmyelinated white matter into account when determining the boundaries of brain structures in very young subjects.

Because of the substantially different approaches used for imaging in the first 3 years of life, this chapter is divided into a section that reviews imaging studies of the fetal and perinatal period and a section on imaging of subjects from ages 4 to 25 years. Most of the data for the second section are from an ongoing brain imaging project being conducted at the Child Psychiatry Branch of the National Institute of Mental Health (CPB/NIMH). The goals of the project are to (1) map the trajectories (i.e., size by age) of anatomical brain development; (2) discern the influences on these trajectories; and (3) use the knowledge of the influences to guide treatment interventions or optimize healthy development.

IMAGING OF BRAIN DEVELOPMENT
FROM CONCEPTION THROUGH AGE 3 YEARS

Key Processes in Early Brain Development

Some knowledge of the processes influencing early brain development is useful in interpreting neuroimaging studies (see Figure 3.1). *Primary neurulation* refers to the development of the neural tube, which is the source of the future central nervous system (CNS) and is usually complete by 3–4 weeks of gestation. Abnormalities in neural tube formation result in birth defects such as spina bifida and meningomyelocele (Victor, Ropper, & Adams, 2001). Development of key forebrain and facial structures, called *prosencephalic development*, occurs during the remainder of the first trimester. The next stage is *proliferation*, which occurs for neurons primarily in the third and fourth months of gestation and for glia through the first year of life (Rakic, 1988). *Migration* occurs during the third through fifth months, in which proliferating neurons migrate from their origins near the ventricles to destinations in the cortex, moving along a "scaffolding" of glial cells (Rakic, 1990). After migration a period of rapid cell death, called *apoptosis*, occurs, which results in the removal of approximately 50% of neurons between 6 months gestation and 1 month after birth.

The remaining processes of brain development include proliferation and organization of synapses and myelination of axons. These processes begin before birth and extend well into postnatal life. Huttenlocher (1979) found that the density of synaptic connections increases rapidly after birth, by 2 years of age reaching a level approximately 50% greater than that typically seen in adults. This growth period is followed by a period of loss, during which synaptic connections are "pruned." This pattern appears to

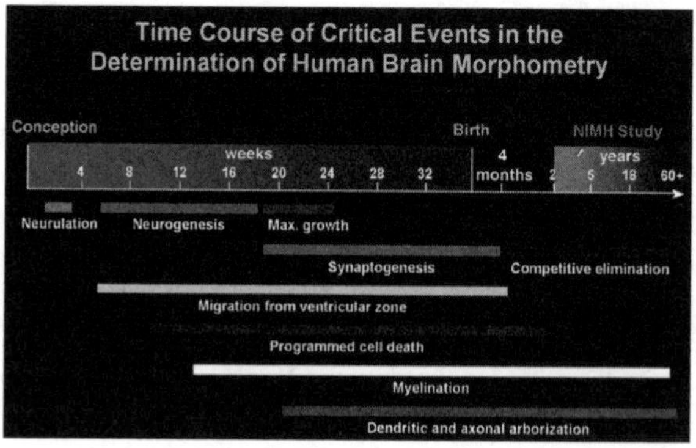

Time Course of Critical Events in the Determination of Human Brain Morphometry

Conception ... Birth ... NIMH Study

weeks | 4 months | years

4 8 12 16 20 24 28 32 | 2 5 18 60+

Neurulation Neurogenesis Max. growth

Synaptogenesis Competitive elimination

Migration from ventricular zone

Programmed cell death

Myelination

Dendritic and axonal arborization

FIGURE 3.1. A summary of the sequence of events in brain maturation.

occur in a similar fashion but at different rates in different brain regions. For example, the period of maximum synaptic density occurs in the visual cortex at 4 months postnatally, but not until 4 years of age in the prefrontal cortex.

Myelination also occurs in an orderly process by region; this process begins in the brainstem at 29 weeks (Inder & Huppi, 2000). Although the most prolific period of myelination occurs in the first year of postnatal life, in postmortem data myelination has been found to continue at least into the second decade of life (Benes, 1989; Yakovlev & Lecours, 1967). In general, myelination appears to proceed from inferior to superior and posterior to anterior. Volpe (2000) has summarized more specific principles regarding which pathways tend to be myelinated first: proximal pathways before distal, sensory before motor pathways, projection before association pathways, and from the central loci toward the frontal and occipital poles, with the occipital poles maturing first. The period of time between the first appearance of myelin in a given region and achievement of mature form in that region varies as well, ranging from 6 weeks in the posterior limb of the interior capsule to 69 weeks in portions of the frontal lobe (Kinney, Brody, Kloman, & Gilles, 1988). Benes (1989) compared myelination in a region along the surface of the hippocampus in young children from birth to 9 years old and older children ages 10–19 and found a 92% increase in myelination with age after correction for increases in total brain volume.

Synaptic development and myelination both contribute to the rapid growth of the brain in the first 2 years of life, by which time the brain has achieved 80% of its adult weight. Growth continues more slowly thereafter, with 90% of brain weight achieved by age 5 (Dekaban & Sadowsky, 1978) and a largely adult appearance of the brain by age 10 (Jernigan, Trauner, Hesselink, & Tallal, 1991).

Imaging Studies of Fetal and Perinatal Brain Development

The earliest neuroimaging studies of brain development using computerized tomography (CT) in the 1970s and MRI in the 1980s focused on qualitative descriptions of gray and white matter during the first 2 years of life (Barkovich, Kjos, Jackson, & Norman, 1988; Holland, Haas, Norman, Brant-Zawadzki, & Newton, 1986; Johnson & Bydder, 1983; Levene et al., 1982; McArdle et al., 1987). A stable developmental sequence of brain appearance in MR images was described, beginning with an infantile stage (less than 6 months) characterized by a contrast pattern opposite to what is seen in adults; that is, on a T1 image the cortex is lighter than the underlying axonal regions. This contrast switches to the "adult" pattern around 12 months of age, with an intervening crossover period showing an isointense pattern in which gray and white matter are not well differentiated. MR studies quantifying T1 and T2 relaxation times have found that both significantly shorten during this period, consistent with a substantial loss of water content in both gray and white matter, in addition to the arrival of macromolecular precursors to myelination and finally myelination itself (Inder & Huppi, 2000; Paus et al., 2001). As may be expected, the crossover occurs at different times in different regions of the brain and becomes evident on images at a time dependent on the nature of the sequence, with changes occurring in T1 weighted sequences prior to T2.

MRI studies of premature infants and fetuses *in utero* have made possible the *in vivo* description of brain structural development from early in pregnancy (Girard, Raybaud, & Poncet, 1995; Rivkin et al., 2000). Although concerns about potential risks to the developing infant limit fetal MRI use, especially during the first trimester, no clear evidence of adverse effects has been found to date, increasing the likelihood that use of MRI will become more common. In addition, current interest in attempting to map developmental abnormalities as early in their trajectory as possible and in delineating the role of adverse birth events in later outcomes is increasing attention to the value of obtaining brain measurements in individuals with normal or suspected abnormal development prior to birth.

As one example of an MRI study in early development, Huppi, Warfield, and colleagues (1998) applied automated methods to the quantification of gray matter, unmyelinated white matter, myelinated white matter, and CSF in preterm infants and infants from 29 to 41 weeks gestational age. They found an increase in brain tissue volume of 22 ml/week and a fourfold linear increase of primarily cortical gray matter. The volume of myelinated white matter increased markedly between 35 weeks and term, whereas CSF did not show significant changes.

Myelination and gyrification are both aspects of brain development that are not easily ascertainable with ultrasonography; gyrification, in particular, is seen as a good index of gestational maturation (Garel, Chantrel, Elmaleh, Brisse, & Sebag, 2003). Fetal MRI studies have described fetal brain maturation from as early as 22 weeks of gestation, including visualization of the intrahemispheric and sylvian fissures by 15 weeks (Levine & Barnes, 1999). The major sulci, except for the occipital lobe, are in place by 28 weeks of gestation, after which secondary and tertiary sulci are elaborated, with nearly all gyri present by birth. The patterns of the sulci and gyri continue to increase in complexity after birth, likely related to changes in cell-packing density and maturation of subcortical tracts. Sulcal folding patterns are highly variable between individuals, and intriguingly, sulcal folding patterns have been shown to be relatively less alike in identical twins than other measures (e.g., total brain volume), suggesting that nongenetic factors may play a significant role in determining sulcal morphology. However, due to the difficulty of quantifying features such as sulcal shapes and the still relatively sparse amount of data regarding prenatal brain development, it is not yet possible to describe exactly what determines these variations and what functional implications they may have (Lohmann, von Cramon, & Steinmetz, 1999; White, Andreasen, & Nopoulos, 2002).

IMAGING OF BRAIN DEVELOPMENT FROM AGES 4 TO 25 YEARS

The first MRI studies of healthy development were cross-sectional and often consisted of data collected from children who were being scanned as part of an evaluation for a clinical complaint and whose scans were subsequently read as normal. Despite these methodological limitations, it became apparent from these data that although overall brain volume was not changing significantly over time, significant remodeling was nevertheless occurring, as reflected in changes in relative volumes of gray matter, white matter, and CSF (Jernigan & Tallal, 1990; Reiss, Abrams, Singer, Ross, & Denckla, 1996; Schaefer et al., 1990).

In 1989 the CPB/NIMH initiated a large longitudinal study of normal and abnormal brain development, which is still ongoing. The study was designed to assess the hypotheses that many of the most severe neuropsychiatric disorders of childhood onset are associated with deviations from normal brain development and that the anatomical substrates of these deviations may be detectable through MRI. The study includes twin and nontwin healthy controls and subjects from a variety of diagnostic groups. Participants are scanned at approximate 2-year intervals, and many have been scanned three or more times, allowing for the assessment of individual trajectories without the limitations of attempting to use cross-sectional data to address longitudinal questions (Kraemer, Yesavage, Taylor, & Kupfer, 2000). As of May 2005 the data set includes approximately 3,600 scans from 1,800 subjects, about half typically developing and half from various diagnostic groups such as attention-deficit/hyperactivity disorder or childhood-onset schizophrenia. In the remainder of this section we focus on results obtained from the CPB/NIMH Brain Imaging Project, a focus that reflects our familiarity with these data and is not meant to minimize or disregard the seminal contributions of others. Because of the emphasis on the CPB/NIMH data, specifics about subject selection, image acquisition, and image analysis are reviewed below.

Subjects

Concerns regarding potential confounds from using controls that had been referred for clinical purposes led to the adoption of a stringent screening process for the CPB/NIMH Brain Imaging Project. Healthy control subjects are recruited from the community and undergo physical and neurological exams, clinical interviews, family history assessment, and an extensive neuropsychologic battery. Further details of the subject screening and assessment are presented elsewhere (Chung et al., 2001; Giedd, Snell, et al., 1996; Giedd et al., 1999; Zijdenbos, Dawant, & Margolin, 1994).

MRI Acquisition

All images are acquired on the same General Electric 1.5 Tesla Signa Scanner located at the NIH clinical center. A three-dimensional spoiled gradient recalled echo in the steady state sequence, designed to optimize discrimination between gray matter, white matter, and CSF, is used to acquire 124 contiguous 1.5 millimeter (mm) thick slices in the axial plane. Imaging parameters are as follows: time to echo = 5 milliseconds (msec); time to repeat = 24 msec; flip angle = 45 degrees; acquisition matrix = 256 × 192; number of excitations = 1; field of view = 24 centimeters (cm); and time of acquisition = 9 minutes, 52 seconds. In addition, a Fast Spin Echo/Proton Density weighted imaging sequence is acquired for clinical evaluation.

Image Analysis

Once the images are acquired, they are analyzed by a variety of automated parcellation and manual tracing techniques through collaboration with several imaging centers around the world.

Validation of MR image analysis techniques is hindered by lack of an absolute "gold standard." Comparison of postmortem data are with MRI data for purposes of validation is less than ideal on several counts. When removed from the intracranial cavity and the cerebrospinal fluid in which it is immersed, the brain collapses on its own weight, distorting *in vivo* morphology. Fixation and drying processes affect different brain structures to various degrees, with gray matter and white matter shrinking at different rates. Also, age itself is a confound, since younger brains have higher water content and are differentially affected by fixation processes. Studies using human-made models that mimic the shape and tissue characteristics of the human brain can be useful, but valid models are difficult to construct. The standard for validation of automated measures for the quantification of many structures remains a comparison to results obtained from manual tracing by expert human raters.

Classification of tissue into different types is usually accomplished by computer algorithms that create an intensity histogram of all of the voxels in the image and then fit Gaussian functions to the distribution to infer the probabilities of a given intensity corresponding to a given type of tissue. This information is sometimes supplemented with probabilistic atlases to help determine whether a given voxel is gray matter, white matter, or CSF based on its location in the brain (Collins, Holmes, Peters, & Evans, 1995).

Once the voxels have been classified, the number of voxels in a given region may be counted to provide volume estimates. Lobar volumes are most commonly reported, but as greater anatomical specification is achieved, increasingly smaller subregions will be accurately quantified.

Another approach to comparing brain anatomy from MR images is to create "average" brains for each group. Geometrical models of the brain or brain substructures can then be constructed, which lend themselves to statistical analysis. The challenge to this approach is to "register" or align the different brains in a standardized way so that a voxel from one brain image corresponds meaningfully to a voxel from another brain image. High individual variation in cortical sulcal and gyral folding patterns make this one-to-one correspondence difficult, although techniques to anchor the average shapes by aligning certain less variant sulci have greatly advanced the utility of this approach (Thompson et al., 2004).

Total Cerebral Volume

Our results show that total cerebral volume peaks at 14.5 years in males and 11.5 years in females (see Figure 3.2). By age 6 years the brain is at approximately 95% of this peak. Male brains are approximately 9% larger, on average, than those of females. This difference is statistically significant, even when controlling for height and weight.

Total brain size differences should not be interpreted as imparting any sort of functional advantage or disadvantage. Gross structural measures may not reflect sexually dimorphic differences in functionally relevant factors such as neuronal connectivity and receptor density. This point is further highlighted by the remarkable degree of variability seen in overall volumes and shapes of individual trajectories in this carefully selected group of healthy children. Healthy, normally functioning children at the same age could have 50% differences in brain volume, highlighting the need to be cautious regarding our conclusions about possible functional implications of absolute brain sizes.

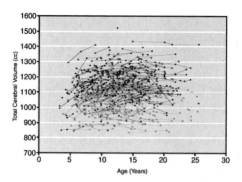

FIGURE 3.2. Total cerebral volume (TCV) by age for 224 females (375 scans) and 287 males (532 scans). Data from Giedd et al. (1999).

Cortical Gray Matter

Cortical gray matter volume tends to follow an inverted U-shape developmental course, with volumes peaking at different times in different lobes (see Figure 3.3). For instance, frontal lobe gray matter reaches its maximal volume at 11.0 years in girls and 12.1 years in boys, temporal lobe cortical gray matter peaks at 16.7 years in girls and 16.2 years in boys, and parietal lobe cortical gray matter peaks at 10.2 years in girls and 11.8 years in boys (Giedd et al., 1999).

To explore cortical gray matter changes at a smaller spatial resolution, we examined the change in gray matter density at the voxel level in a group of 13 subjects scanned four times at approximately 2-year intervals (Gogtay et al., 2004). Manually selected cortical landmarks were used as anchors to aid registration between brains. The changes over time can be viewed as time-lapse movies online (*www.loni.ucla.edu/~thompson/ DEVEL/dynamic.html*). Here it can be seen that cortical gray matter loss occurs earliest in the primary sensorimotor areas and latest in the dorsolateral prefrontal cortex (DLPFC) and superior temporal gyrus (STG). Regions subserving primary functions, such as motor and sensory systems, mature earliest, whereas the higher-order association areas that integrate those primary functions mature later. For example, in the temporal lobes the latest part to reach adult levels of maturation is the superior temporal region, which, along with the prefrontal and inferior parietal cortices, is associated with integrating memory, audiovisual input, and object recognition functions (Calvert, 2001; Martin & Chao, 2001; Mesulam, 1998).

These MRI findings, particularly the relatively late development of the DLPFC (involved in the control of impulses, judgment, and decision mak-

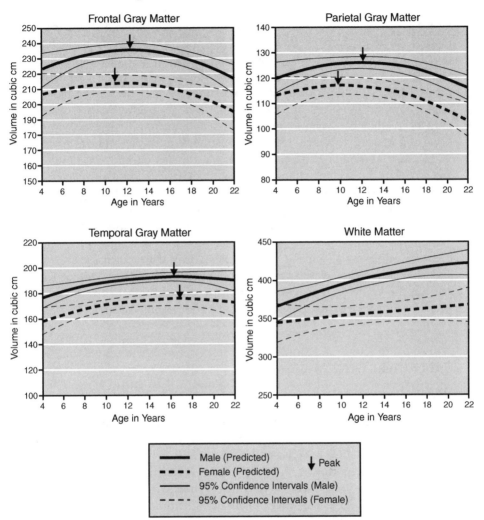

FIGURE 3.3. Frontal GM, parietal GM, temporal GM, and total WM trajectories: 243 scans from 145 subjects (scans acquired at approximately 2-year intervals). The arrows indicate peak volume. Data from Giedd et al. (1999).

ing), have entered educational, social, political, and judicial discourse in matters ranging from whether minors are cognitively mature enough to qualify for the death penalty to the age at which teenagers should be allowed to drive. However, interpretations of the meaning of these structural changes should proceed with great caution because the underlying cellular events are not well understood. The change in gray matter density may be related to synaptic proliferation and pruning, suggested to be occurring during this age range in postmortem studies (Huttenlocher, 1994). Myelination is also occurring during this period and may result in voxel classification being changed from gray matter to white, producing an apparent loss of gray matter. Indirect evidence in support of this possibility has been reported in cross-sectional studies of normal brain development by Sowell and colleagues in an independent sample of healthy children and adolescents using similar voxel based techniques. In this study of 14 children, 11 adolescents, and 10 young adults, gray matter density decrease and volume increase were spatially contemporaneous, interpreted as supporting the contention that myelination may contribute to the observed decrease in gray matter density (Sowell, Thompson, Tessner, & Toga, 2001).

Subcortical Gray Matter

Basal Ganglia

The basal ganglia consist of the caudate, putamen, globus pallidus, subthalamic nucleus, and substantia nigra. Of these, the caudate nucleus is the only structure that we have been able to quantify reliably. The basal ganglia have long been known to play a role in the control of movement and muscle tone but more recently have been shown to be involved in circuits mediating higher cognitive functions, attention, and affective states (Graybiel & Saka, 2004). Like the cortical gray matter structures, the caudate nucleus follows an inverted U-shape developmental trajectory. Caudate size peaks at age 7.5 years in girls and 10.0 years in boys.

Amygdala and Hippocampus

The temporal lobes, amygdala, and hippocampus subserve emotion, language, and memory functions that change markedly between the ages of 4 and 18 years (Diener, Sandvik, & Larsen, 1985; Jerslid, 1963; Wechsler, 1974). Quantification of the amygdala and hippocampus for the longitudinal sample is underway. In a previous cross-sectional study of a subset of these longitudinal data, amygdala volume increased with age significantly only in males, and hippocampal volume increased with age significantly only in females (Giedd, Vaituzis, et al., 1996). This pattern of gender-specific maturational volumetric changes is consistent with nonhuman primate studies, indicating a relatively higher number of androgen receptors in the amygdala (Clark, MacLusky, & Goldman-Rakic, 1988) and a relatively higher number of estrogen receptors in the hippocampus (Morse, Scheff, & DeKosky, 1986), although direct links between receptor density and growth patterns have not yet been established.

White Matter

In contrast to the inverted U shape of gray matter developmental curves, the amount of white matter in the brain generally increases throughout childhood and adolescence. Although the rate of white matter increase varies with age, we have not detected periods of overall white matter reduction for any region within the age range we have examined (Giedd et al., 1999). Gray matter volume peaks and then begins to decrease during the second decade, whereas white matter volume does not begin to decrease until the fourth decade (Bartzokis et al., 2001). Unlike the lobar differences seen in gray matter trajectories, the white matter slopes are similar in frontal, temporal, and parietal lobes.

The differences in gray matter and white matter developmental trajectories belie the inseparable connection among neurons, glial cells, and myelin, which are components of the same neural circuits and share life-long reciprocal relationships (Fields & Stevens-Graham, 2002). Neuron activity influences myelin production and the proliferation and survival of oligodendrocytes (Barres & Barde, 2000; Fields, Eshete, Dudek, Ozsarac, & Stevens, 2001), whereas oligodendrocytes influence neurons via secretion of neuronal growth factors and influence axonal growth and clustering of ion channels (Du & Dreyfus, 2002). As mentioned above, proximal pathways tend to be myelinated before distal, sensory before motor, and projection before association (Volpe, 2000). Later-maturing myelin sheaths, such as those in association tracts and intracortical regions, tend to be thinner, with greater axonal load per oligodendrocyte (Kinney, Karthigasan, Borenshteyn, Flax, & Kirschner, 1994; Yakovlev & Lecours, 1967), which may render them more vulnerable to environmental or aging-related factors (Bartzokis, 2004).

The most prominent white matter structure is the corpus callosum (CC), consisting of approximately 200 million myelinated fibers, most of which connect homologous areas of the left and right cortex. The functions of the CC can generally be thought of as integrating the activities of the left and right cerebral hemispheres, including functions related to the unification of sensory fields (Berlucchi, 1981; Shanks, Rockel, & Powel, 1975), memory storage and retrieval (Zaidel & Sperry, 1974), attention and arousal (Levy, 1985), and enhancement of language and auditory functions (Cook, 1986). Several studies have indicated that CC development continues to progress throughout adolescence (Allen, Richey, Chai, & Gorski, 1991; Cowell, Allen, Zalatimo, & Denenberg, 1992; Pujol, Vendrell, Junque, Marti-Vilalta, & Capdevila, 1993; Rauch & Jinkins, 1994; Thompson et al., 2000), raising the question of whether this structural development may be related to improvements in these cognitive capacities seen during childhood and adolescence. Effects of sex on CC development have been widely debated, with some authors finding gender-related differences (Clarke, Kraftsik, Van Der Loos, & Innocenti, 1989; Cowell et al., 1992; de Lacoste, Holloway, & Woodward, 1986; Holloway & de Lacoste, 1986) whereas many others have not (Bell & Variend, 1985; Byne, Bleier, & Houston, 1988; Oppenheim, Benjamin, Lee, Nass, & Gazzianga, 1987; Weis, Weber, Wenger, & Kimbacher, 1988, 1989; Witelson, 1985a, 1985b). In the NIMH sample, total midsagittal CC area increased robustly from ages 4 to 18 years, but there were no significant gender effects.

The relatively homogeneous appearance of white matter on typical T1 and T2 images after approximately the second year of life does not reflect its highly complex structure and extensive postnatal development. MRI techniques such as relaxometry, magnetization transfer imaging (MTI), and diffusion tensor imaging (DTI) may be of particular utility to characterize nonvolumetric features of white matter. Changes in T1 and T2 relaxation rates associated with maturation were some of the first findings to be reported using MRI in the 1970s, but then received relatively little attention while investigators focused on describing anatomy based on gray–white contrast. The growing interest in being able to use neuroimaging techniques to obtain quantitative measures of myelination as an index of brain maturation and in neural circuits as basic anatomic and functional units has led to a surge of studies using newer MR techniques.

Neuroimaging studies assessing the process of myelination and the maturation of white matter structures have found results consistent with the available postmortem data. Routine T1 and T2 weighted scans show marked changes during the first (approximately) 2 years of life that can be described qualitatively based on visual inspection. As noted above, at birth, contrast between tissue types on T1 weighted images is roughly opposite to what is seen in adults; that is, gray matter appears lighter than white matter. This contrast changes over the first 6 months of life as the water content in the brain decreases and myelination increases, so that by approximately 6 months of age T1 weighted scans appear similar to those of adults.

Contrast in T2 weighted scans changes later and does not gain its adult appearance until approximately 18 months of age. As noted above, there is a variable period of overlap during which gray and white matter are isointense and contrast is lost. A natural extension of these observations was to quantitatively map changes in T1 and T2 signal with development. Hassink and colleagues compared T2 relaxation values in nine children and eight adults and found that the T2 values in the frontal lobe decreased with age (Hassink, Hiltbrunner, Muller, & Lutschg, 1992). The largest decreases were found in the lateral frontal cortex, with smaller decreases in the dorsal frontal cortex, CC, and the head of the caudate. Steen, Ogg, Reddick, and Kingsley (1997) created T1 relaxation maps for 19 children, 31 adolescents, and 20 adults. They calculated T1 relaxation in nine regions of interest in gray and white matter regions. They found that T1 values changed at different rates in gray and white matter. T1 in white matter reached the mean level for adults by 8 years of age in all regions except frontal, which did not reach the mean adult level until 25 years of age. The T1 relaxation value did not reach its adult level in cortical gray matter until 20 years of age. The difference in T1 relaxation between children and adults was nearly twice as large in gray matter as in white. The authors of both of these papers proposed multiple potential contributors to the changes in relaxation values, including decreased water content, increased myelin, or structural changes.

MTI is a variation of relaxometry and appears to be influenced primarily by myelin, at least in white matter (Barkovich, 2000). Several studies of the effects of normal development on MT measures have shown increased MT levels with maturation. Engelbrecht and colleagues found a threefold increase in the magnetic transfer ratio (MTR) in white matter as it went from an unmyelinated to a myelinated state; MTR in gray matter during the same period also rose, but only approximately 25%, thought to be due to myelination within the gray matter (Engelbrecht, Rassek, Preiss, Wald, & Modder, 1998). The more marked changes in MT than had been seen in T2 relaxation studies were thought to reflect a component of the changing T1 as well. Rademacher and colleagues assessed MT measures within particular fiber tracts (Rademacher, Engelbrecht, Burgel, Freund, & Zilles, 1999). They obtained MT measures in children ages 1, 3, 6, and 30 months in several regions of interest, based on fiber tracts determined by a combination of an atlas and postmortem data from 10 adults. They were able to show that MT increased in all regions as a function of age, but that it was higher in projection and commissural fiber tracts than association tracts, as expected from the postmortem studies of Yaklovev and Lecours (1967), who found lingering longest in association tracts. Van Buchem and colleagues (2001) took a slightly different approach, creating a histogram of MTR in each brain tissue voxel and obtaining a peak reflective of the MTR values in the brain as a whole. They found that the peak of the histogram both decreased and widened with age, likely reflecting the increasing heterogeneity of the state of myelination in different parts of the brain with maturation compared to the relatively uniform state at birth.

Studies using DTI have also found that regions of the brain mature at different rates. The most marked effects were found in studies of infants, as might be expected from the rapid rates of brain change seen with other imaging modalities and in postmortem exams during this period. Huppi, Maier, and colleagues (1998) obtained DTI measures in infants born from 26 to 40 weeks of gestation. They found that as infants approached the age of full gestation, their central white matter regions showed features consistent with increased structural organization and myelination of tissues.

McGraw et al. measured mean anisotropy in 66 infants with an average age of 16 months in order to compare maturation in "compact" and "noncompact" areas of white matter (McGraw, Liang, & Provenzale, 2002). Compact white matter areas were defined as the CC, internal capsule, and cerebral peduncle, and noncompact areas were defined as frontal–parietal white matter and the corona radiate. They found that mean anisotropy was higher in the compact regions at all ages, although anisotropy values increased more rapidly after birth in the noncompact regions.

Studies of diffusion characteristics early in life have shown how anisotropy can be affected by factors other than myelination. McKinstry and colleagues (2002) found a transient period of increased anisotropy in cortical gray matter between 26 and 31 weeks gestational age, which then disappeared permanently and was thought to correspond to a period in which radial glial processes were prominent in the cortex, before dendritic arborization obscured the directional tendency. Another group looked at children ages 1 day to 17 years and found that the apparent diffusion coefficient (ADC) decreased and fractional anisotropy increased rapidly over the first few months of life (Morriss, Zimmerman, Bilaniuk, Hunter, & Haselgrove, 1999). However, these changes occurred prior to the stage at which myelination is known to occur (from postmortem studies) and before myelin-associated signal was seen on T1 or T2 weighted images. Others have also observed that anisotropy increased before onset of myelination (Huppi et al., 1998). It is currently thought most likely that these changes are due to "premyelination," the stage in which oligodendroglia are beginning to wrap processes around axons and macromolecule concentrations are increasing in preparation for production of myelin (Prayer & Prayer, 2003; Wimberger et al., 1995).

DTI studies in older children show subtler findings but also support the presence of continued maturation of white matter structures and myelination. Lovblad and colleagues (2003) found prolonged changes in ADC in frontal and temporal white matter. Olesen, Nagy, Westerberg, and Klingberg (2003) combined DTI with fMRI to determine whether maturing myelination in a given tract would correlate with increased blood oxygenation level dependent (BOLD) response in the pertinent cortical regions. They studied 23 children with an average age of 11.9 years, using a working memory task. In order to simplify analysis they first determined in which regions fractional anisotropy values correlated with performance on the working memory task and then looked at levels of cortical activity in these same regions. They found that fractional anisotropy in the frontal–parietal region correlated positively with cortical activity in the superior frontal sulcus and intraparietal lobe. Schneider, Il'yasov, Hennig, and Martin (2004) found that diffusion anisotropy had its sharpest increase during the first 2 years of life, but they also reported that it continued to correlate with age in participants into their 20s. Although fractional anisotropy measures reached adult levels by 2 years of age in most regions of the brain, these measures were still changing in deep white matter structures in the oldest individuals in their study.

Summary of Results

Total brain size is 95% of maximum size by the age of 6 years. Gray matter volumes follow inverted U-shaped developmental curves during childhood and are regionally specific, whereas white matter volume changes tend to be more linear and less variant across regions. Both brain structure size and developmental trajectories are highly variable and sexually dimorphic.

DISCUSSION AND FUTURE DIRECTIONS

Next Steps in Neuroimaging Studies of Brain Development

The field of developmental neuroimaging has made significant progress, including observation of many of the key events in brain development and longitudinal measurements of anatomical developmental trajectories. Future directions will include the quantification of increasingly finer subdivisions of neuroanatomy, characterizing different aspects of tissue composition, combining data from multiple sites to increase sample sizes, employing novel image acquisition techniques, and applying increasingly sophisticated image analysis and statistical modeling methods.

The next major stage in the effort to understand normal brain development is to better identify and understand the key factors that influence developmental trajectories. Although efforts in this direction are underway in this group and others, there is currently little direct evidence of what effects specific genetic or environmental parameters have on specific developmental trajectories. Diet, education, music, sports, video games, bacteria, viruses, sleep, and many other factors may all have a substantial impact, but to date no specific relationships have been established.

One approach to the study of the interplay between nature and nurture on brain development is through longitudinal research with twins. Comparing differences in brain structure between individuals who share differing amounts of genetic material or environmental exposures may help to illuminate which aspects of brain structure are most strongly influenced by genetic factors and whether the relative impact of nature and nurture changes during different stages of development. The effects of specific genes on brain morphometry can be investigated by comparing brain structures, such as regional volumes or cortical thickness between groups that have different alleles for genes important in brain development.

Another factor that has a clear effect on brain development is sex. As noted above, males and females have clear differences in brain structure and developmental trajectories. However, it is not well understood to what extent these differences are due to sex-specific hormonal exposures or to genes on the sex chromosomes. An approach being adopted by our group is to study subjects with anomalous sex chromosome variations (e.g., XXY, XXX, XXXY, XYY) and subjects with anomalous hormone levels (e.g., congenital adrenal hyperplasia, familial male precocious puberty, Cushing syndrome) in order to investigate which aspects of brain structure and function are most affected by the presence of these different factors.

The Role of Imaging in Neuropsychiatric Disorders

Group differences in anatomical MRI have been reported for nearly all neuropsychiatric disorders. However, because of the large overlap in structure sizes and developmental trajectories, MRI is currently not of diagnostic utility for psychiatric disorders (except to rule out possible central nervous system insults, such as tumors, intracranial bleeds, or congenital anomalies, as etiologies for the symptoms). There is no identified "lesion" common to all, or even most, children with the most frequently studied disorders of autism, attention-deficit/hyperactivity disorder, childhood-onset schizophrenia, dyslexia, fragile X syndrome, juvenile-onset bipolar disorder, posttraumatic stress disorder, Sydenham chorea, or Tourette syndrome.

A more immediately useful aspect of anatomical imaging may be to provide endophenotypes in typical or atypical populations. Endophenotypes are biological markers that may serve as intermediaries between genes and behavior or diagnostic syndromes. Endophenotypes related to a disease may be found in milder form in family members without the full-blown syndrome. Current nonimaging examples in schizophrenia research include eye tracking abnormalities (Calkins & Iacono, 2000; Holzman et al., 1974) and deficits in P50 suppression (Braff & Freedman, 2002; Braff, Geyer, & Swerdlow, 2001). Using brain morphometry as an endophenotype has the potential to create more biologically driven subtypes (to address the important issue of heterogeneity in current polythetic diagnostic schemes, such as the *Diagnostic and Statistical Manual of Mental Disorders—Fourth Edition, Text Revised* (DSM-IV-TR), which combines historical tradition, compatibility with the *International Classification of Diseases—10th Edition* (ICD-10), clinical and research data, and consensus of the field) and may be more directly related to specific gene effects.

Another phenomenon of developmental brain trajectories that may lead to more effective interventions is heterochronicity—that is, the brain grows in fits and starts. Speculatively, the periods of most rapid change may relate to critical or sensitive periods of environmental impact.

Future Directions

Remarkable advances in the field of pediatric neuroimaging have opened new windows into our understanding of the living, growing human brain. The mapping of developmental trajectories in typical development lays the groundwork for the next stage of exploring the influences on those trajectories and ultimately using this knowledge to optimize brain development in both healthy and clinical populations.

REFERENCES

Allen, L. S., Richey, M. F., Chai, Y. M., & Gorski, R. A. (1991). Sex differences in the corpus callosum of the living human being. *Journal of Neuroscience, 11*, 933–942.

Barkovich, A. J. (2000). Concepts of myelin and myelination in neuroradiology. *American Journal of Neuroradiology, 21*(6), 1099–1109.

Barkovich, A. J., Kjos, B. O., Jackson, D. E., Jr., & Norman, D. (1988). Normal maturation of the neonatal and infant brain: MR imaging at 1.5T. *Radiology, 166*, 173–180.

Barres, B. A., & Barde, Y. (2000). Neuronal and glial cell biology. *Current Opinions in Neurobiology, 10*(5), 642–648.

Bartzokis, G. (2004). Age-related myelin breakdown: A developmental model of cognitive decline and Alzheimer's disease. *Neurobiology of Aging, 25*(1), 5–18; author reply, 49–62.

Bartzokis, G., Beckson, M., Lu, P. H., Nuechterlein, K. H., Edwards, N., & Mintz, J. (2001). Age-related changes in frontal and temporal lobe volumes in men: A magnetic resonance imaging study. *Archives of General Psychiatry, 58*(5), 461–465.

Bell, A. D., & Variend, S. (1985). Failure to demonstrate sexual dimorphism of the corpus callosum in childhood. *Journal of Anatomy, 143*, 143–147.

Benes, F. M. (1989). Myelination of cortical–hippocampal relays during late adolescence. *Schizophrenia Bulletin, 15*(4), 585–593.

Berlucchi, G. (1981). Interhemispheric asymmetries in visual discrimination: A neurophysiological hypothesis. *Documenta Ophthalmologica: Proceedings Series, 30*, 87–93.

Braff, D. L., & Freedman, R. (2002). Endophenotypes in studies of the genetics of schizophrenia. In K. L. Davis, D. S. Charney, J. T. Coyle, & C. B. Nemeroff (Eds.), *Neuropsychopharmacology: The fifth generation of progress* (pp. 703–716). Philadelphia: Lippincott, Williams & Wilkins.

Braff, D. L., Geyer, M. A., & Swerdlow, N. R. (2001). Human studies of prepulse inhibition of startle: Normal subjects, patient groups, and pharmacological studies. *Psychopharmacology (Berl), 156*(2–3), 234–258.

Byne, W., Bleier, R., & Houston, L. (1988). Variations in human corpus callosum do not predict gender: A study using magnetic resonance imaging. *Behavioral Neuroscience, 102*, 222–227.

Calkins, M. E., & Iacono, W. G. (2000). Eye movement dysfunction in schizophrenia: A heritable characteristic for enhancing phenotype definition. *American Journal of Medical Genetics, 97*(1), 72–76.

Calvert, G. A. (2001). Crossmodal processing in the human brain: Insights from functional neuroimaging studies. *Cerebral Cortex, 11*(12), 1110–1123.

Chung, M. K., Worsley, K. J., Paus, T., Cherif, C., Collins, D. L., Giedd, J. N., et al. (2001). A unified statistical approach to deformation-based morphometry. *NeuroImage, 14*(3), 595–606.

Clark, A. S., MacLusky, N. J., & Goldman-Rakic, P. S. (1988). Androgen binding and metabolism in the cerebral cortex of the developing rhesus monkey. *Endocrinology, 123*, 932–940.

Clarke, S., Kraftsik, R., Van Der Loos, H., & Innocenti, G. M. (1989). Forms and measures of adult and developing human corpus callosum: Is there sexual dimorphism? *Journal of Comparative Neurology, 280*, 213–230.

Cook, N. D. (1986). *The brain code: Mechanisms of information transfer and the role of the corpus callosum.* London: Methuen.

Cowell, P. E., Allen, L. S., Zalatimo, N. S., & Denenberg, V. H. (1992). A developmental study of sex and age interactions in the human corpus callosum. *Developmental Brain Research, 66*, 187–192.

Dekaban, A. S., & Sadowsky, D. (1978). Changes in brain weight during the span of human life: Relation of brain weights to body heights and body weights. *Annals of Neurology, 4*, 345–356.

de Lacoste, M. C., Holloway, R. L., & Woodward, D. J. (1986). Sex differences in the fetal human corpus callosum. *Human Neurobiology, 5,* 93–96.

Diener, E., Sandvik, E., & Larsen, R. F. (1985). Age and sex effects for affect intensity. *Developmental Psychology, 21,* 542–546.

Du, Y., & Dreyfus, C. F. (2002). Oligodendrocytes as providers of growth factors. *Journal of Neuroscience Research, 68*(6), 647–654.

Engelbrecht, V., Rassek, M., Preiss, S., Wald, C., & Modder, U. (1998). Age-dependent changes in magnetization transfer contrast of white matter in the pediatric brain. *American Journal of Neuroradiology, 19*(10), 1923–1929.

Fields, R. D., Eshete, F., Dudek, S., Ozsarac, N., & Stevens, B. (2001). Regulation of gene expression by action potentials: Dependence on complexity in cellular information processing. *Novartis Foundation Symposium, 239,* 160–172; discussion, 172–166, 234–140.

Fields, R. D., & Stevens-Graham, B. (2002). New insights into neuron–glia communication. *Science, 298,* 556–562.

Garel, C., Chantrel, E., Elmaleh, M., Brisse, H., & Sebag, G. (2003). Fetal MRI: Normal gestational landmarks for cerebral biometry, gyration and myelination. *Child's Nervous System, 19*(7–8), 422–425.

Giedd, J. N., Blumenthal, J., Jeffries, N. O., Castellanos, F. X., Liu, H., Zijdenbos, A., et al. (1999). Brain development during childhood and adolescence: A longitudinal MRI study [Letter]. *Nature Neuroscience, 2*(10), 861–863.

Giedd, J. N., Snell, J. W., Lange, N., Rajapakse, J. C., Casey, B. J., Kozuch, P. L., et al. (1996). Quantitative magnetic resonance imaging of human brain development: Ages 4–18. *Cerebral Cortex, 6*(4), 551–560.

Giedd, J. N., Vaituzis, A. C., Hamburger, S. D., Lange, N., Rajapakse, J. C., Kaysen, D., et al. (1996). Quantitative MRI of the temporal lobe, amygdala, and hippocampus in normal human development: Ages 4–18 years. *Journal of Comparative Neurology, 366*(2), 223–230.

Girard, N., Raybaud, C., & Poncet, M. (1995). In vivo MR study of brain maturation in normal fetuses. *American Journal of Neuroradiology, 16*(2), 407–413.

Gogtay, N., Giedd, J. N., Lusk, L., Hayashi, B. S., Greenstein, D., Vaituzis, A. C., et al. (2004). Dynamic mapping of human cortical development during childhood through early adulthood. *Proceedings of the National Academy of Sciences, 101*(21), 8174–8179.

Graybiel, A. M., & Saka, E. (2004). The basal ganglia and the control of action. In M. S. Gazzaniga (Ed.), *The cognitive neurosciences* (3rd ed., pp. 495–510). Cambridge, MA: MIT Press.

Hassink, R. I., Hiltbrunner, B., Muller, S., & Lutschg, J. (1992). Assessment of brain maturation by t2-weighted MRI. *Neuropediatrics, 23,* 72–74.

Holland, B. A., Haas, D. K., Norman, D., Brant-Zawadzki, M., & Newton, T. H. (1986). MRI of normal brain maturation. *American Journal of Neuroradiology, 7,* 201–208.

Holloway, R. L., & de Lacoste, M. C. (1986). Sexual dimorphism in the human corpus callosum: An extension and replication study. *Human Neurobiology, 5,* 87–91.

Holzman, P. S., Proctor, L. R., Levy, D. L., Yasillo, N. J., Meltzer, H. Y., & Hurt,

S. W. (1974). Eye-tracking dysfunctions in schizophrenic patients and their relatives. *Archives of General Psychiatry, 31*(2), 143–151.

Huppi, P. S., Maier, S. E., Peled, S., Zientara, G. P., Barnes, P. D., Jolesz, F. A., et al. (1998). Microstructural development of human newborn cerebral white matter assessed in vivo by diffusion tensor magnetic resonance imaging. *Pediatric Research, 44*(4), 584–590.

Huppi, P. S., Warfield, S., Kikinis, R., Barnes, P. D., Zientara, G. P., Jolesz, F. A., et al. (1998). Quantitative magnetic resonance imaging of brain development in premature and mature newborns. *Annals of Neurology, 43*(2), 224–235.

Huttenlocher, P. R. (1979). Synaptic density in human frontal cortex: Developmental changes and effects of aging. *Brain Research, 163*, 195–205.

Huttenlocher, P. R. (1994). Synaptogenesis in human cerebral cortex. In G. Dawson & K. Fischer (Eds.), *Human behavior and the developing brain* (pp. 137–152). New York: Guilford Press.

Inder, T. E., & Huppi, P. S. (2000). In vivo studies of brain development by magnetic resonance techniques. *Mental Retardation and Developmental Disabilities Research Reviews, 6*(1), 59–67.

Jernigan, T. L., & Tallal, P. (1990). Late childhood changes in brain morphology observable with MRI. *Developmental Medicine and Child Neurology, 32*, 379–385.

Jernigan, T. L., Trauner, D. A., Hesselink, J. R., & Tallal, P. A. (1991). Maturation of human cerebrum observed in vivo during adolescence. *Brain, 114*, 2037–2049.

Jerslid, A. T. (1963). *The psychology of adolescence* (2nd ed.). New York: Macmillan.

Johnson, M. A., & Bydder, G. M. (1983). NMR imaging of the brain in children. *Medical Bulletin, 40*(2), 175–178.

Kinney, H. C., Brody, B. A., Kloman, A. S., & Gilles, F. H. (1988). Sequence of central nervous system myelination in human infancy: II. Patterns of myelination in autopsied infants. *Journal of Neuropathology and Experimental Neurology, 47*(3), 217–234.

Kinney, H. C., Karthigasan, J., Borenshteyn, N. I., Flax, J. D., & Kirschner, D. A. (1994). Myelination in the developing human brain: Biochemical correlates. *Neurochemical Research, 19*(8), 983–996.

Kraemer, H. C., Yesavage, J. A., Taylor, J. L., & Kupfer, D. (2000). How can we learn about developmental processes from cross-sectional studies, or can we? *American Journal of Psychiatry, 157*(2), 163–171.

Lenroot, R. K., Gogtay, N., Greenstein, D., Molloy, E., Wallace, G. L., Vaituzis, A. C., et al. (2005). *Sexual dimorphism of brain developmental trajectories during childhood and adolescence.* Paper presented at the Human Brain Mapping Conference, Toronto, Canada.

Levene, M. I., Whitelaw, A., Dubowitz, V., Bydder, G. M., Steiner, R. E., Randell, C. P., et al. (1982). Nuclear magnetic resonance imaging of the brain in children. *British Medical Journal (Clinical Research Ed.), 285*, 774–776.

Levine, D., & Barnes, P. D. (1999). Cortical maturation in normal and abnormal fetuses as assessed with prenatal MR imaging. *Radiology, 210*(3), 751–758.

Levy, J. (1985). Interhemispheric collaboration: Single mindedness in the asymmetric brain. In C. T. Best (Ed.), *Hemisphere function and collaboration in the child* (pp. 11–32). New York: Academic Press.

Lohmann, G., von Cramon, D. Y., & Steinmetz, H. (1999). Sulcal variability of twins. *Cerebral Cortex, 9*(7), 754–763.

Lovblad, K. O., Schneider, J., Ruoss, K., Steinlin, M., Fusch, C., & Schroth, G. (2003). Isotropic apparent diffusion coefficient mapping of postnatal cerebral development. *Neuroradiology, 45*(6), 400–403.

Martin, A., & Chao, L. L. (2001). Semantic memory and the brain: Structure and processes. *Current Opinion in Neurobiology, 11*(2), 194–201.

McArdle, C. B., Richardson, C. J., Nicholas, D. A., Mirfakhraee, M., Hayden, C. K., & Amparo, E. G. (1987). Developmental features of the neonatal brain: MR imaging: Part I. Gray–white matter differentiation and myelination. *Radiology, 162*, 223–229.

McGraw, P., Liang, L., & Provenzale, J. M. (2002). Evaluation of normal age-related changes in anisotropy during infancy and childhood as shown by diffusion tensor imaging. *American Journal of Roentgenology, 179*(6), 1515–1522.

McKinstry, R. C., Mathur, A., Miller, J. H., Ozcan, A., Snyder, A. Z., Schefft, G. L., et al. (2002). Radial organization of developing preterm human cerebral cortex revealed by non-invasive water diffusion anisotropy MRI. *Cerebral Cortex, 12*(12), 1237–1243.

Mesulam, M. -M. (1998). From sensation to cognition. *Brain, 121*(6), 1013–1052.

Morriss, M. C., Zimmerman, R. A., Bilaniuk, L. T., Hunter, J. V., & Haselgrove, J. C. (1999). Changes in brain water diffusion during childhood. *Neuroradiology, 41*(12), 929–934.

Morse, J. K., Scheff, S. W., & DeKosky, S. T. (1986). Gonadal steroids influence axonal sprouting in the hippocampal dentate gyrus: A sexually dimorphic response. *Experimental Neurology, 94*, 649–658.

Olesen, P. J., Nagy, Z., Westerberg, H., & Klingberg, T. (2003). Combined analysis of DTI and fMRI data reveals a joint maturation of white and grey matter in a fronto-parietal network. *Brain Research: Cognitive Brain Research, 18*(1), 48–57.

Oppenheim, J. S., Benjamin, A. B., Lee, C. P., Nass, R., & Gazzianga, M. S. (1987). No sex-related differences in human corpus callosum based on magnetic resonance imagery. *Annals of Neurology, 21*, 604–606.

Pakkenberg, B., & Gundersen, H. J. (1997). Neocortical neuron number in humans: Effect of sex and age. *Journal of Comparative Neurology, 384*(2), 312–320.

Paus, T., Collins, D. L., Evans, A. C., Leonard, G., Pike, B., & Zijdenbos, A. (2001). Maturation of white matter in the human brain: A review of magnetic resonance studies. *Brain Research Bulletin, 54*(3), 255–266.

Prayer, D., & Prayer, L. (2003). Diffusion-weighted magnetic resonance imaging of cerebral white matter development. *European Journal of Radiology, 45*(3), 235–243.

Pujol, J., Vendrell, P., Junque, C., Marti-Vilalta, J. L., & Capdevila, A. (1993). When does human brain development end?: Evidence of corpus callosum growth up to adulthood. *Annals of Neurology, 34,* 71–75.

Rademacher, J., Engelbrecht, V., Burgel, U., Freund, H., & Zilles, K. (1999). Measuring in vivo myelination of human white matter fiber tracts with magnetization transfer MR. *NeuroImage, 9*(4), 393–406.

Rakic, P. (1988). Specification of cerebral cortical areas. *Science, 241,* 170–176.

Rakic, P. (1990). Principles of neural cell migration. *Experientia, 46,* 882–891.

Rauch, R. A., & Jinkins, J. R. (1994). Analysis of cross-sectional area measurements of the corpus callosum adjusted for brain size in male and female subjects from childhood to adulthood. *Behavioral Brain Research, 64,* 65–78.

Reiss, A. L., Abrams, M. T., Singer, H. S., Ross, J. L., & Denckla, M. B. (1996). Brain development, gender and IQ in children. A volumetric imaging study. *Brain, 119*(5), 1763–1774.

Rivkin, P., Kraut, M., Barta, P., Anthony, J., Arria, A. M., & Pearlson, G. (2000). White matter hyperintensity volume in late-onset and early-onset schizophrenia. *International Journal of Geriatric Psychiatry, 15*(12), 1085–1089.

Schaefer, G. B., Thompson, J. N., Jr., Bodensteiner, J. B., Hamza, M., Tucker, R. R., Marks, W., et al. (1990). Quantitative morphometric analysis of brain growth using magnetic resonance imaging. *Journal of Child Neurology, 5,* 127–130.

Schneider, J. F., Il'yasov, K. A., Hennig, J., & Martin, E. (2004). Fast quantitative diffusion-tensor imaging of cerebral white matter from the neonatal period to adolescence. *Neuroradiology, 46*(4), 258–266.

Shanks, M. F., Rockel, A. J., & Powel, T. P. S. (1975). The commissural fiber connections of the primary somatic sensory cortex. *Brain Research, 98,* 166–171.

Sowell, E. R., Thompson, P. M., Tessner, K. D., & Toga, A. W. (2001). Mapping continued brain growth and gray matter density reduction in dorsal frontal cortex: Inverse relationships during postadolescent brain maturation. *Journal of Neuroscience, 21*(22), 8819–8829.

Steen, R. G., Ogg, R. J., Reddick, W. E., & Kingsley, P. B. (1997). Age-related changes in the pediatric brain: Quantitative MR evidence of maturational changes during adolescence. *American Journal of Neuroradiology, 18,* 819–828.

Thompson, P. M., Giedd, J. N., Woods, R. P., MacDonald, D., Evans, A. C., & Toga, A. W. (2000). Growth patterns in the developing brain detected by using continuum mechanical tensor maps. *Nature, 404,* 190–193.

Thompson, P. M., Hayashi, K. M., Sowell, E. R., Gogtay, N., Giedd, J. N., Rapoport, J. L., et al. (2004). Mapping cortical change in Alzheimer's disease, brain development, and schizophrenia. *NeuroImage, 23,* S2–S18.

van Buchem, M. A., Steens, S. C., Vrooman, H. A., Zwinderman, A. H., McGowan, J. C., Rassek, M., et al. (2001). Global estimation of myelination in the developing brain on the basis of magnetization transfer imaging: A preliminary study. *American Journal of Neuroradiology, 22*(4), 762–766.

Victor, M., Ropper, A. H., & Adams, R. D. (2001). *Adams and Victor's principles of neurology* (7th ed.). New York: McGraw-Hill.

Volpe, J. J. (2000). Overview: Normal and abnormal human brain development. *Mental Retardation and Developmental Disabilities Research Reviews, 6*(1), 1–5.

Wechsler, D. (1974). *Wechsler Intelligence Scale for Children—Revised.* New York: Psychological Corporation.

Weis, S., Weber, G., Wenger, E., & Kimbacher, M. (1988). The human corpus callosum and the controversy about sexual dimorphism. *Psychobiology, 16,* 411–415.

Weis, S., Weber, G., Wenger, E., & Kimbacher, M. (1989). The controversy about sexual dimorphism of the human corpus callosum. *International Journal of Neuroscience, 47,* 169–173.

White, T., Andreasen, N. C., & Nopoulos, P. (2002). Brain volumes and surface morphology in monozygotic twins. *Cerebral Cortex, 12*(5), 486–493.

Wimberger, D. M., Roberts, T. P., Barkovich, A. J., Prayer, L. M., Moseley, M. E., & Kucharczyk, J. (1995). Identification of "premyelination" by diffusion-weighted MRI. *Journal of Computer Assisted Tomography, 19*(1), 28–33.

Witelson, S. F. (1985a). The brain connection: The corpus callosum is larger in left-handers. *Science, 229,* 665–668.

Witelson, S. F. (1985b). On hemisphere specialization and cerebral plasticity from birth. In C. T. Best (Ed.), *Hemisphere function and collaboration in the child* (pp. 33–85). Orlando, FL: Academic Press.

Yakovlev, P. I., & Lecours, A. (1967). The myelogenetic cycles of regional maturation of the brain. In A. Minkowski (Ed.), *Regional development of the brain in early life* (pp. 3–65). Oxford, UK: Blackwell.

Zaidel, D., & Sperry, R. W. (1974). Memory impairment after commissurotomy in man. *Brain, 97,* 263–272.

Zijdenbos, A. P., Dawant, B. M., & Margolin, R. A. (1994). Automatic detection of intracranial contours in MR images. *Computerized Medical Imaging and Graphics, 18*(1), 11–23.

Dynamic Development of Hemispheric Biases in Three Cases

COGNITIVE/HEMISPHERIC CYCLES, MUSIC, AND HEMISPHERECTOMY

Mary Helen Immordino-Yang
Kurt W. Fischer

Vigorous debate about the roles of the two hemispheres in development and behavioral functioning has pervaded research in recent years. Evidence clearly shows that the hemispheres have different properties and functions, especially with regard to processing in specific, narrow domains, such as classical music, intonation in language, and certain aspects of emotional functioning. However, many of these apparent, surface-level differences are also misleading, in that they tend toward prescriptive or oversimplified explanations of the relations between the hemispheres, focusing too much on the localization of particular functions and too little on the distributed organization of different kinds of functioning into adaptive neural patterns through development.

In recent years educators have been looking increasingly to neuroscience to illuminate how learning experiences shape children's brain, cognitive, and social development (Diamond & Hopson, 1998; Fischer, Bernstein, & Immordino-Yang, 2006; Goswami, 2006; Johnson et al., 2005; National Research Council, 1999). In the emerging view, brain development is an active, dynamic process in which a learner's approach to problem solving serves to organize his or her brain over time and a learner's particular neuropsychological strengths, in turn, shape his or her problem-solving approach. Small differences in biases or constraints in system or hemisphere produce different organizations and functions with development over time (Fischer & Bidell, 1998; Ivry & Robertson, 1997). In this chapter, we bring this mindset to the study of hemispheric roles and interactions, moving beyond a strict localization approach to one that sees hemispheric roles as organized developmentally by organic constraints, dynamic experience-based interactions, and contextualized learning. After all, any complete neurobiological or cognitive account of hemispheric roles must be developmentally plausible.

To establish this kind of account, what is needed is a set of specific, empirically grounded examples of hemispheric interactions and reorganizations involving developmental processes. What parallels exist across these examples? What general principles of brain organization apply? Although a full set of examples is not yet available, in this chapter we present three starting points for empirically analyzing and conceptualizing the interactions of the hemispheres through development. These starting points are purposely disparate so that their juxtaposition can spark a different kind of thinking about the development of hemispheric functioning and organization.

We first present a developmental model of growth cycles of cognitive and brain development that includes systematic changes in the relations between the hemispheres (Fischer, in press; Fischer & Rose, 1994, 1996). Major cognitive and emotional reorganizations develop in correspondence with cycles of growth in brain connectivity, as measured by power and coherence in the electroencephalogram (EEG). (Power and coherence provide an indirect measure of functional white-matter connectivity between brain regions and are statistically inferred from the degree of synchrony in electrical potentials recorded over various areas of the scalp.) The series of behavioral and brain reorganizations form a general scale for assessing development and learning. In the general developmental cycle, we propose that a person first analyzes new domains from a more global perspective, relying heavily on the right hemisphere and moving through a developmental sequence within that hemisphere. Then the person analyzes the domains in a more differentiated manner, relying heavily on the left hemisphere and moving through a developmental sequence within that hemisphere. This cycle repeats for each level of cognitive and emotional development, with a continual recycling between more global and more differentiated analysis.

Another example of the global-to-local, right-to-left processing shift is the case of adults learning classical music (Immordino-Yang, 2001). In the course of this activity, a right-to-left processing shift occurs as domain-specific knowledge is built. The shifts could relate to the developmental cycle model mentioned above, or perhaps both patterns could be understood as exemplifying an underlying principle of brain functioning and reorganization through growth and learning.

A third example highlights the enormous adaptability of each of the hemispheres when one is left without the resources of the other, as represented by the cases of two hemispherectomized boys, one without a right hemisphere and one without a left (Immordino-Yang, 2005). The boys show an intriguing pattern of cognition and emotion in which they seem to have compensated remarkably effectively for the functions normally associated with the missing hemisphere. However, a deeper analysis shows that the strategies the boys use seem to be hemisphere dependent and are atypical compared to those of normally developing boys performing the same tasks with both hemispheres intact. This analysis leads to the interesting notion that rather than directly compensating for lost functions or remaining impaired, these boys have transformed the cognitive and emotional problems that they face in order to suit their remaining processing biases, their relative strengths. An empirically grounded example is the boys' production and comprehension of intonation in speech, known as affective prosody.

CASE 1: CYCLICAL GROWTH OF BRAIN AND BEHAVIOR

The growth of neural systems in the brain clearly relates to children's psychological development, but the state of knowledge about brain–behavior relations in development has been primitive, with most research merely establishing global correlations. Fortunately, the substantial neuroscientific knowledge of recent years provides possibilities for moving beyond global correlations to major breakthroughs in understanding. Especially promising is the analysis of patterns of growth in which development of brain and behavior show complex variations that share many characteristics. Based on new findings about development of brain and behavior, we have created a dynamic model of cyclical growth that hypothesizes common developmental mechanisms behind development of skills and brain activity—which we proposed over a decade ago (Fischer & Rose, 1994) and have subsequently elaborated and revised (Fischer, in press; Fischer & Bidell, 2006; Fischer & Rose, 1996). One of the central mechanisms is cyclical growth of cortical connections within and between the right and left hemispheres.

Two characteristics are especially important for analyzing and explaining these common developmental mechanisms. First, both skills and brain activity move repeatedly through periods of rapid change or developmental discontinuity that reflect dynamic underlying processes, such as connections among skills and brain regions. Second, these growth patterns take place in recurring cycles that show similar discontinuities across skills and brain regions over time. Recent advances in methods and concepts for studying and modeling development provide ways of using these two characteristics to analyze the processes of development of brain and behavior.

Discontinuities Mark Emergence of Developmental Levels

The discovery that many growth functions for brain and behavior show marked discontinuities has provided a powerful tool for establishing major developmental changes and for relating changes in brain and behavior (Thatcher, 1994). Brain characteristics such as myelination, synaptic density, dendritic branching, brain mass, pruning of neurons and synapses, and brain electrical activity all change systematically with age during childhood (Conel, 1939–1963; Dawson & Fischer, 1994; Yakovlev & Lecours, 1967; see also various chapters in this volume). Simultaneously, children's actions, speech, problem solving, concepts, social interactions, and emotions likewise change systematically. The result is that growth in all these characteristics necessarily correlates globally, but the nonlinear characteristics of growth make it possible to demarcate when major changes occur and provide tools for relating changes in skills and brain activity (Fischer & Bidell, 1998).

Brain activity evidences a series of discontinuities in growth, as illustrated in Figure 4.1 from a study by Matousek and Petersén (1973). These authors recorded several measures of brain activity that showed patterns of discontinuous growth, including relative power (reflecting level of cortical activation at the neuronal level) in the alpha band of the EEG for the occipital–parietal region of the cortex, as shown in Figure 4.1. Notice that besides the general upward growth, there are regular cycles of rapid growth (spurts) followed by slower growth or even decrease (plateaus).

Similar discontinuities in growth are common for psychological development, as illustrated in Figure 4.2, which shows growth at later stages of a complex kind of reasoning called reflective judgment (Kitchener, Lynch, Fischer, & Wood, 1993). Participants considered complex knowledge dilemmas for which there were no simple answers, such as whether chemical additives (preservatives) to food are helpful (preventing illness, such as

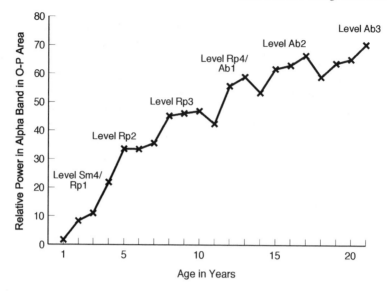

FIGURE 4.1. Development of spurts in relative energy in alpha EEG in the occipital–parietal (O-P) area in Swedish children and adolescents. (Relative energy—also called relative power—is the amplitude [in microvolts] of absolute energy in one region divided by the sum of the amplitudes in all regions, calculated as a percentage.) Data from Matousek and Petersén (1973).

food poisoning) or harmful (producing illness, such as cancer). Prior research with these dilemmas has found that people develop through seven stages of increasing sophistication in their ability to coordinate viewpoint, argument, and evidence. Adolescents and young adults showed spurts in their level of understanding with each new stage of reflective judgment, both in their reasoning at a specific stage (Y2 shows stage 6 in Figure 4.2) and in their reasoning when all stages were combined (Y1). This kind of spurt-and-plateau pattern does not occur for all developing behaviors but is common in people's optimal performance—the most complex skills that they can control with contextual support in a given domain (Fischer & Bidell, 2006).

Figures 4.1 and 4.2 illustrate the kinds of parallels that are often found between discontinuities in development of brain and behavior. There are spurts at approximately 15 and 20 years for both EEG power and reflective judgment. Figure 4.2 shows an additional discontinuity in reflective judgment at approximately age 25, and we posit a discontinuity in brain activity at the same age. However, we have been unable to find EEG research to test this hypothesis, because brain development research typically does not record variations in age in subjects in their 20s.

With these kinds of findings, research on both brain development and skill development (including cognition and emotion) has set the stage for better research and theory about relations between the two. For neural systems, key knowledge about specific growth functions goes beyond global descriptions, on the one hand, and narrow analyses of isolated local brain systems, on the other. For example, across large areas of the cerebral cortex in rhesus monkeys, synapses grow and are pruned in approximately parallel cycles that show clear discontinuities (Goldman-Rakic, 1987; Rakic, Bourgeois, Eckenhoff, Zecevic, & Goldman-Rakic, 1986), and human cortical activity and networks show distinctive patterns of spurts and drops (Fischer, in press; Hudspeth & Pribram, 1992; Thatcher, 1994).

Likewise for behavior, key knowledge about specific growth functions, especially for cognitive development, goes beyond global stage theories, on the one hand, and narrow analysis of one local behavior or knowledge domain, on the other. Evidence is now extensive that skills develop along a systematic scale in which new levels are marked by discontinuities, both in growth functions and in Rasch scaling patterns (Dawson-Tunik, Commons, Wilson, & Fischer, 2005; Fischer & Bidell, 2006). We have pro-

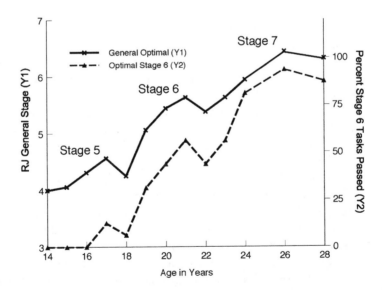

FIGURE 4.2. Development of three stages (levels) of reflective judgment in adolescents and young adults. Optimal performance spurts with the emergence of stages 5, 6, and 7 of reflective judgment. The top line (solid) shows the general score for reflective judgment across all tasks, and the dotted line shows the percentage of correct performance for the subset of tasks assessing stage 6, which is the beginning of true reflective thinking. Based on Kitchener, Lynch, Fischer, and Wood (1993).

posed that this is a universal scale reflecting general processes of skill acqui-sition; a person uses common processes to construct specific skills, yet the skills are distinctive and separate for each domain.

The dynamic skill model describes a growth cycle that repeats with each new developmental level. The coordination of components of brain and behavior into higher-order control systems, which are called dynamic skills, produces clusters of discontinuities in both brain and behavior with each major reorganization. The skills are composed of many elements in brain, body, and environment, all interacting according to the principles of dynamic systems (Fischer & Bidell, 1998; Fischer & Rose, 1994; van Geert, 1991). Before coordination, these elements are mostly independent, with only weak connections as a result of being components in the brain of a person. As coordination develops, the connections become powerful and strongly influence the shapes of growth functions for the dynamic skills, producing clusters of discontinuities. The parallel, distributed networks grow in regular cycles in the sense that each new system starts the coordi-nation process anew, becoming a potential component for a new coordina-tion into a still more complex system. The cycles typically produce periods of rapid growth in alternation with periods of slower growth, and so dis-continuities (sudden changes) are a primary index of a cycle.

The mechanism producing synchronous spurts is the development of a new capacity to build skills at a given level of complexity, which we hypothesize also involves emergence of a new level of neural network. This capacity is not to be confused with the powerful, general competencies hypothesized by Piaget (1957) and Chomsky (1965) (which we argue do not exist). The change in cognitive capacity does not automatically eventu-ate in skill changes (Fischer & Bidell, 1998), but instead, people must take time and effort to actually build the changed skills that the capacity makes possible, and factors such as state and task contribute to the actual skills produced. An individual's skills vary routinely between a higher, optimal level in situations that provide contextual support and a lower, functional level in ordinary situations that provide no support. Discontinuities in level are consistently evident only under optimal assessment conditions. Most conditions in which researchers have traditionally assessed development are nonoptimal and produce evidence for slow, gradual, continuous growth, even when people are performing the same tasks that show discontinuities under optimal conditions.

Finding and interpreting such discontinuities is no simple matter, be-cause in dynamic systems, spurts and drops in growth can occur for many dif-ferent reasons (van Geert, 1991). For example, cognitive and emotional activ-ities can vary abruptly as a result of changes in context, emotional state, social interaction, and many other component factors. However, research shows that the discontinuities are highly robust, appearing not only in development but also within a person's performances at a given time in tests or interviews (Dawson & Stein, in press; Dawson et al., 2005). Rasch scaling of test items, for instance, shows gaps between clusters of items that demonstrate the same skill scale that developmental research has documented.

Although the vagaries of dynamically growing systems make the search challenging, the complex patterns of discontinuities in growth functions for brain and behavior provide a methodological tool for testing relations across skill domains or brain regions and between brain and behavior. Researchers can search for links between specific discontinuities or other characteristics of the shapes of growth functions.

Brain-Growth Hypothesis: Parallel Cycles in Brain and Cognitive Growth

Fortunately, the framework we propose provides clear guidelines about where and how to look for developmental relations between brain and behavior. Emergence of a new level is typically marked by points of discontinuity or sharp change in growth of brain and behavior, such as sharp spurts or drops (Fischer & Bidell, 1998; van der Maas & Molenaar, 1992). Contrary to popular belief, most body organs grow in fits and starts, just like the brain (Lampl, Veldhuis, & Johnson, 1992). Individual growth curves routinely show jumps interspersed with periods of little change, whether in bones, muscles, brain, or skill.

A good model for studying brain–behavior relations in development is changes at approximately 8 months of age, where extensive evidence from multiple indices of behavior and brain development indicates a cluster of discontinuous changes. For behavior, the evidence is vast because so many studies of cognitive and emotional development have focused on the second half of the first year. Included in the behaviors that show discontinuities such as spurts and drops are search for hidden objects, distress at separation from mother, and general infant test performance. There is also substantial knowledge about one of the behavioral mechanisms behind these changes: Campos and his colleagues have shown that self-produced locomotion (crawling with the head up, not dragging on the belly or other less effective forms of locomotion) facilitates development of an array of spatial skills during this period (Campos et al., 2000). The evidence is also extensive for the brain: EEG frequency and power, some aspects of EEG coherence, glucose metabolism, and head circumference all spurt at approximately 8 months (Dawson & Fischer, 1994).

The frontal cortex seems to play a major role in the reorganization at 8 months of age. In searching for hidden objects, infants who exhibited a spurt during this age period in EEG power and coherence involving the frontal cortex also produced an advance in search behaviors, whereas infants who did not exhibit the EEG changes did not produce the cognitive advance (Bell & Fox, 1994). Research with rhesus monkeys likewise pinpoints cortical changes at the age of emergence of these search skills (Goldman-Rakic, 1987; Rakic et al., 1986): a spurt in synaptic density in the frontal area as well as other parts of the cortex. In addition, research has shown that a specific column of frontal cells holds information about the location of the hidden object while the monkey is searching. Removal of these cells prevents correct search.

This cluster of changes at approximately 8 months suggests a hypothesis about brain growth and cognitive development: When there is sudden emergence of a cluster of new cognitive capacities, there will also be sudden changes in indexes of brain growth, including connections between the frontal cortex and other regions. Prefrontal functions facilitate holding information "online" for co-occurrence and coordination of components.

According to the brain-growth hypothesis, each new developmental level for behavioral control systems is supported by growth of a new type of neural network that facilitates construction of skills at that level. Growth of the network is evident in discontinuities in both brain and cognitive development. The new networks are then gradually pruned to form efficient neural systems, during which time some indices of relevant brain growth decrease slowly and some indices of relevant cognitive growth increase gradually. Eventually, as the networks are consolidated, another new type of network begins to grow for the next developmental level, and another cluster of discontinuities begins. Most likely, the cycles are not all or none, with changes occurring everywhere at once, but instead involve a cascade of changes that moves through brain areas systematically, including systematic shifts between the right and left hemispheres. But before we elaborate a model of growth of neural networks, we need to describe the developmental scale for skill and brain that emerges from evidence for discontinuities.

Developmental Scale Marked by Clusters of Discontinuities

Evidence for clusters of discontinuities in behavior indicates development of a series of 10 levels between early infancy and 30 years of age, as shown in Figure 4.3 (Fischer, in press; Fischer & Bidell, 1998; Fischer & Rose, 1994, 1996). (There is some evidence for three additional levels in the first

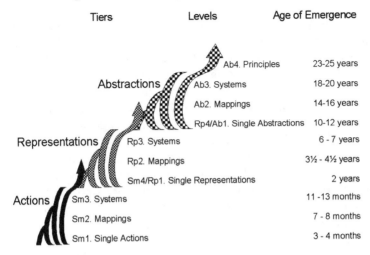

| Tiers | Levels | Age of Emergence |

FIGURE 4.3. Developmental scale of skill levels and tiers. Development moves through 10 skill levels, starting with the tier of actions (solid lines), then representations (lines with small squares), and finally abstractions (lines with large squares). Levels first emerge under optimal conditions, with high social–contextual support, and they move through a recurring cycle of single components, mappings, systems, and systems of systems—which create a new unit for the next tier, as when systems of systems of representations (Rp4) create single abstractions (Ab1). The ages are based on research with middle-class American or European children.

months after birth.) The ages listed for each level mark its emergence— when the person (child or adult) can first control a number of skills at that level. During infancy, levels grow in four rapidly occurring spurts separated by a few months—at approximately 4, 8, 12, and 20 months. Intervals become larger after infancy, with spurts at approximately 4, 7, 11, 15, 20, and 25 years of age.

Of course, individuals vary somewhat in the age of emergence of each level, and skills in specific domains and contexts also vary. There is an approximate synchrony of discontinuities within a definable time interval, along with substantial variation, as a developmental scale of control structures for the coordination of increasingly complex skills is formed. According to the brain-growth hypothesis, each level corresponds to a neural network reorganization reflected in brain-growth discontinuities.

Qualitative changes in development can be described in three different grains of detail. At the finest grain, skills develop through a sequence of small, microdevelopmental steps, which skill theory predicts via a set of transformation rules for explaining skill coordination and differentiation (Fischer, 1980). Most steps do not involve developmental discontinuities but are simply points along a pathway of skill construction. Certain steps in a sequence mark the emergence of a new developmental level; that is, a capacity to construct a new type of control system or skill. As the person enters a new level, he or she shows a stage-like spurt in optimal performance. Each of the developmental levels involves a large, indeterminate number of steps that extends beyond the initial period of developmental discontinuity, and assessment of fine-grained steps greatly facilitates detection of levels via discontinuities.

At the broadest grain, skills develop through a series of tiers, each involving four successive levels, as shown in Figure 4.3. Tiers mark the emergence of a radically new type of unit for controlling behavior—reflexes (not shown), actions, representations, or abstractions, respectively—showing an especially strong discontinuity (marked by the arrow head). For example, the emergence of the representational tier late in the second year produces the onset of complex language and a host of other changes that radically transform children's behavior. Each tier involves the same cycle of development through levels from single units to mappings to systems and finally to systems of systems, shown by the cycle of lines leading to an arrow in Figure 4.3. With the level of systems of systems, a new unit emerges and a new tier begins so that the final level of one tier is also the start of the next tier. For more detailed specification of skill levels and tiers, see Fischer (1980) and Fischer and Bidell (1998); see Fischer and Hogan (1989) for infancy; Fischer, Hand, Watson, Van Parys, and Tucker (1984) for early childhood; and Fischer, Yan, and Stewart (2003) for adolescence and early adulthood.

Growth Cycle of Neural Networks with Shifts between the Right and Left Hemispheres

The few comprehensive studies of brain development show clear growth cycles and provide evidence to help us build a model of developmental cycles of brain growth that shows remarkable parallels with the levels of skill development (Fischer & Rose, 1994, 1996; Marshall, Bar-Haim, & Fox, 2002; Somsen, van 't Klooster, van der Molen, van Leeuwen, & Licht, 1997; Thatcher, 1994). For the first 9 of the 10 developmental levels, evidence shows brain growth spurts at ages that parallel skill levels, as we illustrated for the changes at 8 months of age. As mentioned above, evidence is not available for the 10th level, at approximately 25 years, because there has been little research to assess brain growth in the 20s.

Existing evidence about changes in brain activity suggests a specific model of how cycles of brain change map onto levels of skill development. The most relevant findings come from Swedish studies of development of

EEG power (Hagne, Persson, Magnusson, & Petersén, 1973; Hudspeth & Pribram, 1992; Matousek & Petersén, 1973), Thatcher's (1994) large-sample study of development of EEG coherence as a measure of neural connectivity, Somsen and colleagues' (1997) study of EEG in middle childhood, and a Japanese study of infant brain activity (Mizuno et al., 1970). These studies sample wide age ranges and divide the samples into groups separated by no more than 1 year in age, thus providing data for modeling growth functions of brain activity. With them, we have built a model of how neural networks grow at each developmental level by connecting various cortical regions.

According to the model, each skill level is marked by a similar cycle of growth of connections, as shown in Figure 4.4. Network peak growth begins with growth of front-to-back connections in both hemispheres and then moves primarily to the right hemisphere, where growth of connections gradually contracts, changing from more distant (global) to more local. After a brief period of peak growth of frontal connections in both hemispheres, growth of connections moves to the left hemisphere, where it gradually expands, shifting from more local to more global. Then the cycle completes by returning to front-to-back growth, which begins the cycle again. Figure 4.4 shows the hypothesized growth cycle for the levels that typically emerge at approximately 7 and 11 years of age: representational systems and single abstractions.

The cycle refers to the leading edge of growth—the areas of peak growth in connections; other, less salient changes undoubtedly occur simultaneously in other cortical areas. Based on the nature of cognitive-developmental changes within each level (Fischer & Bidell, 2006) and evidence about differences between the two hemispheres (Immordino-Yang, 2005; Ivry & Robertson, 1997), this cycle would seem to start with a more global, integrative orientation at the beginning of construction of a network and move toward a more focal, differentiated orientation later in the construction.

This model of growth of a neural network is a generalization and modification of Thatcher's (1994) analysis, which was based on his large-sample study. His findings of connection spurts fit the ages, in general, for the levels emerging during childhood and early adolescence, but he has not analyzed his data for the years of infancy or later adolescence. Findings from the other studies listed above support the existence of clusters of discontinuities for each level during infancy and later adolescence, but they provide no evidence concerning growth of connections between specific cortical regions.

Extensive research will be required to discover where this model works and where it does not. In brain development research, the primary empha-

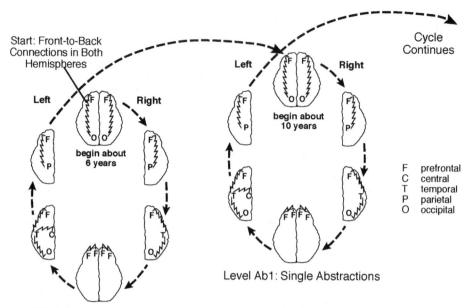

FIGURE 4.4. An illustration of the cortical network cycle for two successive developmental levels: representational systems and single abstractions. Jagged lines mark the leading edge of growth of coherence, which indicates increasing connection between cortical areas. Peak connections move around the cortex, starting with both hemispheres connecting front to back, moving to the right hemisphere, then to the prefrontal cortex in both hemispheres, and finally to the left hemisphere. This growth cycle repeats as a new network grows for each developmental level. The cycle for the level of Rp3, representational systems, lead to a new cycle for level Ab1, single abstractions, which in turn leads to a new cycle for the next level, Ab2, abstract mappings (not shown). (Connections between the middle and back of the left hemisphere are more prevalent than similar connections for the right hemisphere; the temporal–central connection for the left hemisphere is shown as an example of that difference.)

sis has traditionally been placed on measurement of neural functions, with extremely limited assessments of behavior—even when behavior is an explicit focus of investigation. Richer behavioral assessments will be required for strong research on how brain and behavior develop together. Most studies use a single behavioral task, sometimes with a few parametric variations. Psychological development involves much more than actions on a single task. It involves a rich diversity of activities, wide variations in the forms of those activities, and powerful effects of emotions on the activities.

Conclusion: Cycles of Skill Development and Brain Growth

Each developmental level requires a new type of control system to coordinate component skills, and each produces a cluster of discontinuities in behavioral growth and apparently brain growth as well. We hypothesize that each skill level is grounded in a broadly based brain-growth spurt that produces a new type of neural network and thus a new type of control system. The convergence is remarkable between the growth spurts evident in EEG and other brain-growth findings and the spurts for cognitive and emotional developments (summarized in Figure 4.4). Unfortunately, almost all relevant studies have investigated either brain growth or behavior development, not both, so extensive research will be required to test and improve this model of specific connections between brain-growth discontinuities and developmental changes in behavior.

Development is often analyzed as a linear process similar to climbing a ladder. The growth patterns that we have described suggest a different kind of model based on growth cycles. Biology is replete with cycles, and we propose that developmental science needs to move away from linear growth models toward cyclical models (Fischer & Bidell, 2006). The brain has many parts that work together in complicated ways. One part of the brain growth pattern seems to be that new learning and development begin with a bias toward the right hemisphere, with its more global approach, and then gradually move to more involvement with the left hemisphere and a focus on differentiation and specificity. This promising idea can help ground the search for organizational principles of learning, cognitive development, and brain growth. It can help explain how brain components work together to produce an emerging developmental level or an emerging set of expert skills. The growth cycles that we propose for skill and brain development provide a beginning.

CASE 2: CLASSICAL MUSIC

Classical music processing provides an example of this global-to-local, right-to-left hemispheric shift through development of domain-specific analytic skills (Immordino-Yang, 2001). This example differs in an important way from the developmental growth cycle: The research is with adult learners as they acquire musical competence through formal training, not with development of music as the result of normal environmental experience with music in children. Learning deeply about music, including the formal rules that govern the structure of classical music, changes the way people process music neuropsychologically, moving them beyond initial right-hemispheric analysis to syntactic analyses that heavily recruit the left hemisphere.

Dynamic Shifts in Brain Organization

The example of hemispheric biases in music processing is interesting from a historical perspective because it exemplifies a shift in thinking about hemispheric capacities from statically localized functions to more dynamically organized processing biases that reflect and affect learning. Modern attempts to lateralize music processing date from an abundant period of research in the 1960s. It was then widely held that language was relegated to the left hemisphere, whereas the right hemisphere handled other aspects of auditory analysis, including music and environmental sounds. This belief fit well with the notion that language and music represented clear examples of verbal and nonverbal domains (Peretz, 1993) and reflected the dominant paradigm of localization (Caramazza, 1992; Harrington, 1991), in which the role of expertise in organizing neuropsychological functioning was largely overlooked.

Since then, the study of the lateralization of broad functions such as music processing has become more complex, growing to reflect the dynamic interactions between the brain hemispheres and cognitive experience. Rather than assigning music to one hemisphere, it is now recognized that such a large domain involves several smaller functions, some of which are processed in the left hemisphere and many of which are processed differently in novices and experts. For instance, the original relegation of music processing to the right hemisphere came out of a tradition of studying only the organization of either isolated pitches or pitches in melodies and chords (Peretz, 1993), especially in nonmusicians. However, scientists now understand that the processing of pitches and melodies changes with domain-specific learning, as different features come to dominate the analysis. In nonmusicians, the most salient feature is the contour of the musical phrase (Bever & Chiarello, 1974), or the up and down movements of the pitches, akin to "inner singing." Because contour analysis is a relatively global, spatial property, it is generally lateralized to the right hemisphere (Patel, Peretz, Tramo, & Labreque, 1998).

Whereas novice listeners tend to rely more on the overall melodic contour of the musical phrase in comparing passages of music (Balch, 1984), expert musicians rely more on the formal, syntactic structure of the composition (Bever & Chiarello, 1974). Experts rely on such key characteristics as intervals (the relative difference in pitch between notes), harmonic structure (the ways that intervals are combined in a composition), and temporal characteristics of phrasing (divisions of a composition into functional units of musical processing, akin to sentences; Chiappe & Schmuckler, 1997). As musicians develop domain-specific expertise, temporal aspects of music as well as knowledge about the formal harmonic structure become the organizing features of perception and memory (Berz, 1995). Because these features rely heavily on left-hemispheric analysis (Fabbro, Brusaferro, & Bava, 1990; Ohnishi et al., 2001; Peretz, 1993; Schuppert, Munte, Wieringa, & Altenmuller, 2000), expert musicians recruit the left hemisphere for music much more than do novices.

In general, music processing involves not one unitary kind of processing supported by a single neuropsychological system, but several kinds of domain-specific processing that reflect recruitment and specialization of various component skills. As novice musicians become experts, they develop new kinds of processing that include formal analyses of the music. From the beginning, the right hemisphere handles the more global aspects such as contour analysis, and with expertise the left hemisphere is recruited for the formal, rule-bound and syntactic aspects, such as harmonic or temporal analyses. Neuropsychologically, this change is reflected in an increased reliance on left-hemispheric processing, so that music processing in experts shifts from mostly right to bilateral activation patterns.

Evidence for the Hemispheric Shift in Music

Various sources provide neuropsychological evidence for the shift to increased left-hemispheric reliance with formal musical experience. Expert musicians tend to show a right-ear advantage in dichotic listening, indicating a left-hemispheric bias. As revealed by the EEG, they also demonstrate a pattern of approximately equal activations in both hemispheres during music tasks (Davidson & Schwartz, 1977; Hirshkowitz, Earle, & Paley, 1978). In contrast, nonexperts tend to display a different pattern: greater right-hemispheric activation when listening to music and left-ear advantages in dichotic listening tasks. Nonexperts include nonmusicians with high aptitude for music (Fabbro et al., 1990), nonmusicians with average aptitude (Berz, 1995), and infants (Balaban, Anderson, & Wisniewski, 1998). Research in cerebral hemodynamics also supports this trend, demonstrating through transcranial doppler sonography a left-hemispheric dominance in musicians but a right-hemispheric dominance in nonmusicians during various music and melody recognition tasks (Evers, Dannert, Rodding, Rotter, & Ringelstein, 1999; Marinoni, Grassi, Latorraca, Caruso, & Sorbi, 2000; Matteis, Silvestrini, Troisi, Cupini, & Caltagirone, 1997). Similarly, expert musicians, especially those who began musical training before age 7, have been found to have a larger anterior corpus callosi than nonexpert controls (Schlaug, Jancke, Huang, Staiger, & Steinmetz, 1995), presumably related to increased interhemispheric communication.

In addition to syntactic and contour-based processing, other aspects of musical processing are distributed between the two hemispheres in ways that follow the principle of a bias toward basic music processing in the right hemisphere and increased reliance on left-hemispheric processing with expertise. One general finding is that both expert and untrained musicians use the right hemisphere for long-term storage of familiar melodies, probably because contour information is processed more in the right hemisphere (e.g., Berz, 1995; Patel et al., 1998; Peretz, 1993). This store is probably organized by contour of the melodies, because contour has been shown to be equally salient to musicians and novices (Burns & Ward, 1978; Dowling, 1978), and novices have been shown to rely primarily on contour in melody recognition (Sloboda & Parker, 1985). Evidence from stroke patients also supports the existence of an autonomous long-term memory store for familiar melodies in the right hemisphere, dissociated from formal syntactic knowledge. One music patient with right-hemisphere damage largely retained her ability to process pitch and rhythmic patterns but lost her memory for familiar songs (Patel et al., 1998). Another stroke patient largely retained her syntactic knowledge of music and ability to play the piano yet could not recognize well-known tunes (Beatty, Zavadil, Bailly, & Rixen, 1988). By way of a double dissociation, in one professional musician a left-hemispheric lesion to the posterior temporal lobe left her unable to read music or interpret musical syntax, but largely uncompromised in her ability to remember and play both familiar and new melodies (Cappelletti, Waley-Cohen, Butterworth, & Kopelman, 2000). (This woman's case is also evidence for left-hemispheric syntactic store in experts, discussed below.)

With regard to organization, this melodic store seems to be rule-bound in a limited sense, in that even nonmusicians are able to complete unfamiliar melodies in ways that are consistent with Western tonal frameworks (Jones & Yee, 1993). It is also available for relatively nonstrategic rehearsal in the form of chunked mental replay, as is demonstrated by an experiment in which subjects required more time to compare pitches that were further apart in familiar songs. This added time was presumably due to the subjects' mentally singing through the entire melody in real time (Crowder, 1993; Halpern, 1988).

Separate from the long-term store for familiar melodies, the evidence also points to a left-hemispheric, long-term store of syntactic musical information that can be used strategically by trained musicians for memory and other purposes (e.g., Balch, 1984; Berz, 1995; Roberts, 1986). Further evidence for this second long-term store derives from the finding that although novices can transpose familiar melodies (a task that relies on right-hemispheric contour analysis), they have trouble transposing intervals. That is, novices can sing familiar melodies starting on different notes, but are poor at producing intervals on different starting notes (Attneave & Olson, 1971). Apparently they are competent at manipulating the right-hemispheric contour-based store, but they have no well-developed syntactic framework or left-hemispheric strategy with which to process isolated intervals. Expert musicians do not show this difference (Deutsch, 1980; Sigel, McGillicuddy-DeLisi, & Goodnow, 1992).

Another example of musical processing that is organized around the right-to-left hemispheric processing shift with the acquisition of expertise is pitch comparison and categorization. Whereas both musicians and non-musicians share the ability to categorize musical pitches along a continuum, only expert musicians show true "categorical perception" of pitches, especially within intervals and chords (Patel et al., 1998, p. 198). That is, only musicians show the ability to place chords, intervals, and pitches into psychophysically bounded discrete perceptual categories in which "stimulus pairs of a given physical difference . . . are easily discriminated when they straddle a category boundary, but poorly . . . discriminated when they lie within a category" (Matzel et al., 2003, p. 198; see also Repp, 1984). Thus, it appears that knowledge of musical syntax, which defines the previously psychoacoustically arbitrary boundaries between given pitches, influences categorization and learning of pitch stimuli in music. Research with event-related potentials (ERPs, based on EEG to repeated events) compared experts and nonmusicians and found that neuropsychological changes accompanied this cognitive reorganization (Besson & Faieta, 1995). Research with functional magnetic resonance imaging (fMRI) showed enlargement of left-hemispheric sensory activations during presentation of piano tones in musicians compared to novices (Pantev et al., 1998).

These effects of expertise and associated cognitive functions suggest an interhemispheric model of music processing in which a right-to-left processing shift occurs as domain-specific knowledge is acquired (see Figure 4.5). In this model, music processing in both novices and experts likely begins in the right hemisphere, with an analysis of more global or pattern-based features such as contour of the melody. As we have seen, it is likely that the right hemisphere also contains a long-term store for familiar melodies as well as the neuropsychological substrate for pitch comparison. Following this initial processing, experts then perform additional, more differentiated analyses in the left hemisphere based on syntactic knowledge about the music. These analyses probably include constructs such as categorical pitch perception and interval, harmonic, and rhythmic analyses,

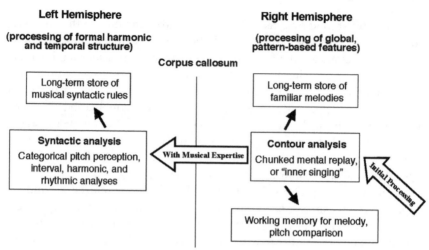

FIGURE 4.5. A schematic diagram of the neuropsychological components of music processing, illustrating a shift with musical training from mainly right-hemispheric processing to strategies associated with the left hemisphere. The boxes on the right contain the processing components normally associated with the right hemisphere, heavily recruited regardless of expertise. The boxes on the left are associated with the left hemisphere and are heavily recruited in experts after initial right-hemispheric processing.

and are likely governed by a long-term store of musical syntactic rules, also housed primarily in the left hemisphere.

Besides the finding that music processing shifts from mainly right-hemispheric analysis to combined right- and left-hemispheric processing with expertise, researchers have found that the neurological processing of music in experts has important commonalities with language processing. Specifically, evidence is accumulating that the classical left-hemispheric language regions—Broca's and Wernicke's areas and nearby locations—are recruited during music processing under certain conditions (Maess, Koelsch, Gunter, & Friederici, 2001). In experts, musical and linguistic processing seems to recruit some of the same neural resources, presumably because both domains involve processing of syntactic (left-hemisphere-related) as well as more global (right-hemisphere-related) features. For example, one study using a combined magnetic resonance imaging (MRI) and positron emission tomography (PET) technique examined the neural correlates of sight reading, playing, and listening to music in 10 professional pianists (Sergent, Zuck, Terriah, & MacDonald, 1992). The authors found a series of asymmetric left-hemispheric activations that paralleled the neural substrates of verbal processing but were partly distinct (Sergent et al., 1992). Since that study, other fMRI (Koelsch, 2005; Koelsch et al., 2002), magnetoencephalography (MEG; Koelsch, Maess, Gunter, & Friederici, 2001), and PET (Brown, Martinez, & Parsons, 2006) studies using chord sequences or other musical stimuli have found activations that overlap significantly with language areas and generally appear to reflect similar aspects of processing in the two domains, such as timing and syntactic processing.

Other evidence also suggests that music and language processing use similar neural networks, with both involving distinct regions for syntactic and nonsyntactic (often more global) processing. For example, a series of ERP studies found that prosodic processing in language elicits patterns of brain waves similar to those elicited by melodic and rhythmic processing in music (Besson, 1997, 1998). Conversely, harmonic analyses of music were similar to those for syntactic processing of language. Other studies with diverse tasks indicate distinct processing of syntactic versus nonsyntactic musical information in musicians versus nonmusicians: discrimination of melodic intervals (Crummer, Hantz, Chuang, Walton, & Frisina, 1988), discrimination of timbre from trumpets of different keys (Hantz, Crummer, Wayman, Walton, & Frisina, 1992), harmonic incongruity (Levett & Martin, 1992), and syntactic reanalysis of a musical phrase (Patel, Gibson, Ratner, Besson, & Holcomb, 1998). Complementary work with stroke patients reinforces the syntactic and nonsyntactic associations between processing in the two domains, indicating that rhythmic and melodic aspects of language and music share neurological substrates (Hofman, Klein, & Arlazoroff, 1993; Patel et al., 1998; Peretz, 1993).

In summary, music processing requires several kinds of domain-specific processing, and thinking about these aspects of music processing is essential for understanding how and why the right-to-left-hemispheric processing shift happens in musical expertise. Initially, the right hemisphere processes information about melody and other global aspects of music and then increasing expertise requires the left hemisphere for the rule-bound, syntactic parts of music such as harmonic analysis. In this way, music processing illustrates how neurological biases and experience interact in learning and development to shape the dynamic organization of the hemispheres. Experience leading to expertise organizes the domain-specific music system and shapes the distribution and organization of processing in the brain. The demands that music processing puts on the brain differ between novices, who focus on contour analysis, and experts, who incorporate syntactic analysis. The processing system for music cannot be treated as cognitively static and neurologically localized. Instead, understanding this system requires analyzing the demands that a particular knowledge domain places on the brain as it recruits various kinds of processing along a continuum of experience. Because experts process according to different criteria from novices, understanding how domain-specific systems are organized and localized in the hemispheres of the brain requires analysis in terms of development and learning.

CASE 3: DEVELOPMENT OF TWO HEMISPHERECTOMIZED BOYS

A third approach to studying the development of hemispheric organization and bias is to examine high-functioning hemispherectomized children with the goal of understanding how they have compensated for their lost functions. In hemispherectomy, one cerebral hemisphere is surgically removed to control the spread of intractable epileptic seizures. Although this drastic procedure is usually associated with profound developmental delays, a few exceptional patients have gone on to function well in mainstream environments, even attaining normal standardized IQs. Studying these individuals affords a unique perspective on hemispheric bias, as all cerebral processing now takes place in the one remaining hemisphere. These rare cases give a glimpse into the adaptive functioning of the hemispheres and provide the opportunity to ask interesting questions about the capabilities and biases of the remaining hemisphere as it acts on its own to control emotion and behavior.

Two Boys: NT and BS

In this section of the chapter, we present the extraordinary cases of NT and BS, two adolescent boys who have compensated remarkably well for the loss of one cerebral hemisphere (Immordino-Yang, 2005). To study such extreme neurological conditions requires the development of new methods that move beyond the identification of deficits on standardized assessments to characterize the ways that such children actively compensate for their brain damage. Immordino-Yang (2005) created a comparative case method in which each subject with brain damage was compared to a group of neurologically normal matched peers. The results from these analyses provided a means of comparing the hemispherectomized participants in relation to their respective groups of peers. This method illuminates the ways that each hemispherectomized person performs focal tasks relative to normal peers and allows for comparisons across the two cases that partly control for many differences in individual histories, such as the local language and culture.

NT is a 12-year-old Argentine who at age 3 years 7 months underwent a complete functional right hemispherectomy, sparing only right subcortical structures and basal ganglia, to control intractable epilepsy from polymicrogyria (see Battro, 2000, for a complete medical history and personal account). NT was born with a congenital left hemiplegia but walked at 19 months old and spoke in sentences just before age 2. His first seizures were recorded at age 22 months and were relatively mild, after which followed an 8-month seizure-free period, before he commenced with much more serious seizures involving loss of consciousness. Following surgery, he experienced no loss of language and began walking within a few days.

NT lives with his parents and younger siblings and attends a mainstream middle school at grade level, where his favorite subjects are language arts and chorus. He presents as a charming and persistently pleasant adolescent who loves reading books, and, despite a mild hemiplegia, greatly enjoys swimming, soccer, and fencing. At the time of our testing, he had a standardized Verbal IQ of 75, a Full Scale IQ of 68, and a Performance IQ of 65, although he scored much higher on some verbal measures than on others. For example, he scored at the 98th percentile on the word associations subtest of the Clinical Evaluation of Language Fundamentals–3 (CELF-3) and at the 89th percentile on the Woodcock–Muñoz Language Survey picture vocabulary test, but at the 25th percentile on the CELF-3 concepts and directions subtest.

BS is an 18-year-old American who underwent a complete left functional hemispherectomy at age 10 years, 10 months, sparing only the left basal ganglia and below. As a child he suffered from small stature and was diagnosed with pituitary dwarfism but was otherwise cognitively normal. His seizures began at age 9 years, 7 months and became severe shortly thereafter, when he was diagnosed with Rasmussen syndrome. BS was mute following his surgery and regained his language over a period of about 18 months. A few months after our testing, he graduated from high school and began attending college part time, while continuing his job bagging groceries at a local supermarket. He lives with his grandmother and presents as a very friendly and sociable young man, although stubborn and easily frustrated at times. At the time of our testing, he had a standardized Verbal IQ of 80, a Full Scale IQ of 87, and a Performance IQ of 98.

Boys such as NT and BS are extremely rare, and we will never know how much their successful compensation for extensive brain damage resulted from individual differences in their presurgery neurological profiles and how much from their supportive educational environments. Nonetheless, their success begs for exploration of the broader principles governing the ways that they have adapted. How have these boys compensated and what can we learn from them about how a person uses his or her developing hemispheres to make sense of emotional and cognitive experience, given an extreme profile of strengths and weaknesses? In this section we investigate these questions by analyzing the boys' emotional development and their use of affective prosody (intonation) in speech.

Different Ways of Processing Emotion and Language

One major way that emotion is expressed in language is through prosody, which is the intonational contour or melody and the stress pattern of speech (Crystal, 1997; Monrad-Krohn, 1948; Ross, 2000). Through manipulating the contour of an utterance, speakers can convey various emotional states and pragmatic intents, from the rising pitch of a question to the exaggerated emphasis of sarcasm:

> Person A: "I'm going to Timbuktu next summer."
> Person B: "YOU'RE going?"
> Person C: "You're GOING?"

In this example, both B and C are incredulous about A's travel plans, but B thinks that someone else should go, or that A, in particular, is not fit to go, whereas C had been under the impression that A had previously decided not to go. These nuances of meaning and affect are conveyed through linguistic intonation and accompanying paralinguistic cues, such as the facial expressions of B and C.

Although there is continuing debate about the specifics of the neurological mechanisms supporting affective prosody, it is becoming increasingly clear that an integrative process between the two hemispheres must take place for appropriate affective intonation to be incorporated into the syntax and meaning of speech. The question then arises as to how both NT and BS have fully functional language when each is missing half of the neural hardware normally relied upon for affectively appropriate language use. With careful observation, might we find evidence for systematic hemispheric biases in their prosodic profiles that could be revealing of their compensatory strategies?

As this question suggests, clues to understanding NT's and BS's good outcomes may lie in examining not only the cognitive skills but also, concurrently, the motivations and strategies they use to construct skills for using and understanding affective prosody. In assessments of their affective prosody, the boys' compensatory strategies were organized around the emotional and cognitive biases or strengths associated with the remaining hemisphere. In other words, they did not compensate by using their hemisphere to do "double duty" by taking on the processing attributes of the missing half of the brain. Instead, each boy seemed to use his remaining hemisphere to adapt the cognitive problem to suit his brain's strengths. These findings imply that brain plasticity and development arise, in part, from the brain's adaptation of behavioral needs to fit available strengths and biases. It appears that, at least in this case, the boy adapts the task to fit his brain more than he adapts his brain to fit the task.

One important example of this adaptation involves the use of intonational contours in speech. In most adults, the syntactic, temporal, and semantic aspects of language are mainly localized to the left hemisphere of the brain, whereas affective prosody and its associated skills, including control of intonational contour, are mainly handled by the right hemisphere (Kandel, Schwartz, & Jessell, 2000; Ross, 2000; Ross, Thompson, & Yenkowsky, 1997). In general, then, right-hemispheric damage in adults is associated with flattened intonational contours or monotonic speech (Cohen, Riccio, & Flannery, 1994; Heilman, Leon, & Rosenbek, 2004; Pell, 1999), whereas left-hemispheric damage is associated only with minor affective prosodic difficulties, usually attributed to speech timing rather than intonational problems (Danly & Shapiro, 1982; Gandour, Petty, & Dardarananda, 1989; Schirmer, Alter, Kotz, & Friederici, 2001; Van Lancker & Sidtis, 1992). Thus, the neuropsychological literature suggests that NT should have flat contour because he lacks a right hemisphere, and BS should have close to normal contours. Surprisingly, both boys produced atypical contours, but not in the way that the literature would have predicted.

To assess prosody regulation in NT and BS, Immordino-Yang (2005) measured the amount of pitch fluctuation each boy produced in his spontaneous speech compared to matched peers. (See Table 4.1 for a summary of NT's and BS's performance on a selection of prosody and emotion tasks.) Quite interestingly, both NT, missing his right hemisphere, and BS, missing his left hemisphere, exhibited more intonational variation than their peers. Whereas this variation was fairly subtle for NT, BS's speech at times sounded hypermelodic, with exaggerated and almost humorous intonation, especially when he was enjoying himself. Both NT's and BS's mean pitch ranges were significantly higher than those of their peers, and at times they produced utterances with wildly fluctuating range unlike anything produced by their peers in this experimental context. In addition, neither boy appeared to produce intonation as systematically as his peers and some of both boys' most prosodically atypical utterances were quite banal in content, such as BS's "to go to the park" and NT's "because I just heard it."

TABLE 4.1. Summary of NT's and BS's Performance on a Selection of Prosodic and Emotional Tasks, with Hypothesized Compensatory Strategies

Task	Hemispheric roles in normals	NT's behavior (retains LH)	BS's behavior (retains RH)
Clinical emotional interview—Participant reflected on his own emotions and thoughts about important personal relationships (e.g., how he feels with his mother).	The RH is thought to be more emotional overall and more negative than the LH. RH damage can be associated with severe emotional disturbances.	Remained quite concrete in describing his relationships and hardly mentioned emotions. Appeared uncomfortable/bored with the task.	Strongly avoided emotional topics at first, then opened up to explain effortful cognitive strategies for maintaining positive and avoiding negative emotion.
Prosodic production—Measured intonation fluctuation in participants' spontaneous speech, both for the whole utterance and for a shorter, grammatical unit.	The LH is thought to contribute mainly to linguistic prosody for grammar/words, and the RH to utterance-level prosody for emotion/conversational intent.	Defied expectation—used more intonation than peers and compensated best at the utterance level. Hypothesis: recruited the unemotional LH grammatical tonal system for an affective purpose, in order to sound socially engaging.	Used more intonation than peers and was less systematic in assigning intonation to utterances. Hypothesis: a regulatory role for the LH in prosodic production, and both hemispheres may be necessary for true competence.
Comprehending sarcastic tone of voice—Participants listened and responded to tape-recorded vignettes involving sarcastic or sincere remarks from one character to another.	Comprehending sarcasm is thought to require an intact brain and to heavily recruit the RH.	Defied expectation—identified sarcastic and sincere tones of voice as well as peers. Used a very atypical strategy, making correct snap judgments with little insight into the source of his knowledge. Hypothesis: recruited LH pseudo-grammatical categorization for a normally social and affective task.	Performed better than peers at recognizing sarcastic and sincere tone of voice. Used a very atypical strategy, in which he explicitly analyzed intonation contours and pause patterns and made connections to emotions and social contexts.
Pitch contour matching—Participants heard two utterances with different intonation patterns, and chose the one that matched the intonation pattern of a syllable string of "na na na . . . "	Thought to heavily recruit RH systems for intonation contour analysis at the utterance level.	Defied expectation—performed perfectly and better than peers. May have capitalized on the unemotional nature of the task to recruit LH strengths for pseudo-grammatical categorization.	Defied expectation—performed worse than peers, despite being able to recognize sarcastic tone (above). Persisted in describing emotional attributes of the stimuli, despite their irrelevance.

Note. Both boys' strategies appeared to be organized by the emotional and cognitive characteristics of their retained hemisphere, which for NT is the left and for BS is the right. LH signifies the left hemisphere; RH signifies the right hemisphere.

This is in contrast to the normal boys, whose most intonationally varied utterances were generally jokes or sound effects.

Clearly, these results defy prediction from traditional models of brain functioning about the boys' cognitive abilities and likely are attributable to developmental compensatory mechanisms not available to adults with brain damage. But what is the nature of these compensatory mechanisms? When analyzed in terms of each boy's emotion profile, some sense begins to emerge, providing a set of clues to how each boy's independent hemisphere is handling affective prosodic problem solving. In short, the emotion characteristics of each hemisphere appear to be an important factor driving the boys' cognitive compensation by organizing their adaptive processing shifts.

Although hemispheric specialization for emotion processing remains less clear than for language processing, the emotion profiles associated with left- and right-hemispheric damage are distinct (Lezak, 1995). Extensive work over the past decades has attempted to divine the emotion profiles of the two intact hemispheres, with varying success. Despite continuing debate, it is widely accepted that the right hemisphere is more strongly implicated in emotion (Adolphs, Damasio, Tranel, Cooper, & Damasio, 2000; Compton, Heller, Banich, Palmieri, & Miller, 2000; Perry et al., 2001), especially facial expression of affect (Borod, Koff, Yecker, Santschi, & Schmidt, 1998; Corina, Bellugi, & Reilly, 1999) and the ability to feel and perceive negative emotions (Campbell, 1982; Jansari, Tranel, & Adolphs, 2000). Although certain types of left-hemispheric damage can produce subtle emotion defects, extensive right-hemispheric damage, especially to the parietal or temporal lobe, can result in severe and at times bizarre emotion syndromes (Damasio, 2003), including notable concreteness of emotion or denial of illness or tragedy (Ramachandran, 1998). Following from this, we would expect BS to be particularly emotional and NT to be relatively less so. In fact, the findings turn out to follow this logic quite closely.

In a clinical interview, BS was reluctant to discuss his emotions and personal relationships, despite the fact that most adolescents greatly enjoy this interview protocol. Also, although patients with extensive left-hemispheric damage are prone to depression, he described himself as "always happy." However, toward the end of the interview, BS revealed that he is, in fact, strategic about managing his thoughts and emotions and keeping them exclusively positive. As the conversation worked around again to negative feelings, BS explained:

> "I put those questions away in the back of my head. . . . I really don't want to [pull them out]. . . . It's like a locked door. . . . All those things

you are saying, that I don't want to do, 'cause I try to hide those things. I don't open it up. That's my theory. That's why I'm always happy."

Overall, BS's strategy with regard to emotion seemed to be to actively avoid negative emotions at all cost and to effortfully cultivate positive emotion states. He explained, "I just do things that make me happy. . . . [You] just got to open up one of those boxes in your head to think about the fun thing you did. And when you are done with your happiness, you close the box again to save." In describing how he "gets out of the dumps," he stated, "there's different kinds of methods I use to get out. . . . I got to think of it, think of it hard, and sometimes it doesn't click till, like, 2 hours later."

As these statements reveal, BS seemed to modulate any potentially overwhelming emotions by consciously controlling the situations he allowed himself to think about, cultivating positive emotions and refusing to think about negative emotions. It could be that BS's neurological condition has left him less able to modulate or control his own emotional states, a condition for which he compensates by strategically manipulating his thoughts. BS's strong tendency toward heightened emotionality may play a role in his exaggerated use of intonation, especially as BS seemed to greatly enjoy the testing session. In a happy mood, his emotions and thus his prosody were unfettered by the regulatory capacity of the left hemisphere.

In summary, given that the right hemisphere is heavily implicated in prosodic functioning in normal adults, BS's prosodic processing was predicted to be normal. Contrary to this prediction, his approach to the tasks led to exaggerated prosody, apparently reflecting the emotional–cognitive profile of his right hemisphere as well as a lack of regulation by his absent left hemisphere.

NT, on the other hand, remained very concrete in his emotion interview and appeared uninspired by the topic of emotions in personal relationships. Rather than talk even in rudimentary ways about his emotions and feelings, as a younger child might, he instead provided concrete descriptions of activities he shares with family and friends, such as going to the cinema. How, then, is he compensating so effectively for emotional prosody in his language? The answer may lie in his remaining left hemisphere's ability to handle another type of prosody, linguistic prosody, which is strikingly unemotional.

Languages use tone to mark nonemotional aspects of speech, including syntactic characteristics such as the ends of sentences in English and the tones that distinguish words in tonal languages such as Mandarin Chinese.

The left hemisphere seems to play a major role in this kind of prosody—the relatively unemotional analysis of syntactically salient prosodic features (Gandour et al., 2000; Hughes, Chan, & Su, 1983; Moen & Sundet, 1996; Packard, 1986). Prosody is used to express both grammatical/lexical information and affective information. In tonal language speakers, whereas the right hemisphere is heavily recruited for affective prosodic processing, the left hemisphere specializes in processing prosodic grammatical information (Gandour, Ponglorpisit, & Dardarananda, 1992; Gandour, Wong, & Hutchins, 1998), such as distinguishing between words. It is conceivable that NT has approximated the affective intonation patterns of the language around him by learning and imitating through a nonaffective, "pseudo-grammatical" mechanism; in effect, perhaps he has memorized particular pitch patterns with affective significance in the same way that a Mandarin speaker memorizes a list of differently intoned words. If this were the case, his hyperprosodic tendencies may come from overcompensating for a left-hemispheric propensity for flatter intonation, perhaps in order to sound more socially engaging.

Further evidence for these interpretations comes from a study of NT's and BS's comprehension of other people's use of intonation for sarcasm. Although impaired comprehension of nonliteral language and sarcasm have been associated with prefrontal damage, especially in the right hemisphere (McDonald, 1999, 2000, 2004; Shamay-Tsoory, Tomer, & Aharon-Peretz, 2005), both NT and BS performed comparably to their peers on recognizing that counterfactual final statements in a story context signaled a sarcastic intent on the part of the story character. Clearly both boys understood the concept of sarcasm.

However, detection of a sarcastic tone of voice showed a different pattern. For a task that used the speaker's tone of voice to differentiate sarcasm versus sincerity, the boys' hemispheric biases became pronounced, affecting their strategies for inferences. Both boys could recognize a sarcastic tone as signaling a joking intent on the part of the story character, but BS's and NT's uses of social, emotional, and cognitive strategies to make inferences about the tonal information were strikingly different and hemisphere specific. BS focused strongly on intonation patterns and emotions, whereas NT never dealt explicitly with intonation or emotion and gave vague explanations for his choices.

Overall, BS's strategies relied heavily on imitating or alluding to a speaker's tone of voice, building connections between tone and its underlying emotion, and noting the implications that a particular tone and emotion would have for the story. For instance, in a story in which an older sister sarcastically tells her younger sister, "Yeah, I'm sure you have *lots* of homework!" BS responded:

"She was probably joking around. But I think she was serious at the same time. It's like two things at once . . . joking around is like, 'you don't have no homework' [said in a joking tone]. That's joking around. Serious is like, 'you have homework? That's a drag' [said in an exaggeratedly serious tone]. That's serious. So it's like a little mix."

In this example, BS justifies his decision that the story character's intent was sarcastic by talking as the character would sound were she sarcastic or serious, and then explaining that the character's original statement was, in his opinion, a mix between these two tones.

BS's interest in both emotion and intonation also extended to a set of pitch discrimination tasks requiring categorical judgments of matching pitch contours. Unlike the normal boys, in these tests he often spontaneously volunteered descriptions of the pitch contours, the relative amplitude (stress), or an emotion, often musing excessively about the speaker's intent or feelings. In doing this, he sometimes provided detailed descriptions of tonal patterns and their emotional implications, as in "Because [that choice] goes up and then down and then up again. Because it's the anger going on. It sounds meaner, but the other [choice] goes up at the last word, which is nicer." In this example, BS explicitly analyzes the pitch contour of the utterance and then assigns emotions to these contours, even though emotional considerations were not relevant to the task.

On the other hand, in justifying and reasoning about his decisions, NT never mentioned tone of voice or discussed emotion beyond simply labeling the speaker's intent as sarcastic or sincere. Instead, he tended to merely reiterate his original choice, giving answers such as, "How do I know that [she is joking]? Because I just heard it." His accuracy at categorizing the statements and inferring the story outcomes notwithstanding, he showed little awareness of the source of his tone judgment. This was true despite his generally talkative nature and evident engagement with the task. His lack of access to his strategies in these tasks fits the hypothesis that, using his left hemisphere, he has managed to transform the interpretation of emotional tone into a different kind of "pseudo grammatical" categorization task. Typical people do not naturally verbalize the bases for their grammatical usage either, except after extensive schooling about grammar. To categorize in this way, NT appears to have learned to associate different pitch contours with sarcasm or sincerity in an automatic, unemotional way—a strategy that leaves him with accurate judgments but little access to the emotional implications of the sarcastic or sincere tone for the story.

In addition to the information that this work provides about the independent functioning of each cerebral hemisphere, these findings have two main implications for the dynamic development and functioning of the two halves of the brain. First, they suggest that the cognitive and emotional biases associated with each hemisphere's normal processing remain even in the extreme circumstances of developmental compensation after hemispherectomy. This important finding suggests that these biases should be a focus of neuropsychological research on all people and underscores the importance of dynamic adaptation of not only the brain but also the tasks taken on by the hemispheres in regulating normal behavior and emotion. A fascinating question that we could not address with NT and BS is how their cycles of brain and cognitive growth might have changed as a result of having only one hemisphere.

Second, these findings emphasize the importance of emotion in organizing the development of the hemispheres. Too often neuropsychological researchers focus entirely on the cognitive aspects of processing and ignore the emotional and motivational aspects of subjects' behavior. Although the brain's cognitive aspects are undoubtedly important, NT's and BS's cases remind us of the fundamental and pervasive emotional properties of neurological processing (Damasio, 1999, 1994; Panksepp, 1998). After all, had we not analyzed in depth the emotional and motivational aspects of NT's and BS's strategies, we would not have seen important differences between them, and we may have concluded, for example, that their prosodic comprehension was similar to other children's—although analysis of emotions showed it to be strikingly and informatively atypical.

CONCLUSION: HEMISPHERIC SPECIALIZATION AND DYNAMIC INTERACTION

The three cases—growth cycles in brain–behavior development, a hemispheric shift in mastering music, and development of surprising skills by hemispherectomized children—together provide a jumping off point for thinking about hemispheric relations and developmental reorganizations in a manner that goes beyond overly simplistic localization models and moves toward understanding the dynamics of hemispheric collaboration, specialization, development, and learning. As further interesting approaches and examples accrue, our hope is to build a unifying model that moves beyond oversimplifications and prescriptions to describe, both qualitatively and empirically, the interactions between the hemispheres as well as other brain regions. Overly simplistic models of brain and behavior cannot possibly explain the remarkable adaptations (1) that people construct as they develop skills and brain structures from infancy to adulthood, (2) that musicians create as they master the complexities of music perception and performance, and (3) that NT and BS built as they recovered from hemispherectomies and created skills that they needed to live effectively, many of which they were not "supposed" to be able to produce (based on classical neurological concepts).

A cycle that moves between global analysis and differentiation in association with the two hemispheres is likely to be a central part of any model that explains these remarkable adaptations. More generally, growth processes are likely to be cyclical in nature, with people adapting their cycles for different functions as they build skills and master them in different contexts. Other central themes will include the organizing effects of biases of several kinds—from emotions, from the processing characteristics of the hemispheres and other brain components, and from experience. In all plausible models, both experience (cognitive, social, emotional, and biological) and environmental/cultural support for specific pathways will play essential roles in shaping and directing the plasticity and limitations of the hemispheres and other brain regions. Undoubtedly, there will be many surprises along the way.

ACKNOWLEDGMENTS

We thank NT, BS, and their anonymous agemates for their generous participation in the research on hemispherectomy. We are grateful to Dr. Antonio Battro for suggesting this line of research and providing sage advice as we proceeded. Funding was provided by grants from the Harvard Graduate School of Education, the Harvard Interfaculty Initiative on Mind, Brain, and Behavior, the Spencer Foundation Predoctoral Fellowship Program, the American Association of University Women Dissertation Support Fellowships Program, and Mr. and Mrs. Frederick and Sandra Rose. We express appreciation to the following people whose research and ideas have contributed to this chapter: Robbie Case, Donna Coch, Samuel P. Rose, Robert Thatcher, and Paul van Geert.

REFERENCES

Adolphs, R., Damasio, H., Tranel, D., Cooper, G., & Damasio, A. (2000). A role for somatosensory cortices in the visual recognition of emotion as revealed by three-dimensional lesion mapping. *Journal of Neuroscience, 20*(7), 2683–2690.

Attneave, F., & Olson, R. (1971). Pitch as a medium: A new approach to psychophysical scaling. *American Journal of Psychology, 84,* 147–166.

Balaban, M., Anderson, L., & Wisniewski, A. (1998). Lateral asymmetries in infant melody perception. *Developmental Psychology, 34*(1), 39–48.

Balch, W. (1984). The effects of auditory and visual interference on the immediate recall of melody. *Memory and Cognition, 12*(6), 581–589.

Battro, A. (2000). *Half a brain is enough: The story of Nico.* Cambridge, UK: Cambridge University Press.

Beatty, W., Zavadil, K., Bailly, R., & Rixen, G. (1988). Preserved musical skill in a severely demented patient. *International Journal of Clinical Neuropsychology, 10*(4), 158–164.

Bell, M. A., & Fox, N. A. (1994). Brain development over the first year of life: Relations between electroencephalographic frequency and coherence and cognitive and affective behaviors. In G. Dawson & K. W. Fischer (Eds.), *Human behavior and the developing brain* (pp. 314–345). New York: Guilford Press.

Berz, W. (1995). Working memory in music: A theoretical model. *Music Perception, 12*(3), 353–364.

Besson, M. (1997). Electrophysiological studies of music processing. In I. Deliege & J. Sloboda (Eds.), *Perception and cognition of music* (pp. 217–250). Hove, UK: Psychology Press/Erlbaum.

Besson, M. (1998). Meaning, structure, and time in language and music. *Cahiers de Psychologie Cognitive, 17*(4–5), 921–950.

Besson, M., & Faieta, F. (1995). An event-related potential (ERP) study of musical expectancy: Comparison of musicians with nonmusicians. *Journal of Experimental Psychology: Human Perception and Performance, 21*(6), 1278–1296.

Bever, T., & Chiarello, R. (1974). Cerebral dominance in musicians and non musicians. *Science, 185,* 537–539.

Borod, J. C., Koff, E., Yecker, S., Santschi, C., & Schmidt, J. M. (1998). Facial asymmetry during emotional expression: Gender, valence, and measurement technique. *Neuropsychologia, 36*(11), 1209–1215.

Brown, S., Martinez, M., & Parsons, L. (2006). Music and language side by side in the brain: A PET study of the generation of melodies and sentences. *European Journal of Neuroscience, 23*(10), 2791–2803.

Burns, E., & Ward, W. (1978). Categorical perception—phenomenon or epiphenomenon: Evidence from experiments in the perception of melodic musical intervals. *Journal of the Acoustical Society of America, 63,* 456–468.

Campbell, R. (1982). The lateralization of emotion: A critical review. *International Journal of Psychology, 17*(Suppl. 2–3), 211–229.

Campos, J. J., Anderson, D. I., Barbu-Roth, M. A., Hubbard, E. M., Hertenstein, M. J., & Witherington, D. (2000). Travel broadens the mind. *Infancy, 1,* 149–219.

Cappelletti, M., Waley-Cohen, H., Butterworth, B., & Kopelman, M. (2000). A selective loss of the ability to read and to write music. *Neurocase, 6*(4), 321–331.

Caramazza, A. (1992). Is cognitive neuropsychology possible? *Journal of Cognitive Neuroscience, 4,* 80–95.

Chiappe, P., & Schmuckler, M. (1997). Phrasing influences the recognition of melodies. *Psychonomic Bulletin and Review, 4*(2), 254–259.

Chomsky, N. (1965). *Aspects of the theory of syntax.* Cambridge, MA: MIT Press.

Cohen, M. J., Riccio, C. A., & Flannery, A. M. (1994). Expressive aprosodia following stroke to the right basal ganglia: A case report. *Neuropsychology, 8*(2), 242–245.

Compton, R. J., Heller, W., Banich, M. T., Palmieri, P. A., & Miller, G. A. (2000). Responding to threat: Hemispheric asymmetries and interhemispheric division of input. *Neuropsychology, 14*(2), 254–264.

Conel, J. L. (1939–1963). *The postnatal development of the human cerebral cortex.* Cambridge, MA: Harvard University Press.

Corina, D. P., Bellugi, U., & Reilly, J. (1999). Neuropsychological studies of linguistic and affective facial expressions in deaf signers. *Language and Speech, 42*(2–3), 307–331.

Crowder, R. (1993). Auditory memory. In S. McAdams & E. Bigand (Eds.), *Thinking in sound: The cognitive psychology of human audition* (pp. 113–145). Oxford, UK: Oxford University Press.

Crummer, G., Hantz, E., Chuang, S., Walton, J., & Frisina, R. (1988). Neural basis for music cognition: Initial experimental findings. *Psychomusicology, 7,* 117–126.

Crystal, D. (1997). *The Cambridge encyclopedia of language* (2nd ed.). Cambridge, UK: Cambridge University Press.

Damasio, A. R. (1994). *Descartes' error: Emotion, reason and the human brain.* New York: Avon Books.

Damasio, A. R. (1999). *The feeling of what happens.* New York: Harcourt Brace.

Damasio, A. R. (2003). *Looking for Spinoza: Joy, sorrow and the feeling brain.* Orlando, FL: Harcourt.

Danly, M., & Shapiro, B. (1982). Speech prosody in Broca's aphasia. *Brain and Language, 16,* 171–190.

Davidson, R., & Schwartz, G. (1977). The influence of musical training on patterns of EEG asymmetry during musical and non-musical self-generation tasks. *Psychophysiology, 9,* 412–418.

Dawson, G., & Fischer, K. W. (Eds.). (1994). *Human behavior and the developing brain.* New York: Guilford Press.

Dawson, T. L., & Stein, Z. (in press). Cycles of research and application in science education. In K. W. Fischer & T. Katzir (Eds.), *Building usable knowledge in mind, brain, and education.* Cambridge, UK: Cambridge University Press.

Dawson-Tunik, T. L., Commons, M., Wilson, M., & Fischer, K. W. (2005). The shape of development. *European Journal of Developmental Psychology, 2,* 163–195.

Deutsch, D. (1980). The processing of structured and unstructured tonal sequences. *Perception and Psychophysics, 28,* 381–389.

Diamond, M., & Hopson, J. (1998). *Magic trees of the mind: How to nurture your child's intelligence, creativity, and healthy emotions.* New York: Plume.

Dowling, J. (1978). Scale and contour: Two components of a theory of memory for melodies. *Psychological Review, 85,* 341–354.

Evers, S., Dannert, J., Rodding, D., Rotter, G., & Ringelstein, E. (1999). The cerebral hemodynamics of music perception: A transcranial Doppler sonography study. *Brain, 122,* 75–85.

Fabbro, F., Brusaferro, A., & Bava, A. (1990). Opposite musical-manual interference in young versus expert musicians. *Neuropsychologia, 28*(8), 871–877.

Fischer, K. W. (1980). A theory of cognitive development: The control and construction of hierarchies of skills. *Psychological Review, 87,* 477–531.

Fischer, K. W. (in press). Dynamic cycles of cognitive and brain development: Measuring growth in mind, brain, and education. In A. M. Battro & K. W. Fischer (Eds.), *The educated brain.* Cambridge, UK: Cambridge University Press.

Fischer, K. W., Bernstein, J. H., & Immordino-Yang, M. H. (Eds.). (2006). *Mind, brain, and education in reading disorders.* Cambridge, UK: Cambridge University Press.

Fischer, K. W., & Bidell, T. R. (1998). Dynamic development of psychological structures in action and thought. In W. Damon & R. M. Lerner (Eds.), *Handbook of child psychology: Theoretical models of human development* (5th ed., Vol. 1, pp. 467–561). New York: Wiley.

Fischer, K. W., & Bidell, T. R. (2006). Dynamic development of action, thought, and emotion. In W. Damon & R. M. Lerner (Eds.), *Handbook of child psychology: Theoretical models of human development* (6th ed., Vol. 1, pp. 313–399). New York: Wiley.

Fischer, K. W., Hand, H. H., Watson, M. W., Van Parys, M., & Tucker, J. (1984). Putting the child into socialization: The development of social categories in preschool children. In L. Katz (Ed.), *Current topics in early childhood education* (Vol. 5, pp. 27–72). Norwood, NJ: Ablex.

Fischer, K. W., & Hogan, A. E. (1989). The big picture for infant development: Levels and variations. In J. J. Lockman & N. L. Hazen (Eds.), *Action in social context: Perspectives on early development* (pp. 275–305). New York: Plenum Press.

Fischer, K. W., & Rose, S. P. (1994). Dynamic development of coordination of components in brain and behavior: A framework for theory and research. In G. Dawson & K. W. Fischer (Eds.), *Human behavior and the developing brain* (pp. 3–66). New York: Guilford Press.

Fischer, K. W., & Rose, S. P. (1996). Dynamic growth cycles of brain and cognitive development. In R. Thatcher, G. R. Lyon, J. Rumsey, & N. Krasnegor (Eds.), *Developmental neuroimaging: Mapping the development of brain and behavior* (pp. 263–279). New York: Academic Press.

Fischer, K. W., Yan, Z., & Stewart, J. (2003). Adult cognitive development: Dynamics in the developmental web. In J. Valsiner & K. Connolly (Eds.), *Handbook of developmental psychology* (pp. 491–516). Thousand Oaks, CA: Sage.

Gandour, J., Petty, S. H., & Dardarananda, R. (1989). Dysprosody in Broca's aphasia: A case study. *Brain and Language, 37,* 232–257.

Gandour, J., Ponglorpisit, S., & Dardarananda, R. (1992). Tonal disturbances in Thai after brain damage. *Journal of Neurolinguistics, 7*(1–2), 133–145.

Gandour, J., Wong, D., Hsieh, L., Weinzapfel, B., Van Lancker, D., & Hutchins, G. (2000). A crosslinguistic PET study of tone perception. *Journal of Cognitive Neuroscience, 12*(1), 207–222.

Gandour, J., Wong, D., & Hutchins, G. (1998). Pitch processing in the human brain is influenced by language experience. *NeuroReport, 9*(9), 2115–2119.

Goldman-Rakic, P. S. (1987). Connectionist theory and the biological basis of cognitive development. *Child Development, 58*, 601–622.

Goswami, U. (2006). Neuroscience and education: From research to practice? *Nature Reviews Neuroscience, 7*(5), 406–411.

Hagne, I., Persson, J., Magnusson, R., & Petersén, I. (1973). Spectral analysis via fast Fourier transform of waking EEG in normal infants. In P. Kellaway & I. Petersén (Eds.), *Automation of clinical electroencephalography* (pp. 103–143). New York: Raven.

Halpern, A. (1988). Mental scanning in auditory imagery for songs. *Journal of Experimental Psychology: Learning, Memory and Cognition, 14*, 434–443.

Hantz, E., Crummer, G., Wayman, J., Walton, J., & Frisina, R. (1992). Effects of musical training and absolute pitch on the neural processing of melodic intervals: A P3 event-related potential study. *Music Perception, 10*, 25–42.

Harrington, A. (1991). Beyond phrenology: Localization theory in the modern era. In P. Corsi (Ed.), *Enchanted loom: Chapters in the history of neuroscience* (pp. 207–239). London: Oxford University Press.

Heilman, K. M., Leon, S. A., & Rosenbek, J. C. (2004). Affective aprosodia from a medial frontal stroke. *Brain and Language, 89*, 411–416.

Hirshkowitz, M., Earle, J., & Paley, B. (1978). EEG alpha asymmetry in musicians and non-musicians: A study of hemispheric specialization. *Neuropsychologia, 16*, 125–128.

Hofman, S., Klein, C., & Arlazoroff, A. (1993). Common hemisphericity of language and music in a musician: A case report. *Journal of Communication Disorders, 26*(2), 73–82.

Hudspeth, W. J., & Pribram, K. H. (1992). Psychophysiological indices of cerebral maturation. *International Journal of Psychophysiology, 12*, 19–29.

Hughes, C., Chan, J., & Su, M. (1983). Aprosodia in Chinese patients with right cerebral hemisphere lesions. *Archives of Neurology, 40*, 732–736.

Immordino-Yang, M. H. (2001). *Working memory for music and language: Do we develop analogous systems based on similar symbolic experience?* Unpublished qualifying paper, Harvard Graduate School of Education, Cambridge, MA.

Immordino-Yang, M. H. (2005). *A tale of two cases: Emotion and affective prosody after left and right hemispherectomy.* Doctoral dissertation, Harvard University Graduate School of Education, Cambridge, MA.

Ivry, R. B., & Robertson, L. C. (1997). *The two sides of perception.* Cambridge, MA: MIT Press.

Jansari, A., Tranel, D., & Adolphs, R. (2000). A valence-specific lateral bias for discriminating emotional facial expressions in free field. *Cognition and Emotion, 14*(3), 341–353.

Johnson, M., Griffin, R., Csibra, G., Halit, H., Farroni, T., De Haan, M., et al. (2005). The emergence of the social brain network: Evidence from typical and atypical development. *Development and Psychopathology, 17*, 599–619.

Jones, M. R., & Yee, W. (1993). Attending to auditory events: The role of temporal organization. In S. McAdams & E. Bigand (Eds.), *Thinking in sound: the cog-*

nitive psychology of human audition (pp. 69–112). Oxford, UK: Oxford University Press.

Kandel, E., Schwartz, S., & Jessell, T. (2000). *Principles of neural science* (4th ed.). New York: McGraw-Hill.

Kitchener, K. S., Lynch, C. L., Fischer, K. W., & Wood, P. K. (1993). Developmental range of reflective judgment: The effect of contextual support and practice on developmental stage. *Developmental Psychology, 29,* 893–906.

Koelsch, S. (2005). Neural substrates of processing syntax and semantics in music. *Current Opinion in Neurobiology, 15*(2), 207–212.

Koelsch, S., Gunter, T., Cramon, D., Zysset, S., Lohmann, G., & Friederici, A. (2002). Bach speaks: A cortical "language-network" serves the processing of music. *NeuroImage, 17*(2), 956–966.

Koelsch, S., Maess, B., Gunter, T., & Friederici, A. (2001). Neapolitan chords activate the area of Broca: A magnetoencephalographic study. *Annals of the New York Academy of Science, 930,* 420–421.

Lampl, M., Veldhuis, J. D., & Johnson, M. L. (1992). Saltation and stasis: A model of human growth. *Science, 258,* 801–803.

Levett, C., & Martin, F. (1992). The relationship between complex musical stimuli and the late components of the event-related potential. *Psychomusicology, 11,* 125–140.

Lezak, M. D. (1995). *Neuropsychological assessment* (3rd ed.). New York: Oxford University Press.

Maess, B., Koelsch, S., Gunter, T., & Friederici, A. (2001). Musical syntax is processed in Broca's area: An MEG study. *Nature Neuroscience, 4*(5), 540–545.

Marinoni, M., Grassi, E., Latorraca, S., Caruso, A., & Sorbi, S. (2000). Music and cerebral hemodynamics. *Journal of Clinical Neuroscience, 7*(5), 425–428.

Marshall, P., Bar-Haim, Y., & Fox, N. (2002). Development of the EEG from 5 months to 4 years of age. *Clinical Neurophysiology, 113,* 1199–1208.

Matousek, M., & Petersén, I. (1973). Frequency analysis of the EEG in normal children and adolescents. In P. Kellaway & I. Petersén (Ed.), *Automation of clinical electroencephalography* (pp. 75–102). New York: Raven Press.

Matteis, M., Silvestrini, M., Troisi, E., Cupini, L., & Caltagirone, C. (1997). Transcranial doppler assessment of cerebral flow velocity during perception and recognition of melodies. *Journal of the Neurological Sciences, 149*(1), 57–61.

McDonald, S. (1999). Exploring the process of inference generation in sarcasm: A review of normal and clinical studies. *Brain and Language, 68,* 486–506.

McDonald, S. (2000). Neuropsychological studies of sarcasm. *Metaphor and Symbol, 15*(1–2), 85–98.

McDonald, S. (2004). Social perception deficits after traumatic brain injury: Interaction between emotion recognition, mentalizing ability, and social communication. *Neuropsychology, 18*(3), 572–579.

Mizuno, T., Yamauchi, N., Watanabe, A., Komatsushiro, M., Takagi, T., Iinuma, K., et al. (1970). Maturation of patterns of EEG: Basic waves of healthy infants under 12 months of age. *Tohoku Journal of Experimental Medicine, 102,* 91–98.

Moen, I., & Sundet, K. (1996). Production and perception of word tones (pitch accents) in patients with left and right hemisphere damage. *Brain and Language, 53*(2), 267–281.

Monrad-Krohn, G. H. (1948). Dysprosody or altered "melody of language." *Brain, 70*, 405–415.

National Research Council. (1999). *How people learn: brain, mind, experience, and school.* Washington, DC: National Academy Press.

Ohnishi, T., Matsuda, H., Asada, T., Aruga, M., Hirakata, M., Nishikawa, M., et al. (2001). Functional anatomy of musical perception in musicians. *Cerebral Cortex, 11*(8), 754–760.

Packard, J. (1986). Tone production deficits in nonfluent aphasic Chinese speech. *Brain and Language, 29*(2), 212–223.

Panksepp, J. (1998). *Affective neuroscience: The foundation of human and animal emotions.* New York: Oxford University Press.

Pantev, C., Oostenveld, R., Engelien, A., Ross, B., Roberts, L. E., & Hoke, M. (1998). Increased auditory cortical representation in musicians. *Nature, 392*, 811–814.

Patel, A., Gibson, E., Ratner, J., Besson, M., & Holcomb, P. (1998). Processing syntactic relations in language and music: An event related potential study. *Journal of Cognitive Neuroscience, 10*(6), 717–733.

Patel, A., Peretz, I., Tramo, M., & Labreque, R. (1998). Processing prosodic and musical patterns: A neurosychological investigation. *Brain and Language, 61*, 123–144.

Pell, M. D. (1999). Fundamental frequency encoding of linguistic and emotional prosody by right hemisphere-damaged speakers. *Brain and Language, 69*, 161–192.

Peretz, I. (1993). Auditory agnosia: A functional analysis. In S. McAdams & E. Bigand (Eds.), *Thinking in sound: The cognitive psychology of human audition* (pp. 199–230). Oxford, UK: Clarendon Press.

Perry, R. J., Rosen, H. R., Kramer, J. H., Beer, J. S., Levenson, R. L., & Miller, B. L. (2001). Hemispheric dominance for emotions, empathy and social behaviour: Evidence from right and left handers with frontotemporal dementia. *Neurocase, 7*(2, Pt. 2), 145–160.

Piaget, J. (1957). *Logique et équilibre dans les comportements du sujet* [Logic and equilibrium in subjects' behavior]. *Études d'Épistémologie Génétique, 2*, 27–118.

Rakic, P., Bourgeois, J.-P., Eckenhoff, M. F., Zecevic, N., & Goldman-Rakic, P. (1986). Concurrent overproduction of synapses in diverse regions of the primate cerebral cortex. *Science, 232*, 232–235.

Ramachandran, V. (1998). *Phantoms of the brain: Probing the mysteries of the human mind.* New York: Morrow.

Repp, B. (1984). Categorical perception: Issues, methods and findings. In N. J. Lass (Ed.), *Speech and language: Advances in research and practice* (pp. 243–335). New York: Academic Press.

Roberts, L. (1986). Modality and suffix effects in memory for melodic and harmonic musical materials. *Cognitive Psychology, 18*, 123–157.

Ross, E. D. (2000). Affective prosody and the aprosodias. In M.-M. Mesulam (Ed.), *Principles of behavioral and cognitive neurology* (2nd ed., pp. 316–331). London: Oxford University Press.

Ross, E. D., Thompson, R. D., & Yenkowsky, J. (1997). Lateralization of affective prosody in the brain and the collosal integration of hemispheric language functions. *Brain and Language, 56,* 27–54.

Schirmer, A., Alter, K., Kotz, S., & Friederici, A. D. (2001). Lateralization of prosody during language production: A lesion study. *Brain and Language, 76,* 1–17.

Schlaug, G., Jancke, L., Huang, Y., Staiger, J., & Steinmetz, H. (1995). Increased corpus callosum size in expert musicians. *Neuropsychologia, 33*(8), 1047.

Schuppert, M., Munte, T., Wieringa, B., & Altenmuller, E. (2000). Receptive amusia: Evidence for cross-hemispheric neural networks underlying music processing strategies. *Brain, 123,* 546–559.

Sergent, J., Zuck, E., Terriah, S., & MacDonald, B. (1992). Distributed neural network underlying musical sight-reading and keyboard performance. *Science, 257,* 106–109.

Shamay-Tsoory, S. G., Tomer, R., & Aharon-Peretz, J. (2005). The neuroanatomical basis of understanding sarcasm and its relationship to social cognition. *Neuropsychology, 19*(3), 288–300.

Sigel, I. E., McGillicuddy-DeLisi, A. V., & Goodnow, J. J. (1992). *Parental belief systems: The psychological consequences for children* (2nd ed.). Hillsdale, NJ: Erlbaum.

Sloboda, J., & Parker, D. (1985). Immediate recall of melodies. In I. Cross, P. Howell, & R. West (Eds.), *Musical structure and cognition* (pp. 143–167). London: Academic Press.

Somsen, R. J. M., van 't Klooster, B. J., van der Molen, M. W., van Leeuwen, H. M. P., & Licht, R. (1997). Growth spurts in brain maturation during middle childhood as indexed by EEG power spectra. *Biological Psychology, 44,* 187–209.

Thatcher, R. W. (1994). Cyclic cortical reorganization: Origins of human cognitive development. In G. Dawson & K. W. Fischer (Eds.), *Human behavior and the developing brain* (pp. 232–266). New York: Guilford Press.

van der Maas, H., & Molenaar, P. (1992). A catastrophe-theoretical approach to cognitive development. *Psychological Review, 99,* 395–417.

van Geert, P. (1991). A dynamic systems model of cognitive and language growth. *Psychological Review, 98,* 3–53.

Van Lancker, D., & Sidtis, J. J. (1992). The identification of affective prosodic stimuli by left- and right-hemisphere-damaged subjects: All errors are not created equal. *Journal of Speech and Hearing Research, 35,* 963–970.

Yakovlev, P. I., & Lecours, A. R. (1967). The myelogenetic cycles of regional maturation of the brain. In A. Minkowsky (Ed.), *Regional development of the brain in early life* (pp. 3–70). Oxford, UK: Blackwell.

PART II

THE DEVELOPING BRAIN
AND BEHAVIOR IN INFANCY
AND TODDLERHOOD

CHAPTER 5

The Social Brain in Infancy

A DEVELOPMENTAL COGNITIVE NEUROSCIENCE APPROACH

Mark H. Johnson

One of the most prominent characteristics of the human brain is its processing of social stimuli. Although in most adults regions of the brain are specialized for processing and integrating sensory information about the appearance, behavior, and intentions of other humans, how these specializations emerge during development remains largely unknown. Indeed, one of the major debates in cognitive neuroscience concerns the origins of the "social brain" in humans, and the importance of experience in the development of the social brain is a particularly controversial topic.

Perhaps the most obvious answer to the above issue is that specific genes are expressed in particular parts of cortex and consequently "code for" patterns of wiring specific to certain computational functions. Whereas this type of explanation appears to be valid for specialized computations within subcortical structures, a variety of genetic, neurobiological, and cognitive neuroscience evidence indicates that it is, at best, only part of the story for many human cognitive functions dependent on the cerebral cortex (see Johnson, 2005a, for a review). As just one example, in human adults experience or practice in certain domains can change the extent of cortical tissue activated during performance of a task. In this chapter I consider the development of the human social brain network from the point of view of three general perspectives that have been taken on the postnatal development of human brain function.

THREE PERSPECTIVES ON THE FUNCTIONAL DEVELOPMENT OF THE HUMAN BRAIN

Relating evidence on the neuroanatomical development of the brain to the remarkable changes in motor, perceptual, and cognitive abilities that occur during the first decade or so of a human life presents a considerable challenge. I have identified three distinct, but not necessarily incompatible, approaches to this issue (Johnson, 2001): (1) a maturational perspective, (2) interactive specialization, and (3) a skill learning viewpoint. I will now briefly introduce these three approaches before examining their assumptions and predictions in more detail.

Much of the research attempting to relate brain to behavioral development in humans has come from a maturational viewpoint, in which the goal is to relate the maturation of particular regions of the brain, usually regions of cerebral cortex, to newly emerging sensory, motor, and cognitive functions. Evidence concerning the differential neuroanatomical development of brain regions can be used to determine an age when a particular region is likely to become functional. Success in a new behavioral task at this age may then be attributed to the maturation of a new brain region. From this perspective, functional brain development is essentially the reverse of adult neuropsychology, with the difference that specific brain regions (and their corresponding computational modules) are added in instead of knocked out. With regard to the social brain network, different components or modules would come "online" at different postnatal ages.

Despite the intuitive appeal of the maturational approach, it does not successfully explain some aspects of human functional brain development. For example, recent evidence suggests that some of the regions that are slowest to develop by neuroanatomical criteria show activity from shortly after birth (for a review, see Johnson, 2005b). Furthermore, where functional activity has been assessed by fMRI during a behavioral transition, multiple cortical and subcortical areas appear to change their response patterns (e.g., Luna et al., 2001), rather than one or two previously silent regions becoming active (mature). Finally, associations between neural and cognitive changes based on age of onset are theoretically somewhat unconstrained, due to the great variety of different neuroanatomical and neurochemical measures that change at different times in different regions of the brain.

In contrast to the maturational approach, an alternative viewpoint, interactive specialization (IS), assumes that postnatal functional brain development, at least within the cerebral cortex, involves a process of organizing patterns of interregional interactions (Johnson, 2001, 2005a). According to this view, the response properties of a specific region are partly determined by its patterns of connectivity to other regions and their patterns of activity. During postnatal development changes in the response properties of cortical regions occur as they interact and compete with each other to acquire their role in new computational abilities. From this perspective, some cortical regions may begin with poorly defined functions and are consequently partially activated in a wide range of different contexts and tasks. During development, activity-dependent interactions between regions sharpen the functions of regions, such that their activity becomes restricted to a narrower set of circumstances (e.g., a region originally activated by a wide variety of visual objects may come to confine its response to upright human faces). The onset of new behavioral competencies during infancy will therefore be associated with changes in activity over several regions and not just by the onset of activity in one or more additional region(s).

A third perspective on human functional brain development, skill learning, states that the changes in neural activity seen during functional brain development in infants and children, as they acquire new perceptual or motor abilities, are similar to those involved in complex perceptual and motor skill acquisition in adults. For example, Gauthier, Tarr, Anderson, Skudlarski, and Gore (1999) have shown that extensive training of adults with artificial objects (called *greebles*) eventually results in activation of a cortical region previously associated with face processing, the fusiform face area. This example of neural changes associated with perceptual expertise suggests that this region is normally activated by faces in adults not because it is prespecified for faces but due to our extensive expertise with that class of stimulus. Furthermore, it encourages parallels with the development of face processing skills in infants (see Gauthier & Nelson, 2001). Although the extent to which parallels can be drawn between adult expertise and infant development remains unclear, to the extent that the skill learning hypothesis is correct, it presents a possible view of continuity of mechanisms throughout the lifespan.

ASSUMPTIONS UNDERLYING THE THREE APPROACHES

Different key assumptions underlie the three approaches outlined above. With regard to one assumption, Gottlieb (1992) distinguished between two approaches to the study of development: (1) "deterministic epigenesis," in which it is assumed that there is a unidirectional causal path from genes to structural brain changes to psychological function; and (2) "probabilistic epigenesis," in which interactions among genes, structural brain changes, and psychological function are viewed as bidirectional, dynamic, and emergent. In many ways it is a defining feature of the maturational approach that it assumes deterministic epigenesis; region-specific gene expression is assumed to effect changes in intraregional connectivity that, in turn, allow new functions to emerge. A related assumption commonly made within the maturational approach is that there is a one-to-one mapping between cortical regions and particular cognitive functions, such that specific computational modules come online following the maturation of circuitry intrinsic to the corresponding cortical region. In some respects, this view parallels "mosaic" development at the cellular level in which simple organisms (e.g., *C. elegans*) are constructed through cell lineages that are largely independent of each other (Elman et al., 1996). Similarly, different cortical regions are assumed to have different and independent maturational timetables, thus enabling new cognitive functions to emerge at different ages in relative isolation.

IS (Johnson, 2001, 2005a) has a number of different underlying assumptions. Specifically, a probabilistic epigenesis assumption is coupled with the view that cognitive functions are the emergent product of interactions between different brain regions, and between the whole brain and its external environment. Brain regions do not develop independently; rather, they are heavily constrained by interactions with their neighboring regions. With regard to the latter of these assumptions, IS follows recent trends in adult functional neuroimaging. For example, Friston and Price (2001) point out that the response properties of a region are determined by its patterns of connectivity to other regions, and it may be an error to assume that particular functions can be localized within a certain cortical region. By this view, "the cortical infrastructure supporting a single function may involve many specialised areas whose union is mediated by the functional integration among them" (p. 276). Similar views have been expressed by Carpenter and collaborators, who have argued that "in contrast to a localist assumption of a one-to-one mapping between cortical regions and cognitive operations, an alternative view is that cognitive task performance is subserved by large-scale cortical networks that consist of spatially separate computational components, each with its own set of relative specializations, that collaborate extensively to accomplish cognitive functions" (Carpenter et al., 2001, p. 360). Applying these ideas to development, the IS approach emphasizes changes in interregional connectivity as opposed to the maturation of intraregional connectivity. Whereas the maturational approach may be analogous to mosaic cellular development, the IS view corresponds to the "regulatory" development seen in higher organisms, in which cell–cell interactions are critical in determining developmental fate. Just as the brain is shaped by its bodily environment (*embodiment*), the development of each brain region is constrained by its location within the whole brain (*embrainment*) (Johnson, 2005a; Mareschal et al., 2007).

In addition to the mapping between structure and function at one age, we can consider how this mapping might change during development. When discussing functional imaging of developmental disorders, Johnson, Halit, Grice, and Karmiloff-Smith (2002) point out that many laboratories have assumed that the relation between brain structure and cognitive function is static during development. Specifically, in accordance with a maturational view, when new structures come online, the existing (already mature) regions continue to support the same functions they did at earlier developmental stages. The "static assumption" is partly why it is acceptable to study developmental disorders in adulthood and then extrapolate back in time to early development. Contrary to this view, the IS approach suggests that when a new computation or skill is acquired, there is a reorganization of interactions between different brain structures and regions. This reorganization process could even change how previously acquired cognitive functions are represented in the brain. Thus, the same behavior could be supported by different neural substrates at different ages during development.

Stating that structure–function relations can change with development is all very well, but it lacks the specificity required to make all but the most general predictions. Fortunately, the view that there is competitive specialization of regions during development gives rise to more specific predictions about the types of changes in structure–function relations that should be observed. Specifically, as regions become increasingly selective in their response properties during infancy, the overall extent of cortical activation during a given task may decrease. The reason for this decrease is that regions that previously responded to a range of different stimuli (e.g., complex animate and inanimate objects) come to confine their activity to a particular class of objects (e.g., upright human faces) and therefore do not respond in situations in which they previously responded. Evidence in support of this view is discussed below.

A basic assumption underlying the skill learning approach is that there is a continuity of the circuitry underlying skill acquisition from birth through adulthood. This circuitry is likely to involve a network of structures that retains the same basic function across developmental time (a static brain–cognition mapping). However, other brain regions may respond to training with dynamic changes in functionality that are similar or identical to those hypothesized within the IS framework.

Another way in which the skill learning view differs from the other perspectives is with regard to "plasticity." Plasticity in brain development is a phenomenon that has generated much controversy, with several different conceptions and definitions having been presented (Johnson, 2005a). The three perspectives we have discussed provide different viewpoints on plasticity. According to the maturational framework, plasticity is a specialized mechanism that is activated following brain injury. According to the IS approach, plasticity is simply the state in which a region's function is not yet fully specialized; that is, there is still remaining scope for developing more finely tuned responses. This definition corresponds well with the view of developmental biologists that development involves the increasing "restriction of fate." Finally, according to the skill learning hypothesis, plasticity is the result of specific circuitry that remains in place throughout the lifespan. Unlike the IS approach, according to this view plasticity does not necessarily decrease during development.

Now that we have reviewed the three basic perspectives on human functional brain development, we can return to the topic of the social brain and examine which of these perspectives best accounts for the existing evidence. We begin with one of the most basic aspects of social cognition: the detection and perception of faces.

FACE PERCEPTION

Several cortical regions within the social brain, including regions of the fusiform gyrus, lateral occipital area, and superior temporal sulcus (Adolphs, 2003; Kanwisher, McDermott, & Chun, 1997) have all been implicated in neuroimaging studies as face-sensitive regions that are involved in aspects of encoding and detecting facial information. The stimulus specificity of response has been most extensively studied for the "fusiform face area" (FFA), a region that is more activated by faces than by many other comparison stimuli, including houses, textures, and hands (Kanwisher et al., 1997). Whereas the greater activation of the FFA to faces than other objects has led some to propose that it is a face module (Kanwisher et al., 1997), others call this view into question. In particular, investigations demonstrating that (1) the distribution of response across the ventral cortex may be more stimulus specific than the strength of response of a particular region such as FFA (Haxby et al., 2001; Ishai, Ungerleider, Martin, Schouten, & Haxby, 1999; but see Spiridon & Kanwisher, 2002), and (2) activation of the FFA increases with increasing expertise in discriminating members of nonface categories (Gauthier et al., 2000), suggest that this region may play a more general role in object processing. However, the observations remain that faces activate the FFA more than any other object and that the distribution of activity over the ventral cortex for faces differs from other objects in that it is more focal and less influenced by attention (Haxby et al., 2001). How do such specializations arise and why do face-sensitive regions tend to be located in particular regions of cortex? The three viewpoints outlined above provide different answers to these questions.

According to the maturational view, specific genes are expressed within particular cortical regions (such as the fusiform "face area") and prewire those areas for face processing. One of several problems with this argument is that differential gene expression within the mammalian cerebral cortex tends to be on a much larger scale than the functional regions identified in imaging studies (for a review, see Johnson, 2005a). According to the skill learning view, much of the adult social brain network is better characterized as a perceptual skill network that coincides with social processing, because most human adults are experts with this type of stimulus. Finally, according to the interactive specialization view, the social brain emerges from other (nonsocial) brain networks as a result of interactions between brain regions and between the brain and the child's external world.

When considering different accounts of the origins of the social brain network, it is useful to begin at birth. A number of studies have shown that newborn infants (in some studies, within the first hour of life) preferentially look toward face-like patterns (e.g., Johnson, Dziurawiec, Ellis, & Morton, 1991; Valenza, Simion, Cassia, & Umiltà, 1996). There has been considerable debate over the specificity of the mechanisms (or representations) that underlie this behavior. At one extreme is the view that such preferences are simply due to the fact that the visual psychophysical properties of faces match those most ideal for the newborn visual system (consistent with a skill learning viewpoint). At the other extreme is the view that newborns' processing of faces is substantially similar to that in adults, including fully specified representations of individual faces (consistent with one version of the maturational perspective). An intermediate view was advanced by Johnson and Morton (1991), who proposed that newborn face representations could contain the minimum necessary information to elicit adaptive behavior. Specifically, they argued for a mechanism termed *Conspec* that might contain a representation as simple as three high-contrast blobs in the locations of the eyes and mouth. This skeletal representation may be sufficient to "bootstrap" other developing systems by providing them with the appropriate input—a view that in this respect is consistent with the IS approach.

Since these original proposals, several laboratories have focused on determining, through empirical investigation and neural network modeling, the representation that underlies the tendency of newborns to orient to faces. With regard to the latter, results from neural network simulations suggest that a representation for Conspec as simple as three high-contrast blobs can account for most of the newborn data collected to date, involving a variety of schematic and naturalistic face stimuli (see Bednar & Miikkulainen, 2003). Current debate centers on whether the minimal representation supporting Conspec involves the three high-contrast blobs, as originally proposed by Johnson and Morton (1991), or involves a preference for arrays with a greater number of elements in the upper half of a stimulus (Turati, Simion, Milani, & Umiltà, 2002). However, in both cases the representation is probably close to the minimum sufficient to elicit orienting to faces within the natural environment of the newborn, given the constraints of the newborn visual system.

Several lines of evidence suggest that this newborn preference is not mediated by the same cortical structures as are involved in face processing in adults and may be due to subcortical structures such as the amygdala, superior colliculus, and pulvinar (Johnson, 2005b). One purpose of this early bias to fixate on faces may be to elicit bonding from adult caregivers. However, I suggest that an equally important purpose is to bias the visual input to plastic cortical circuits. This biased sampling of the visual environment over the first days and weeks of life may ensure the appropriate specialization of later developing cortical circuitry (Johnson, 2005b; Morton & Johnson, 1991). Specifically, parts of the fusiform cortex become specialized for processing faces partly as a result of the subcortical route ensuring that newborns preferentially orient to faces and therefore foveate them, thus providing input to cortical visual pathways. The cortical projection patterns of the subcortical route may enhance activation of specific areas, including the fusiform cortex, when faces are within the visual field of the young infant. The parts of the fusiform cortex that become face sensitive receive foveal cortical visual input and are at the "object level" of visual stimulus processing in the ventral pathway. Thus, information from both face routes may converge in the FFA. These and other possible constraints, such as multimodal inputs and general biases in gene expression levels between the right and left cerebral cortex, combine to ensure that certain developing cortical circuits become specialized for face-related stimuli. By this developmental account it is inevitable, barring some disruption to the normal constraints, that parts of the fusiform cortex will specialize for faces. However, this inevitable outcome is achieved without genetically decreed domain-specific patterns of connectivity with the FFA (Johnson, 2005b).

While the current evidence on newborn face preferences is difficult to reconcile with a strictly skill learning view of functional brain development, it is not entirely inconsistent with either the maturational or IS approaches. According to at least some versions of the maturational approach, primitive abilities in the newborn would be elaborated by more sophisticated modules maturing at later ages. According to the IS approach, a primitive brain system such as Conspec "bootstraps" later developing experience-dependent systems by providing the appropriate input for them.

Given that newborn behavior alone cannot help us discriminate between at least two of the perspectives on functional brain development, I now consider developmental changes over the first few months of life. Specifically, I address the question of whether subsequent development looks more like the addition of new components or the gradual specialization of circuitry for processing of social stimuli.

Although attempts to study changes in brain activity during development are still in their infancy, several labs have examined changes in event-related potentials (ERPs) in face processing (see de Haan, Johnson, & Halit, 2003, for a review). In particular, attention has focused on the N170, an ERP component that has been strongly associated with face processing in a number of studies with adults (see de Haan et al., 2003, for a review). More specifically, the amplitude and latency of this component vary according to whether or not faces are present in the visual field of the adult volunteer under study. An important aspect of the N170 in adults is that it has a highly selective response; for example, we observed that the N170 showed a different response to human upright faces than to very closely related stimuli, such as inverted human faces and upright monkey faces (de Haan, Pascalis, & Johnson, 2002). Although the exact underlying brain generators of the N170 are currently still debated, the specificity of response of the N170 can be taken as an index of the degree of specialization of cortical processing for human upright faces. For this reason we have undertaken a series of studies on the development of the N170 over the first weeks and months of postnatal life.

The first issue we addressed in our developmental studies concerned the age at which the face-sensitive N170 emerged. In a series of experiments we identified a component in the infant ERP that has many of the properties associated with the adult N170 but that is of a slightly longer latency (240–290 ms; de Haan et al., 2002; Halit, de Haan, & Johnson, 2003). In studying the response properties of this potential at 3, 6, and 12 months of age, we discovered that (1) the component is present from at least 3 months of age (although its development continues into middle childhood), (2) the component becomes more specifically tuned to human upright faces with increasing age, and (3) there is stronger evidence for adult-like lateralization of the component at older ages. Thus, study of the component is consistent with the idea of increased specialization and localization resulting from development.

More direct evidence for increased localization comes from a recent fMRI study of the neural basis of face processing in 10- to 12-year-old children compared to adults (Passarotti et al., 2003). In this study, children activated a larger extent of cortex around face-sensitive areas than did adults during a face-matching task. Similar conclusions can be drawn from a PET study conducted on 2-month-old infants, in which a large network of cortical areas was activated when infants viewed faces compared to a moving dot array (Tzourio-Mazoyer et al., 2002).

Thus, with regard to face perception, the available evidence from newborns allows us to rule out the skill learning hypothesis, whereas the evidence of the neurodevelopment of face processing over the first months and years of life is consistent with the kinds of dynamic changes in processing expected from the IS, and not the maturational, approach. Evidence from this initial case study of face processing is therefore consistent with the view that a variety of constraints operates on a process of emerging specialization, such that cortical regions specialized for face processing are the inevitable result of the typical developmental trajectory.

BEYOND FACE PROCESSING

What about specialization for more complex social–cognitive functions, beyond the early stages of face processing? One of the more complex attributes of the adult social brain is the ability to process information about the eyes of other humans. There are at least two important aspects of processing information about the eyes. The first is detecting the direction of another's gaze in order to direct your own attention to the same object or spatial location. Perception of averted gaze can elicit an automatic shift of attention in the same direction in adults (Driver et al., 1999), allowing the establishment of "joint attention" (Butterworth & Jarrett, 1991). Joint attention to objects is thought to be crucial for a number of aspects of cognitive and social development, including word learning. The second critical aspect of gaze perception is the detection of direct gaze, enabling mutual gaze between the viewer and the perceived face. Mutual gaze (eye contact) provides the main mode of establishing a communicative context between humans and is believed to be important for normal social development (e.g., Kleinke, 1986; Symons, Hains, & Muir, 1998). It is commonly agreed that eye gaze perception is important for mother–infant interactions and that it provides a vital foundation for social development (e.g., Jaffe, Stern, & Peery, 1973; Stern, 1974).

With regard to the social brain network, the superior temporal sulcus (STS) has been identified in several imaging studies of eye gaze perception and processing in adults (for a review, see Adolphs, 2003). The involvement of this region in eye gaze perception is not surprising, given its general involvement in biological motion. As with cortical face processing, in adults the response properties of this region are highly tuned (specialized) in that the region does not respond to nonbiological motion (Puce, Allison, Bentin, Gore, & McCarthy, 1998). Thus, the region potentially provides a good example of specialization *within* the cortical social brain network. Several lines of evidence lead us to propose that eye gaze processing and more general aspects of face processing initially (in development) share common processing. With increasing specialization of functions within the social brain network, eye gaze processing becomes increasingly differentiated from other aspects of face processing during postnatal development. This may become evident as differential patterns of activation within the social brain when information about the eyes is being processed. The lines of evidence in question include the following: (1) direct eye gaze is important for several other aspects of face processing and social cognition and attention in young infants; (2) ERP evidence indicates that eye gaze modulates other aspects of the neural processing of faces in young infants but not in adults; and (3) the partial neural dissociation between eye gaze processing and other aspects of face processing seen in older children and adults is not observed in children with autism.

In the first of these lines of work we studied the importance of a period of direct (mutual) gaze with a face for two key developmental functions in infants: the cueing of attention by gaze direction and the recognition of individual faces. Several studies have demonstrated that gaze cues are able to trigger an automatic and rapid shifting of the focus of an adult viewer's visual attention (Driver et al., 1999; Friesen & Kingstone, 1998; Langton & Bruce, 1999). When does the ability to use eye gaze direction as an attentional cue start? Previous work with human infants indicates that they start to discriminate and follow adults' direction of attention at the age of 3 or 4 months (Hood, Willen, & Driver, 1998; Vecera & Johnson, 1995). In our studies we examined further the visual properties of the eyes that enable infants to follow the direction of the gaze. We tested 4-month-olds using a cueing paradigm adapted from Hood and colleagues (1998). Each trial began with the stimulus face eyes blinking (to attract attention) before the pupils shifted to either the right or the left for a period of 1,500 ms (see Plate 5.1). A target stimulus was then presented either in the same position where the stimulus face eyes were looking (congruent position) or in a location incongruent with the direction of gaze. By measuring the saccadic reaction time of infants to orient to the target, we demonstrated that the infants reacted more rapidly to look at the location congruent with the direction of the face gaze.

In a series of several experiments, we (Farroni, Johnson, Brockbank, & Simion, 2000) found that a variety of types of lateral motion induced cueing effects in infants, but only when preceded by a short period of direct gaze. Taken together with other findings, these results suggest that it is only following a period of mutual gaze with an upright face that cueing effects are observed. In other words, mutual gaze (eye contact) with an upright face may engage mechanisms of attention, such that the viewer is more likely to be cued by subsequent motion. Furthermore, the finding that infants are as effectively cued by lateral motion of features other than the eyes provides preliminary evidence that infants' STS may be less finely tuned in its response properties in comparison to adults'.

Recent behavioral studies in adults have demonstrated that direct gaze can modulate other aspects of face processing. For example, perceived eye contact can affect both the speed of online gender face judgments and the accuracy of incidental recognition memory for faces (Vuilleumier, Gorge, Lister, Armoni, & Driver, 2005), and performance in face memory tasks can be influenced by gaze direction both at the encoding and retrieval levels (Hood, Macrae, Cole-Davies, & Dias, 2003). Hood and colleagues (2003) tested 6- and 7-year-old children and adults on a forced-choice face recognition task, in which the direction of eye gaze was manipulated over the course of the initial presentation and subsequent test phase of the experiment. To establish whether there were any effects of direct gaze on the encoding or retrieval of individual faces, participants were presented with faces displaying either direct or averted gaze and with their eyes closed during the test phase (i.e., encoding manipulation) or with faces presented initially with eyes closed and tested with either direct or averted gaze (i.e., retrieval manipulation). The results demonstrated that direct gaze facilitated the encoding process in both children and adults. Faces with direct gaze also enhanced the retrieval process, although this effect was stronger for adults.

In a follow-up to this work, we (Farroni, Massaccesi, Menon, & Johnson, in press) investigated whether direction of gaze had any effect on face recognition in 4-month-old infants. These infants were shown faces with both direct and averted gaze and were subsequently given a preference test involving the same face and a novel one. A novelty preference during testing was found only following initial exposure to a face with direct gaze. Furthermore, face recognition was also generally enhanced for faces with both direct and averted gaze when the infants started the task with the direct gaze condition. Together, these results indicate that the direction of the gaze modulates face recognition in early infancy. In a further series of experiments, we attempted to gain converging evidence for the differential processing of direct gaze in infants by recording ERPs as infants viewed faces. We studied 4-month-old babies with stimuli similar to those described above and found a difference between the two gaze directions at the time and scalp location of the previously identified face-sensitive component of the infant ERP (N240/N290, de Haan et al., 2002). As reviewed above, this component of the infant ERP is thought to be the equivalent of a well-studied adult face-sensitive component, and in infants is sensitive to changes in the orientation and species of a face by at least 12 months of age (Halit et al., 2003). Thus, our conclusion from these studies was that direct eye contact enhances the neural processing of faces in 4-month-old infants. Further experiments demonstrated that this modulating effect of gaze direction is only found when gaze occurs within the context of an upright face.

Whereas modulation of face-sensitive components of the ERP is observed in infants, as described above, when we used the same paradigm with adult participants, we did not find any modulation of the ERP by gaze direction (Grice et al., 2005). This negative result was confirmed when we tested a group of young children ages 2–5 years old. Why did we find an effect in infants that then disappeared at older ages? One possibility is that although mechanisms related to face processing are relatively unspecialized, eye gaze processing and other aspects of face processing share common mechanisms and are heavily intertwined. As a result of development (and increased specialization) eye gaze processing becomes partially distinct and thus ceases to modulate more general aspects of face processing. If this is the case, it is possible that certain disorders of development will entail a delay or aberrant specialization process. In this case, we may observe gaze direction modulation of the ERP at ages at which such modulation does not occur in typical development. Grice and colleagues (2005) tested this prediction in a group of young children with autism (2–5 years old). These children showed modulation of the N170 in response to direct gaze in a very similar way to that previously observed in typically developing 4-month-old infants. This modulatory effect was not seen in age-matched controls.

The empirical evidence that we and others have gathered on the development and neural basis of eye gaze processing in infants is consistent with the IS perspective on functional brain development (Johnson, 2001, 2005b). Specifically, we (Farroni, Csibra, Simion, & Johnson, 2002) suggest that a primitive representation of high-contrast elements (such as Johnson & Morton's [1991] Conspec) would be sufficient to direct orienting in newborns toward faces with eye contact. Therefore, the more frequent orienting to direct gaze in newborns could be mediated by the same mechanism that underlies newborns' tendency to orient to faces in general. Specifically, Johnson and Morton (1991) hypothesized that subcortical circuits support a primitive representation of high-contrast elements relating to the location of the eyes and mouth. A face with direct gaze would better fit the spatial relation of elements in this template than one with gaze averted, suggesting that the functional role of this putative mechanism is more general than previously supposed. This primitive bias ensures a biased input of human faces with direct gaze to the infant over the first days and weeks of life.

According to the IS view, a network as a whole becomes specialized for a particular function. Therefore, we suggest that the "eye region" of the STS does not develop in isolation, or in a modular fashion, but that its functionality emerges within the context of interacting regions involved in either general face processing or in motion detection. Viewed from this perspective, the STS may be a region that integrates motion information with the processing of faces (and other body parts). Although the STS may be active in infants, we propose that it is not yet efficiently integrating motion and face information. In other words, while the 4-month-old has good face processing and general motion perception, she has not yet integrated these two aspects of perception together into adult eye gaze perception. By this account, making eye contact with upright faces fully engages face processing, which then facilitates the orienting of attention by lateral motion. At older ages, eye gaze perception becomes a fully integrated function in which even static presentations of averted eyes are sufficient to facilitate gaze.

THE PERCEPTION OF ACTION

Whereas the face and eyes are important for interpersonal communication, another function of the social brain network is to perceive and predict the behavior of other humans on the basis of their actions. A developmental cognitive neuroscience approach is emerging with regard to two aspects of the perception of action: biologically possible versus impossible actions and goal-directed versus incomplete actions.

The question of whether young infants can detect biologically impossible human action promises to inform us about the extent to which learning processes are involved in the perception of human action. Behavioral studies of infant perception of biomechanical motion have been conducted for over 20 years. Initial studies such as the one conducted by Bertenthal, Profitt, and Cutting (1984) utilized point-light displays (PLDs), first introduced by Johansson (1973). Using such stimuli, infants as young as 3 months have been shown to be sensitive to configural information relating to movement (Bertenthal et al., 1984). Infants of 5 months have also been shown to discriminate PLDs in the configuration of a human when compared with a scrambled PLD, despite movement in each condition containing the same mathematical constraints between individual points of light. The biomechanics of limb motion have also been investigated with simple

PLDs. Bertenthal, Profitt, Kramer, and Spetner (1987) presented three light points to 5-month-old infants, with each point of light representing the shoulder, elbow, and wrist, respectively. In one condition, all three light points moved in a rigid transformation, appearing biomechanically possible. Another condition moved the PLD out of phase, such that the arm display appeared to look disjointed or biomechanically impossible. The infants successfully discriminated the locally rigid display from the out-of-phase display, suggesting some sensitivity to the biomechanical constraints of the human body. What is clear about research with PLDs is that there is considerable change in infant perception of point-light motion throughout the first year. Even though such stimuli may be useful in investigating the perception of movement, PLDs are unnatural and intrinsically novel for infants. Recent developments in computer technology facilitate the manipulation of still frames from video, thereby allowing for the creation of realistic human movements that are nonetheless biologically impossible.

Adult cognitive neuroscience studies have also investigated the perception of action. PET and fMRI studies with adults indicate that the STS and medial temporal (MT) area are activated during the perception of biological motion (e.g., Castelli, Happe, Frith, & Frith, 2000; Grossman et al., 2000). Research has also investigated adult gamma band EEG activity (30–50 Hz) underpinning the perception of stable and nonstable body postures (Slobonov, Tutwiler, Slobounova, Rearick, & Ray, 2000). The rationale for investigating this frequency was that gamma-band activity increases during sustained attention, with previous studies indicating that this is a physiological correlate of selective attention (Muller, Gruber, & Keil, 2000). Slobonov and colleagues (2000) presented adult participants with an animated human body rocking backward and forward on the ankle joint. Swaying movements were presented as either stable or nonstable, with participant reaction times indicating stability. Results from passive viewing showed that increases in gamma over frontal-central regions and parietal sites correlated with the recognition of postural instability. The change from baseline was shown to be slightly higher in the right hemisphere in the gamma frequencies. These results suggest that during visual perception there are thresholds within human movement that are detectable using EEG technology.

Reid, Belsky, and Johnson (2005) investigated infant perception of possible and impossible movements of the human body and attempted to relate this perception to the perceptual experience and motor abilities of the individual infants. To assess potential differences in individual experience, they measured the extent of "motionese" displayed by the mother during play interaction with the infant. Recent research suggests that parents present objects to infants in a different manner from which they present objects to adults. This activity is characterized by a deliberate enhancing of structure in object manipulation in order to allow infants greater understanding of the action involved in the object manipulation: "motionese" (Brand, Baldwin, & Ashburn, 2002). Such results suggest that the amount of exaggerated object manipulation, or motionese, that is displayed to infants is variable among infants, though the results do not provide information about what aspect of visual experience is critical for the perception of biomechanical movement.

Reid and colleagues (2005) used both behavioral (visual preference) and electrophysiological (EEG) measures because the former provided an overt measure of how infants differed in their responses to the stimuli, whereas the latter provided information about the timing and approximate location of the neurophysiological events that led up to the behavioral response. Specifically, Reid and colleagues examined (1) the environment provided by mothers (as indexed by maternal motionese), (2) infant motor abilities, (3) infant mental and motor abilities assessed via standardized measures of development, and (4) infant processing of biological movement (as indexed by looking times and gamma-band time-frequency analysis of EEG). In their first experiment it was found that, as a group, 8-month-old infants looked longer at video clips of impossible body movements than possible movements. However, this effect was mainly due to the subset of infants with relatively good fine motor skills. In a second experiment the contribution of general developmental maturation was assessed by repeating the first experiment with the addition of the Bayley Scales of Infant Development. The overall looking time effect was replicated from the first experiment, but this effect did not correlate with Bayley mental or motor scores, allowing for the exclusion of general maturational factors. In a third experiment, gamma frequency analysis of EEG resulting from passive viewing of possible and impossible actions indicated that it was only those infants with relatively good fine motor skills who processed these stimuli differently. When taken together, these studies suggest a relation between the infant's own ability to perform fine motor actions and the perception of biologically possible human movement.

Beyond the evaluation of the biological possibility (or otherwise) of a single action, there is the need to segment sequences of actions into appropriate chunks and to use this information to predict the intentions of others. In adults, parsing of action sequences is partly based upon understanding the intentions of the actor and the goals of the action. One study with adults that has investigated neural activity associated with action parsing found bilateral activation in the posterior regions of cortex (Brodmann's areas 19/37) and in a small region in the right frontal cortex, the precentral sulcus (Zacks et al., 2001). In addition, during the perception of action, it has been suggested that the right STS is vital to the processing of human movement (see Blakemore & Decety, 2001, for a review). Frontal regions have also been shown to play a role in the taking of an intentional stance toward an agent in a visual display (Gallagher, Jack, Roepstorff, & Frith, 2002).

The issue of what cues infants use to parse action has produced some debate, with recent behavioral research suggesting that markers of intentionality may be critical. Certainly by 14 months infants are capable of discerning intentional from accidental action (Carpenter, Akhtar, & Tomasello, 1998). Results from other behavioral studies suggest that infants of 9 months can detect intentions in actions and take an intentional stance toward an agent (Gergely, Nadasdy, Csibra, & Bíró, 1995), although this skill is not evident at 6 months (Csibra, Bíró, Koós, & Gergely, 2003). This research also suggests that infants do not require the presentation of the end state of an action in order to attribute a goal to an action.

Reid, Csibra, Belsky, and Johnson (2007) initially conducted a behavioral study in which they established that 8-month-old infants looked longer at an incomplete action involving a pouring event than they did at the complete action. In the latter action, the goal of the actress involved was clear, whereas in the former action sequence it was not. A subsequent gamma-range EEG analysis revealed a significant difference between conditions over left frontal regions shortly after the complete and incomplete action sequences diverged. The direction of the difference indicated that the incomplete condition yielded greater power in the same frequency range than the complete condition.

There are at least two classes of explanation for the neural differences observed in this study. The first of these is that increased gamma power in the incomplete condition reflects greater attention to that sequence. Müller and colleagues (2000) suggest that increases in gamma frequency power in adults are related to task demands involving visual attention. These authors have shown that induced gamma responses are attentionally modulated during visual search tasks when the task involves following a moving cue. In the present experiment infants' increased looking in the incomplete condition is consistent with a violation of expectation encountered by the infants. The consequence of the expectancy violation was an increase in attention that, in turn, may be related to the greater gamma power observed.

A second line of explanation for the results of the EEG experiment is that the increased gamma over left frontal channels reflects a more specific basis for the perception of an action sequence by infants. For example, increased gamma may reflect infant brain processes resetting to prepare for new information once action resumes. Another potential explanation along this line is that the infant brain attempts to continue the action despite visual cues suggesting that the action is not taking place ("forward mapping"). This latter explanation may be consistent with research into object permanence indicating that gamma power in infants increases when an object unexpectedly disappears (Kaufman, Csibra, & Johnson, 2003).

Whatever the precise explanation of the neural correlates of the effect observed in the electrophysiological experiment of Reid and colleagues (2007), the overall finding of increased gamma-band activity for an incomplete action as compared to a complete action promises to provide an important first step in investigating and understanding issues relating to the perception of human action in infancy.

CONCLUSIONS AND FUTURE PROSPECTS

In this chapter I have considered evidence on the development of the social brain network in relation to three perspectives on human functional brain development. In the relatively well-studied case of face perception, when evidence from several developmental ages is taken into account, I argued that the IS view can best account for the data. In the less well-studied case of eye gaze processing, the evidence obtained so far is also consistent with the IS approach (without ruling out alternatives). In the third section of the chapter I reviewed preliminary developmental studies on the perception and parsing of sequences of human action. Future work will be needed to determine which view of human postnatal functional development is most applicable in this case.

There are very exiting days ahead for developmental cognitive neuroscience, as theoretical advances (such as those described in this chapter) combine with recent technical and methodological advances (such as those associated with brain imaging, genetics, and neural network modeling). Perhaps one of the most immediate challenges for the future will be to take the cognitive neuroscience approach away from the static stimuli and repeated trials characteristic of current laboratory studies of infant cognition and move instead to studying brain function during perception of dynamic stimuli in more natural contexts, such as while interacting with other human beings. Another challenge will be to move away from our current dependence on group-averaged data and develop sufficiently sensitive measurement and analytical techniques that will allow us to correlate gene, neural, and cognitive functions within an individual infant. It is not surprising that many governmental agencies and leading charities have identified this field as one of the hottest topics in neuroscience. A cognitive neuroscience approach to development over the early years may shed light on the combinations of factors that contribute to individual differences and thus eventually lead to "tailor-made" preschool and educational provisions.

ACKNOWLEDGMENTS

I acknowledge financial support from the Medical Research Council (United Kingdom) (Grant No. G9715587) and Birkbeck, University of London. This chapter is a revised and updated version of Johnson (2005a).

REFERENCES

Adolphs, R. (2003). Cognitive neuroscience of human social behaviour. *Nature Reviews Neuroscience, 4,* 165–178.

Batki, A., Baron Cohen, S., Wheelwright, S., Connellan, J., & Ahluwalia, J. (2000). Is there an innate gaze module?: Evidence from human neonates. *Infant Behaviour and Development, 23,* 223–229.

Bednar, J. A., & Miikkulainen, R. (2003). Learning innate face preferences. *Neural Computation, 15,* 1525–1557.

Bertenthal, B., Profitt, D., & Cutting, J. (1984). Infant's sensitivity to figural coherence in biochemical motions. *Journal of Experimental Child Psychology, 37,* 213–230.

Bertenthal, B., Profitt, D. R., Kramer, S. J., & Spetner, N. B. (1987). Infant's encoding of kinetic displays varying in relative coherence. *Developmental Psychology, 23,* 171–178.

Blakemore, S. J., & Decety, J. (2001) From the perception of action to the understanding of intention. *Nature Reviews Neuroscience, 2,* 561–567.

Brand, R. J., Baldwin, D. A., & Ashburn, L. A. (2002). Evidence for "Motionese": Modifications in mothers' infant-directed action. *Developmental Science, 5*(1), 72–83.

Butterworth, G., & Jarrett, N. (1991). What minds have in common is space: Spatial mechanisms serving joint visual attention in infancy. *British Journal of Developmental Psychology, 9,* 55–72.

Carpenter, M., Akhar, N., & Tomasello, M. (1998). Fourteen- through 18-month-old infants differentially imitate intentional and accidental actions. *Infant Behavior and Development, 21,* 315–330.

Carpenter, P. A., Just, M. A., Keller, T., Cherkassky, V., Roth, J. K., & Minshew, N. (2001). Dynamic cortical systems subserving cognition: fMRI studies with typical and atypical individuals. In J. L. McClelland & R. S. Siegler (Eds.), *Mechanisms of cognitive development: Behavioral and neural perspectives* (pp. 353–383). Mahwah, NJ: Erlbaum.

Castelli, F., Happe, F., Frith, U., & Frith, C. (2000). Movement and mind: A functional imaging study of perception and interpretation of complex intentional movement patterns. *NeuroImage, 12*(3), 314–325.

Csibra, G., Bíró, S., Koós, S., & Gergely, G. (2003). One-year-old infants use teleological representations of actions productively. *Cognitive Science, 27,* 111–133.

de Haan, M., Johnson, M. H., & Halit, H. (2003). Development of face-sensitive event-related potentials during infancy: A review. *International Journal of Psychophysiology, 51*(1), 45–58.

de Haan, M., Pascalis, O., & Johnson, M. H. (2002). Specialization of neural mechanisms underlying face recognition in human infants. *Journal of Cognitive Neuroscience, 14,* 199–209.

Driver, J., Davis, G., Ricciardelli, P., Kidd, P., Maxwell, E., & Baron-Cohen, S. (1999). Gaze perception triggers reflexive visuospatial orienting. *Visual Cognition, 6,* 509–540.

Elman, J., Bates, E. A., Johnson, M. H., Karmiloff-Smith, A., Parisi, D., & Plunkett, K. E. (1996). *Rethinking innateness: A connectionist perspective on development.* Cambridge, MA: MIT Press.

Farroni, T., Csibra, G., Simion, F., & Johnson, M. H. (2002). Eye contact detection in humans from birth. *Proceeding of the National Academy of Sciences USA, 198,* 9602–9605.

Farroni, T., Johnson, M. H., Brockbank, M., & Simion, F. (2000). Infant's use of gaze direction to cue attention: The importance of perceived motion. *Visual Cognition, 7,* 705–718.

Farroni, T., Massaccesi, S., Menon, E., & Johnson, M. H. (in press). Direct gaze modulates face recognition in young infants. *Cognition.*

Friesen, C. K., & Kingstone, A. (1998). The eyes have it! Reflexive orienting is triggered by nonpredictive gaze. *Psychonomic Bulletin and Review, 5,* 490–495.

Friston, K. J., & Price, C. J. (2001). Dynamic representations and generative models of brain function. *Brain Research Bulletin, 54,* 275–285.

Frith, U. (2001). Mind blindness and the brain in autism. *Neuron, 32,* 969–979.

Gallagher, H., Jack, A., Roepstorff, A., & Frith, C. (2002). Imaging the intentional stance in a competitive game. *NeuroImage, 16,* 14–21.

Gauthier, I., & Nelson, C. A. (2001). The development of face expertise. *Current Opinion in Neurobiology, 11,* 219–224.

Gauthier, I., Tarr, M. J., Anderson, A. W., Skudlarski, P., & Gore, J. C. (1999). Activation of the middle fusiform "face area" increases with expertise in recognizing novel objects. *Nature Neuroscience, 2,* 568–573.

Gauthier, I., Tarr, M. J., Moylan, J., Skudlarski, P., Gore, J. C., & Anderson, A. W. (2000). The fusiform "face area" is part of a network that processes faces at the individual level. *Journal of Cognitive Neuroscience, 12,* 495–504.

Gergely, G., Nadasdy, Z., Csibra, G., & Bíró, S. (1995). Taking the intentional stance at 12 months of age. *Cognition, 56,* 165–193.

Gottlieb, G. (1992). *Individual development and evolution: The genesis of novel behavior.* London: Oxford University Press.

Grice, S. J., Halit, H., Farroni, T., Baron-Cohen, S., Bolton, P., & Johnson, M. H. (2005). Neural correlates of eye-gaze detection in young children with autism. *Cortex, 41,* 342–353.

Grossman, E., Donnelly, M., Price, R., Pickens, D., Morgan, V., Neighbor, G., et al. (2000). Brain areas involved in perception of biological motion. *Journal of Cognitive Neuroscience, 12*(5), 711–720.

Halit, H., de Haan, M., & Johnson, M. H. (2003). Cortical specialisation for face processing: Face-sensitive event-related potential components in 3- and 12-month-old infants. *NeuroImage, 19*, 1180–1193.

Haxby, J. V., Gobbini, M. I., Furey, M. L., Ishai, A., Schouten, J. L., & Pietrini, P. (2001). Distributed and overlapping representations of faces and objects in ventral temporal cortex. *Science, 293*, 2425–2430.

Hood, B. M., Macrae, C. N., Cole-Davies, V., & Dias, M. (2003). Eye remember you: The effects of gaze direction on face recognition in children and adults. *Developmental Science, 6*(1), 67–71.

Hood, B. M., Willen, J. D., & Driver, J. (1998). Adults' eyes trigger shifts of visual attention in human infants. *Psychological Science, 9*, 131–134.

Ishai, A., Ungerleider, L. G., Martin, A., Schouten, J. L., & Haxby, J. V. (1999). Distributed representation of objects in the human ventral visual pathway. *Proceedings of the National Academy of Sciences USA, 96*, 9379–9384.

Jaffe, J., Stern, D. N., & Peery, J. C. (1973). "Conversational" coupling of gaze behavior in prelinguistic human development. *Journal of Psycholinguistic Research, 2*, 321–329.

Johansson, G. (1973). Visual perception of biological motion and a model of its analysis. *Perception and Psychophysics, 14*, 201–211.

Johnson, M. H. (2001). Functional brain development in humans. *Nature Reviews Neuroscience, 2*, 475–483.

Johnson, M. H. (2005a). *Developmental cognitive neuroscience: An introduction* (2nd ed.). Oxford, UK: Blackwell.

Johnson, M. H. (2005b). The ontogeny of the social brain. In U. Mayr, E. Awh, & S. W. Keele (Eds.), *Developing individuality in the human brain: A tribute to Michael Posner* (pp. 125–140). Washington, DC: American Psychiatric Press.

Johnson, M. H. (2005c). Sub-cortical face processing. *Nature Reviews Neuroscience, 6*, 766–774.

Johnson, M. H., & de Haan, M. (2001). Developing cortical specialization for visual–cognitive function: The case of face recognition. In J. L. McClelland & R. S. Seigler (Eds.), *Mechanisms of cognitive development: Behavioral and neural perspectives* (pp. 253–270). Mahwah, NJ: Erlbaum.

Johnson, M. H., Dziurawiec, S., Bartrip, J., & Morton, J. (1992). The effects of movement of internal features on infants' preferences for face-like stimuli. *Infant Behavior and Development, 15*, 129–136.

Johnson, M. H., Dziurawiec, S., Ellis, H., & Morton, J. (1991). Newborns' preferential tracking of face-like stimuli and its subsequent decline. *Cognition, 40*, 1–19.

Johnson, M. H., Halit, H., Grice, S. J. & Karmiloff-Smith, A. (2002). Neuroimaging of typical and atypical development: A perspective from multiple levels of analysis. *Development of Psychopathology, 14*, 521–536.

Johnson, M. H., & Morton, J. (1991). *Biology and cognitive development: The case of face recognition.* Oxford, UK: Blackwell.

Kanwisher, N., McDermott, J., & Chun, M. M. (1997). The fusiform face area: A module in human extrastriate cortex specialized for face perception. *Journal of Neuroscience, 17*, 4302–4311.

Kaufman, J., Csibra, G., & Johnson, M. H. (2003). Representing occluded objects in the human infant brain. *Proceedings of the Royal Society B: Biology Letters, 270*(Suppl. 2), 140–143.

Kleinke, C. L. (1986). Gaze and eye contact: A research review. *Psychological Bulletin, 100,* 78–100.

Krubitzer, L. A. (2000). How does evolution build a complex brain? In G. R. Bock & G. Cardew (Eds.), *Evolutionary developmental biology of the cerebral cortex* (pp. 206–220). Chichester, UK: Wiley.

Langton, S. R. H., & Bruce, V. (1999). Reflexive visual orienting in response to the social attention of others. *Visual Cognition, 6,* 541–567.

Luna, B., Thulborn, K. R., Munoz, D. P., Merriam, E. P., Garver, K. E., Minshew, N. J., et al. (2001). Maturation of widely distributed brain function subserves cognitive development. *NeuroImage, 13,* 786–793.

Mareschal, D., Johnson, M. H., Sirois, S., Spratling, M., Thomas, M., & Westermann, G. (2007). *Neuroconstructivism: Vol. 1. How the brain constructs cognition.* Oxford, UK: Blackwell.

Meltzoff, A. N., & Moore, M. K. (1977). Imitation of facial and manual gestures by human neonates. *Science, 198,* 74–78.

Morton, J., & Johnson, M. H. (1991). Conspec and Conlern: A two-process theory of infant face recognition. *Psychological Review, 98,* 164–181.

Müller, M. M., Gruber, T., & Keil, A. (2000). Modulation of induced gamma band activity in the human EEG by attention and visual information processing. *International Journal of Psychophysiology, 38,* 283–299.

Passarotti, A. M., Paul, B. M., Bussiere, J. R., Buxton, R. B., Wong, E. C., & Stiles, J. (2003). The development of face and location processing: An fMRI study. *Developmental Science, 6,* 100–117.

Posner, M. I. (1980). Orienting of attention. *Quarterly Journal of Experimental Psychology, 32,* 3–25.

Puce, A., Allison, T., Bentin, S., Gore, J. C., & McCarthy, G. (1998). Temporal cortex activation in humans viewing eye and mouth movements. *Journal of Neuroscience, 18,* 2188–2199.

Reid, V. M., Belsky, J., & Johnson, M. H. (2005). Infant perception of human action: Towards a developmental cognitive neuroscience of individual differences. *Cognition, Brain, and Behavior, 9,* 193–210.

Reid, V., Csibra, G., Belsky, J., & Johnson, M. H. (2007). Neural correlates of the perception of goal-directed action in infants. *Acta Psychologica, 124,* 129–138.

Schuller, A. M., & Rossion, B. (2001). Spatial attention triggered by eye gaze increases and speeds up early visual activity. *NeuroReport, 12,* 2381–2386.

Slobonov, S., Tutwiler, R., Slobounova, E., Rearick, M., & Ray, W. (2000). Human oscillatory brain activity within gamma band (30–50 Hz) induced by visual recognition of non-stable postures. *Cognitive Brain Research, 9,* 177–192.

Spiridon, M., & Kanwisher, N. (2002). How distributed is visual category information in human occipito-temporal cortex? An fMRI study. *Neuron, 35,* 1157–1165.

Stern, D. N. (1974). Mother and infant at play: The dyadic interaction involving facial, vocal, and gaze behaviors. In N. M. Lewis & L. Rosenblum (Eds.), *The effect of the infant on its caretaker* (pp. 187–213). New York: Wiley.

Symons, L. A., Hains, S. M. J., & Muir, D. W. (1998). Look at me: Five-month-old infants' sensitivity to very small deviations in eye-gaze during social interactions. *Infant Behavior and Development, 21,* 531–536.

Turati, C., Simion, F., Milani, I., & Umiltà, C. (2002). Newborns' preference for faces: What is crucial? *Developmental Psychology, 38,* 875–882.

Tzourio-Mazoyer, N., De Schonen, S., Crivello, F., Reutter, B., Aujard, Y., & Mazoyer, B. (2002). Neural correlates of woman face processing by 2-month-old infants. *NeuroImage, 15,* 454–461.

Valenza, E., Simion, F., Cassia, V. M., & Umiltà, C. (1996). Face preference at birth. *Journal of Experimental Psychology: Human Perception and Performance, 22,* 892–903.

Vecera, S. P., & Johnson, M. H. (1995). Eye gaze detection and the cortical processing of faces: Evidence from infants and adults. *Visual Cognition, 2,* 101–129.

Vuilleumier, P., Gorge, N., Lister, V., Armoni, J., & Driver, J. (2005). Effects of perceived mutual gaze and gender on face processing and recognition memory. *Visual Cognition, 12,* 85–101.

Zacks, J. M., Braver, T. S., Sheridan, M. A., Donaldson, D. I., Snyder, A. Z., Ollinger, J. M., et al. (2001). Human brain activity time-locked to perceptual event boundaries. *Nature Neuroscience, 4,* 651–655.

CHAPTER 6

Recognition Memory

BRAIN–BEHAVIOR RELATIONS FROM 0 TO 3

Sara Jane Webb

Much of human development involves memory functions, whether explicit recall and use of prior information, improved behavior during repeated motor actions, unconscious changes in behavior based on past exposure, or generalization of an event into a schema. The young child orients and attends to novel items in his or her environment, with salient items becoming familiar and further influencing behavior. Our understanding of the memory abilities of the young child reflects a relatively long and rich tradition in child psychology. However, it is only recently that researchers have begun to seek a mechanistic account of these behaviors by examining changes in brain–behavior relations. Although the behavioral repertoire of the infant and young child is limited, comparative studies of nonhuman primates as well as noninvasive neuroimaging methods such as the recording of event-related potentials (ERPs) provide insight into the mechanisms of brain development that underlie these behaviors. This chapter examines research on memory functions in adult humans and nonhuman primates on infant behavioral tasks as well as studies using ERPs with young children in order to better understand the neural systems that underlie novelty preference, familiarity, and recognition memory during the first 3 years of life.

138

DEFINING MEMORY

How do we characterize the memory abilities of preverbal children? *Memory* refers to the retention of learned information and is related to all cognitive and emotional functioning. In the young infant or toddler, the complex processes related to acquisition, storage, and retrieval are less well defined than those in the adult animal due to the behavioral limitations of preverbal children. Much of what we know about adult memory derives from subtle manipulations of task parameters that can either direct the subject's attention to the memory task (e.g., "Remember these words") or away from the memory requirements (e.g., "Respond if the word is written in capitals") during encoding as well as during retrieval (e.g., "Write down all the words you remember"; "Complete the word fragment with the first word that comes to mind"). However, these same manipulations are not viable in the young child. In addition, infants and toddlers lack the semantic knowledge base that adults have and thus encoding often involves truly novel information for which the child has no a priori stored representation or category. Due to the complexities of these issues, characterizing the memory abilities of young children has drawn on diverse fields of research, including developmental psychology, cognition, perception, neuroscience, and comparative biology.

Memory Systems Perspective

Although the study of memory is not a new undertaking (e.g., Ebbinghaus, 1885), how memory is defined, the classification of the processes involved, and an understanding of the critical neural circuitry have undergone significant modifications in the last quarter century. Schacter (1987) defines a memory system as an interaction among acquisition, retention, and retrieval mechanisms that is characterized by certain rules of operation. Currently, there are several different proposals as to the system and subsystem divisions within memory. Proposals of multiple memory systems have included dichotomous divisions into short-term versus long-term memory (e.g., Atkinson & Shiffrin, 1968), taxon versus locale (Nadel, 1994), hippocampal versus nonhippocampal (e.g., Nadel & O'Keefe, 1974), and declarative versus nondeclarative (Cohen & Eichenbaum, 1991; Cohen & Squire, 1980; Squire, 1987), as well as divisions that include a procedural, perceptual representation, semantic, primary/working, and episodic systems (Schacter & Tulving, 1994).

Despite multiple taxonomies, the simple descriptive terms *explicit* and *implicit* are often used to differentiate memory processes. As a caveat, explicit memory and implicit memory refer to the retrieval conditions rather than the memory systems (Schacter & Tulving, 1994). Explicit memories are often referred to as memories (or representations) that can be declared, can be brought to mind, exist in some time frame, are characterized by recognition and recall of past experiences, and for which we are consciously aware of either the encoding or the retrieval. Furthermore, Eichenbaum, Mathews, and Cohen (1989) suggest that explicit (declarative) memories are defined by relational representations that allow flexible responding in novel situations (see also Squire, 1994). Implicit memories are defined as those for which the subject does not need to recall the specific learning episode and may have no conscious awareness of, or may perform in an unconscious manner; those that are procedural; and those that involve rigid and inflexible representations and responses (Cohen & Squire, 1980; Squire, 1994; Tulving & Schacter, 1990).

If the mature adult memory system consists of functional dissociations as described above, how do we arrive at that point? Should we use the same definitions in developmental models as in adult models? Is there conservation in memory type across species and across age? Or do our definitions change as the organism matures? Further complicating matters, the specificity and selectivity of neural involvement in each system is unclear. For example, the medial temporal lobe is often considered to be the seat of explicit/declarative memories. Thus, are explicit memories defined by hippocampal involvement? Or, conversely, are all tasks that involve the hippocampus explicit or declarative in nature? To add another layer of complexity, functional specificity at the neural level in the adult animal does not necessitate dependence on the same mechanisms in the developing animal. For example, area TEO plays a transient role in early performance on recognition memory tasks such as the visual paired comparison task, but later performance is dependent on the functional integrity of area TE (Bachevalier, 1990; Bachevalier & Mishkin, 1992).

In regard to the development of functional and neural dissociations in memory, several proposals have been put forward that focus on the period of infancy. Piaget (1952) originally proposed that infants have limited perceptual capabilities that dissociated into a conceptual system. Piaget's theory holds that the infant's original state is one of sensory motor reflexes with no representational system; over the first 18 months, the infant undergoes conceptual restructuring (for discussion, see Meltzoff & Moore, 1999). The "sensorimotor" infant is born with the ability to represent the world through perceptual and motor schemas but lacks the ability to form representations that can be used for recall. A symbolic or conceptual system is built upon these early sensorimotor systems. A variation of this proposal is that memory abilities reflect processing stages that develop simultaneously (Rovee-Collier, 1997) or reflect the parallel development of conceptual and sensorimotor systems (Mandler, 1988, 1992). Rovee-Collier (1997) argues that the implicit/explicit dissociation used in adulthood "is untenable from a developmental and comparative perspective" because of its basis in conscious awareness (p. 469). This is primarily due to the inability to directly test whether or not the infant has a conscious awareness of the learning episode and is intentionally utilizing that information. Furthermore, Rovee-Collier has demonstrated that many of the same variables that influence "explicit" memory tasks also influence "implicit" tasks in infancy and that both types of tasks share commonalities in their developmental timelines. In a contrasting proposal, Mandler (1988) suggests that infants have a sensorimotor system that includes sensorimotor procedures (e.g., perceptual recognition, motor schemas) and does not require conscious access to information, as well as a conceptual knowledge system that is available to conscious thought and recall. Infants can engage in a perceptual analysis process by which one perception is actively compared with another. It is this comparative process that is stored in an accessible conceptual knowledge system and is available for recall. In this proposal, habituation and dishabituation are mediated by learning that is characteristic of a perceptual input system and do not require representation.

Lastly, Nelson has proposed that memory functions can be dissociated at the level of both behavior and anatomy early in development and that these early dissociable systems are the precursors to explicit and implicit memory systems in adults (Nelson, 1994; Nelson & Webb, 2003). Nelson proposes that a "pre-explicit" memory system appears within the first 6 months of life and reflects the infant's response to novelty. As the infant approaches the first year, a more integrative form of explicit memory develops, allowing the child to perform more complex tasks such as the delayed non-match-to-sample (DNMS) task, cross-modal memory tasks, and deferred imitation. These tasks likely involve the maturation as well as integration of regions within the inferior temporal cortex and prefrontal cortex. In contrast, implicit memory refers to a more heterogeneous set of abilities, within which each subdivision may have its own developmental trajectory. Nelson and Webb (2003) proposed that by 2–3 months of age, the perceptual representation system (PRS; Mandler, 1992; Schacter, 1992) underlies behavior in priming and instrumental conditioning paradigms in which the infant makes use of similarities between learning and test. Schacter (1994) has argued that the PRS operates at a presemantic level and is based within the modality of the test item. By 2 months, infants are also able to take advantage of contingencies in the environment and show expectation for events. This procedural system is guided by rule-based behavior without the necessity to possess awareness of the relations between concepts.

At the center of the debate surrounding explicit and pre-explicit memory and memory systems is the role of the hippocampus and other medial temporal lobe structures. It has been proposed that the hippocampus is critical for the binding of memory traces from the parahippocampal structures (Eichenbaum, Schoenbaum, Young, & Bunsey, 1996; Squire, Knowlton, & Musen, 1993). Whereas the hippocampus may be mature relatively early in nonhuman primates, the dentate, which connects the parahippocampus and the hippocampus, matures throughout the second year (Serres, 2001). Bauer (2002) suggests that it is the process of consolidation and storage of memory traces that may be compromised in infancy, resulting in the prolonged maturation of declarative memory. In contrast, Liston and Kagan (2002) suggest that retrieval errors resulting from immaturity of the frontal cortex account for age-related development in declarative memory.

In addition to these factors, the modality in which the memory is expected to be demonstrated may contribute to developmental patterns of performance and further confound the definition of the type of memory being indexed. Diamond (1990) suggests that cognitive abilities may first be demonstrated in one response system before becoming accessible to others. The visual system matures earlier than the reaching system because reaching involves the visual system, the arm movement system, and the integration of the two. Thus, tasks that assess memory via reaching show a different developmental timeline and involve additional neural systems than tasks that involve looking behaviors. Whether or not memories assessed via looking and reaching reflect the same system may depend on how that system is defined.

METHODOLOGICAL APPROACHES

Whereas behavioral studies of memory processes in the young child have a long history, the empirical investigation of the neural mechanisms underlying these processes has followed from work in adult cognitive neuroscience. Previously, many of these findings came from lesion studies in adult humans and nonhuman primates. Within the last 20 years, technical advancements have led to the downward applicability of neuroimaging methods to child populations, concurrent with increased attention to the relation between the developing brain and memory. Many of the tasks developed for use with nonhuman primates and infants have also been upwardly extended to adulthood, when applicable, to provide information about the nature of functional activation within similar testing paradigms.

The studies of brain–behavior relations reviewed in this chapter high-light two approaches. The first approach involves studies that investigate or manipulate a particular neural structure in order to understand its relation to behavioral performance on recognition memory tasks. One example is the manipulation of the hippocampus through an induced lesion or a lesion due to disease or injury. Comparative behavioral performance pre- and post-lesion may provide insight into the functional role of a given brain structure on memory tasks. Moreover, this neural manipulation may occur either early or late in development. Early insults provide information not only about the influence of that structure at that point in development but also about how that structure may interact with and influence the develop-mental trajectory of other brain regions and skills over the lifespan. This perspective captures the formation of brain–behavioral relations. In con-trast, the same insult in adulthood may result in a different pattern of skills and deficits. There are three assumptions underlying these studies. The first is that the study of atypical or abnormal development can provide informa-tion about typical development. The second is that lesions have a narrow or limited impact on brain functioning and that disruptions in the lesioned area cause impairment on the task. The third is that the same structures that subserve memory functioning in the adult or mature animal also medi-ate memory behaviors in the developing animal.

The second approach utilizes neuroimaging methods while the child performs a task. These studies provide information about the ongoing pro-cesses in both typical and atypical development. Functional neuroimaging methods, such as functional magnetic resonance imaging (fMRI) and ERPs, have provided a window into neural functioning during experimental con-ditions. fMRI provides detailed information about the spatial domain (on the scale of 5–7 millimeter (mm) slice thickness for whole brain imaging) but less temporal resolution due to the lag in the hemodynamic response (on the scale of 5–7 seconds). In contrast, ERPs provide detailed informa-tion about the temporal domain (on the scale of ms) but less spatial resolu-tion due to extracellular propagation and scalp impedance.

Whereas there are behavioral and experimental limitations of fMRI studies with young populations, ERPs can be used with individuals of all ages because they do not require motor or verbal responses, can be recorded in short epochs, and require less behavioral compliance than fMRI. ERPs reflect the summated postsynaptic potentials of a population of neurons in the cortex; the activity then propagates through extracellular space and can be recorded noninvasively at the surface of the scalp. ERPs are a subset of EEG (electroencephalogram) signals and are generated in response to an external event, such as the appearance of a stimu-lus. Components—deflections in the activity measured at the scalp—are thought to reflect the summation of multiple concurrent processes in the brain. For a methodological review of ERP recording in infants and young children, see Nelson (1996) or deBoer, Scott, and Nelson (2005).

NOVELTY, FAMILIARITY, AND THE MEDIAL TEMPORAL LOBE

Habituation–Dishabituation and Visual Paired Comparison

The habituation–dishabituation (H-D) and visual paired comparison (VPC) tasks comprise a class of behavioral tasks that rely on a subject's preference for viewing a novel stimulus. The H-D and VPC tests have several variables in common: In both, an infant is exposed to a stimulus repeatedly until he or she meets a predetermined learning criterion (familiarization or habituation), a delay is imposed, and then learning or memory is inferred from the child's preference for the novel versus familiarized stimulus (i.e., novelty preference). Unlike most adult tests of memory wherein the subject demonstrates memory by identifying the "old" or remembered item, memory for the familiar stimulus in the H-D and VPC is inferred from looking longer at, or demonstrating a visual preference for, the novel stimulus. Preference for the familiar stimulus or no preference (equal looking at the novel and familiar stimulus) have been treated as failures of memory (but see Courage & Howe, 1998). Thus, it is the child's preference at test that reflects the status of the memory.

Despite their similarities, these two experimental paradigms differ in a number of details. In the H-D protocol, the child is presented with a single repeated stimulus until his or her looking decreases to a preset criterion (habituation). This decrement in looking is often defined as a decline in looking time by less than half of that observed at initial presentation (e.g., the average of the two shortest looks is less than 50% of the average of the two longest looks). Immediately or after a delay, the infant is presented with the same stimulus and a novel stimulus in random serial order. In the VPC procedure, the infant is presented with a novel stimulus until he or she looks for a set period of time (e.g., 10–60 seconds depending on age; familiarization). Again, either immediately or after a delay, the infant is presented (for a fixed amount of time) with the familiarized stimulus and a novel stimulus concurrently, to the right and left of a fixation point. The presentation order is reversed on the second trial. Due to the paired presentation of novel and familiar at test, the VPC task allows the infant to actively compare the two stimuli and may be more sensitive to subtle differences between the familiar and novel (Cohen & Gelber, 1975). Thus, the VPC provides perceptual support for the memory process. In contrast, the H-D procedure presents the test items serially and thus no direct comparative process occurs and there is no perceptual support for comparison.

Novelty preferences are found in human infants shortly after birth (e.g., Pascalis & de Schonen, 1994; Pascalis, de Schonen, Morton, & Deruelle, 1995). On the VPC task, infants at 4 months of age who met the familiarization criteria (looked away three times for at least 3 seconds each time) demonstrated a novelty preference after delays of 10 seconds but not longer; infants age 9 months showed a novelty preference at delays up to 10 minutes (Diamond, 1990). In addition, the length of the familiarization time required to demonstrate a novelty preference shortens with age (e.g., Pascalis, de Haan, Nelson, & de Schonen, 1998), and this decrease in necessary exposure has been attributed to age-related changes in information-processing speed (e.g., Rose, 1983). Memory on the VPC task is also context dependent during the first year of life, with 6- and 12-month-olds failing to show a novelty preference when the background is changed; by 18 and 24 months of age, contextual change does not disrupt novelty preference (Haaf, Lundy, & Codren, 1996; Robinson & Pascalis, 2004). In monkeys, the preference for novelty is present at 1 month of age at delays of 10 seconds and 120 seconds but becomes "stronger" with age (Resende, Chalan-Fourney, & Bachevalier, 2002, as cited in Bachevalier & Vargha-Khadem, 2005).

The neural systems underlying performance on the VPC task are derived from animal models of the medial temporal lobe (MTL). A summary of results from the VPC task in nonhuman primates is presented in Table 6.1. Bachevalier and colleagues found that MTL lesions (hippocampal formation, entorhinal cortex, perirhinal cortex, parahippocampal gyrus, and amygdala) led to impaired performance on the VPC task in both infant and adult monkeys at short delays (Bachevalier, Brickson, & Hagger, 1993). The authors interpreted their findings as reflecting the involvement of the hippocampus in novelty preference. Pascalis and Bachevalier (1999) reported that adult monkeys with neonatal aspiration lesions of the hippocampal formation (including the dentate gyrus, CA fields, subicular complex, and portions of the parahippocampal gyrus) showed intact performance in the VPC paradigm at short delays (10 seconds), but impaired performance at longer delays (30 seconds to 24 hours). In adult monkeys, lesions of the hippocampus (24–33% ablation of the hippocampus, including hippocampal cell fields, dentate gyrus, and subiculum) also disrupt performance on the VPC task with delays of 10 seconds, 1 minute, and 10 minutes but not at a delay of 1 second (Zola et al., 2000).

**TABLE 6.1. Summary of Performance on the VPC Task
in Animal Models**

	Performance over delay					
	1 sec	10 sec	30 sec	1 min	10 min	24 hr
Lesions in adult animals						
H (Zola et al., 2000)	+	–/+ *	NA	–/+ *	–/+ *	NA
H (Pascalis & Bachevalier, 1999)	NA	+	–	–	–	–
PRh (Nemanic et al., 2004)	+	–	–	–	NA	NA
Th/Tf (Nemanic et al., 2004)	NA	+	–	–	NA	NA
H (Nemanic et al., 2004)	NA	+	+	–	NA	NA
TE (Buffalo et al., 1999)	–	–	NA	–	–	NA
PRh (Buffalo et al., 1999)	+	–	NA	–	–	NA
H-A (Bachevalier, 1990)	NA	–	NA	NA	NA	NA
TE (Bachevalier, 1990)	NA	–	NA	NA	NA	NA
Lesions in neonatal animals						
TE (Bachevalier, 1990)	NA	+	NA	NA	NA	NA
H-A (Bachevalier, 1990)	NA	–	NA	NA	NA	NA
H (Resende et al., 2002) at 1 month	NA	+	+	+	NA	–
H (Resende et al., 2002) at 6 months	NA	+	+	+	NA	+

Note. H, hippocampal formation; PRh, perirhinal cortex; TE, area TE; A, amygdala; Th/Tf, parahippocampus; +, similar to controls; NA, not tested; –, impaired; *, performance above chance but significantly worse than control animals.

However, these animals also had unintentional damage to the caudate nucleus (38–73%), limiting the interpretation of the effects of the hippocampal lesions.

In order to tease apart the contribution of specific MTL structures, Nemanic, Alvarado, and Bachevalier (2004) lesioned the perirhinal cortex, parahippocampal gyrus, or hippocampus. Adult monkeys with perirhinal lesions were impaired on the VPC task at delays greater than 10 seconds; animals with parahippocampal lesion were impaired on the task at delays of 30 seconds or more; animals with hippocampal lesion were impaired at delays of 60 seconds and longer. Given that prior reports included lesions to all of these structures, one interpretation is that VPC task impairments at short delays could be attributed to damage to the perirhinal cortex. In summary, hippocampal lesions do not appear to create deficits until delays reach 60 seconds; thus, the hippocampus may not underlie novelty preference in the adult animal.

Visual recognition memory can also be disrupted by lesions or damage to the inferior temporal cortex. Area TE is the last stage of the ventral stream that is engaged solely in visual processing and has reciprocal connections with the perirhinal cortex. Infant lesions in area TE do not disrupt novelty preference but late (adult) lesions do (Bachevalier, 1990). Adult monkeys with lesions in TE were impaired on the VPC task at all delays, including 1 second; in contrast, a perirhinal lesion group did demonstrate novelty preferences at 1 second but not at longer delays (Buffalo et al., 1999). Of note, there is some degree of error in creating lesions such that damage to a particular area is variable across animals and experiments. With this limitation in mind, the pattern of results presented in Table 6.1 suggests that the VPC task involves a number of areas within the MTL; the degree of involvement of any one area reflects the specifics of the task used.

Adult human studies utilizing individuals with typical development and patients with MTL damage have also helped to define the VPC task. One noticeable difference between infant and adult performance on the test is that adults spend the majority of the exposure time fixating on the stimulus. Thus, adults given 15 seconds or 60 seconds of familiarization will look at the stimulus approximately 85–90% of the available time (Richmond, Sowerby, Colombo, & Hayne, 2004). When Richmond and colleagues (2004) familiarized adults to novel stimuli for 15, 20, or 60 seconds, all subjects exhibited a novelty preference at test, but novelty preferences were greatest for those subjects in the 60-second condition. The magnitude of the novelty preference also decreased as the delay between familiarization and test increased, although all groups demonstrated a novelty preference even at delays of 1 month. Adults who were tested in a novel context after a 2-week delay did not demonstrate novelty preferences, whereas testing in a novel context after a delay of 3 minutes did not disrupt novelty preferences. Richmond et al. concluded that because the same factors (familiarization time, delay, and context) similarly affect adult and infant performance, the VPC task likely involves the same memory skills in infants and adults.

McKee and Squire (1993) found that 11 patients with amnesia (four with hippocampal damage, four with Korsakoff syndrome, one with damage to the thalamus, and two with unknown damage) were impaired, relative to controls, in the VPC task at delays of 2 minutes and 1 hour, and concluded that performance on the VPC task likely reflects a form of declarative memory mediated by the MTL memory system. Furthermore, Pascalis tested a patient with discrete hippocampal damage and parietal lobe atrophy who performed as well as controls at the 0-second delay but was impaired relative to controls at delays of 5 and 10 seconds. In contrast, the patient was able to succeed on a forced-choice recognition memory test, regardless of delay. One caveat is of note: The task used in the adult version of the VPC paradigm differs from that employed with infants; during the habituation phase, adults are often familiarized to multiple stimuli versus one exemplar with infants, the exposure period (criterion for familiarization) is often shorter, and adults most likely have semantic representations of the stimuli prior to testing.

Although the VPC paradigm has been important in describing the developmental trajectory of recognition memory, two concerns must be raised. First, recent work has revealed that, at least in adults, novelty preferences and recognition memory can be dissociated. For example, Manns, Stark, and Squire (2000) reported that performance in the visual paired-comparison task declines rapidly over time, such that normal adults do not show novelty preferences after a delay of 1 hour between familiarization and test (but see Richmond et al., 2004). However, these same adults show very high recognition memory (~84%) even after a 24-hour retention interval. Similarly, Hayne and Richmond (2002) found that novelty preferences declined as a function of delay interval, whereas recognition accuracy for the same stimuli did not. These findings may suggest dissociation between novelty preferences and recognition memory in adults.

What processes and mechanisms underlie novelty preference? Lesion work suggests that the hippocampus may not be critical to performance on the VPC task under some conditions (see Table 6.1). Animals with adult lesions of the hippocampus are able to demonstrate novelty preferences at very short delays (1–10 seconds) but not at longer delays. Animals with neonatal lesions show novelty preferences at delays equal to or less than 1 minute, but performance at longer delays depends on the age at which the animals are tested. Thus, the roles of the hippocampus, TE, and other structures in the VPC paradigm depend on the age at which lesions are performed, suggesting that there are developmental alterations in the circuitry that underlies this task.

These results do not preclude the involvement of the hippocampus in novelty detection. Several adult fMRI and single-cell animal studies suggest that the hippocampus becomes active under certain novel conditions, such as responding to stimuli that are more contextually novel (i.e., unusual or unexpected). The hippocampal formation, medial dorsal thalamus, anterior

cingulate, and medial and ventral regions of the prefrontal cortex are activated more to novel (first presentation) than familiar (second presentation)
stimuli (e.g., Dolan & Fletcher, 1997; Tulving & Markowitsch, 1997;
Tulving et al., 1994). In single-cell studies in monkeys, neurons that
respond more to novel than familiar stimuli have been found in the
amygdala, hippocampus, perirhinal cortex, and ventral striatum (Brown,
Wilson, & Riches, 1987; Fahy, Riches, & Brown, 1993b; Rolls, Cahusac,
Feigenbaum, & Miyashita, 1993; Wilson & Rolls, 1993; Wilson, Rolls,
Leonard, & Stern, 1993).

Further exploration into how the acquisition, retention, and retrieval
mechanisms underlying the VPC task reflect the definitions of explicit
memory is needed. Robinson and Pascalis (2004) found that it was not
until 18 months that performance in the VPC paradigm becomes independent of context (background). Context-independent performance on the
mobile conjugate reinforcement paradigm also undergoes a prolonged
period of development during the first year, during which changes in context disrupt performance (see Rovee-Collier, 2001, for a review), and
context-independent performance on the deferred imitation task is not
expressed until after 12 months of age (Barnat, Klein, & Meltzoff, 1996;
Hayne, Boniface, & Barr, 2000). If we use the definition of declarative
memories put forward by Eichenbaum and colleagues (1989), performance
on the VPC before 18 months of age does not represent declarative memory. Disruptions of memory based on context changes during infancy suggest that these memories do not allow flexible responding in novel situations (see also Squire, 1994). Furthermore, several infant/toddler tasks,
including one that involves conditioning (mobile conjugate reinforcement),
show characteristics of declarative memory (flexible responding) after 1
year of age, despite infants' ability to perform them much earlier. Whether
or not this finding reflects differences in how the infant is performing the
task, greater neural connectivity, or both is unknown. Again, whether or
not these tasks reflect "explicit memory" depends on the definition.

Delayed Non-Match-to-Sample (DNMS)

In the DNMS, the participant is presented with a sample object, and the
sample object is placed on a food reward such that displacement of the
object reveals the reward. Either immediately or after a delay, the subject is
then presented with the same sample object and a novel object. On this test
trial, the novel object is rewarded. Each trial has a unique sample and novel
item. The participant must learn to reach for the sample to get the reward
but then to inhibit reaching for the sample and reach for the novel item on
the next presentation. Thus, this task involves learning a non-match–

reward-rule association. The delayed *match*-to-sample paradigm involves the same procedures except that the sample item is rewarded at both learning and test. The task demands can be increased by imposing a delay between sample and test or by presenting multiple samples and then multiple test trials. Unlike the VPC and H-D paradigms, the criterion for learning in DNMS paradigms is often set at 90% correct responses on 2 consecutive days of 15–40 trials per day (e.g., Overman, 1990) or correct responses on five consecutive trials (Dawson, Meltzoff, Osterling, & Rinaldi, 1998; Diamond, 1990).

Nonhuman primates begin to learn the DNMS task by 4 months of age but do not reach mature performance until 1 year of age (Bachevalier & Mishkin, 1994). Human infants can begin to have success on the task at 6 months when the stimulus is the reward (single action; Diamond, 1990), by 12 months when the reward is attached to the sample/novel stimulus or when praise is used as the reward, and by 21–44 months on the standard task in which the sample is displaced to get the reward (Diamond, 1990; Overman, 1990). However, it is not until 45–81 months that young children are able to learn the task quickly and perform reliably, although still significantly worse than adults (Overman, Bachevalier, Turner, & Peuster, 1992).

Similar to the VPC task, what we know about the neuroanatomy supporting the DNMS task derives mainly from lesion studies of nonhuman primates. Neonatal lesions of the MTL lead to reduced rule learning as well as recognition memory at 3 months and 2 years of age (Bachevalier & Mishkin, 1994; Malkova, Mishkin, & Bachevalier, 1995). When the hippocampus and amygdala are lesioned independently, animals with neonatal lesions to the amygdaloid complex are impaired on performance of the DNMS task at 10 months and 6–7 years of age. In contrast, early lesions of the hippocampal formation do not lead to impairments at 10 months and 6 or 7 years on the standard version of the task but do impair performance on the 10-item list version of the DNMS task at the older ages (Bachevalier, Beauregard, & Alvarado, 1999). Although this result would suggest a role for the amygdala in DNMS task performance, the authors attribute the impact of the amygdaloid lesions to the unintended concurrent entorhinal and perirhinal cortex damage rather than to the amygdala proper.

Similar to performance on the VPC task, late but not early lesions of area TE in the inferior temporal cortex disrupt performance on the DNMS task (Bachevalier, 1990). In infant monkeys, there are transient projections from area TEO to the limbic structures that retract by 2 months of age (Webster, Bachevalier, & Ungerleider, 1991, 1995). Early lesions of area TE may have less impact than late lesions due to the redundancy in the connections between TE–limbic system and TEO–limbic system.

Mishkin and Appenzeller (1987) propose that the DNMS task involves the occipitotemporal visual information pathways, inferior temporal cortex (areas TEO and TE), limbic structures (amygdala, hippocampus, and entorhinal cortex), areas of the diencephalon (anterior and medial dorsal nuclei of the thalamus and mamillary bodies), basal forebrain, and ventromedial prefrontal cortex. However, as proposed above, the structures involved in the task in the mature animal may not be the same as the structures necessary in the young animal, and the same structure may not play the same role in early and late development. Bachevalier and colleagues (e.g., Bachevalier & Mishkin, 1994; Malkova, Bachevalier, Webster, & Mishkin, 2000) have concluded that the MTL may be sufficient for supporting rule learning early in development, but increased circuitry provides supplementary routes for learning later in life. For example, neonatal lesions of the inferior convexity induce moderate impairments at 2 years of age on rule learning, suggesting that regions of the frontal lobe play a specific role in DNMS performance later in development.

In adult monkeys, lesions of the MTL, inferior temporal lobe, and prefrontal cortex disrupt performance on the DNMS task. Lesions of the amygdala and hippocampus cause impairments when delays exceed 10 seconds (Mishkin, 1978; see also Bachevalier, 1990). However, Alvarado and Bachevalier (2005) found that there were no differences between adult animals with specific hippocampal lesions and controls in reaching the learning criterion and reported that the lesioned animals were only mildly, or not, impaired on the DNMS task. In contrast, animals with perirhinal or parahippocampal lesions took significantly longer to reach the learning criterion. Lesions to the perirhinal cortex impair animals on delays greater than 8 seconds on the visual DNMS task and a tactile version (Buffalo et al., 1999; Nemanic et al., 2004) but not on delayed non-match-to-location (DNML; Nemanic et al., 2004). Nemanic and colleagues (2004) also found that the perirhinal group was significantly impaired compared to controls and hippocampal lesion animals at all delays, and performance also worsened with increasing delay and list length. The parahippocampus lesion group was only mildly impaired on the DNMS task but showed worse performance with increasing delays; this group was severely affected on the DNML task. When lesions to the inferior prefrontal cortex were combined with amygdala and hippocampal lesions, performance was ablated (Mishkin, 1978). These results further suggest that the type of information (item vs. location) is important in defining the needed neural circuitry; moreover, different areas may be necessary for learning the non-match rule versus performing with a delay.

Lesions of TE do not impair animals on delays of 8 seconds but do cause impairment at delays greater than 15 seconds on the standard visual

DNMS task. Animals with TE lesions performed similarly to controls on a tactile version of the DNMS task (Buffalo et al., 1999), suggesting a specific role for TE in visual memory. In general, animals with perirhinal and TE lesions did not differ from each other in degree of impairment at delays greater than 15 seconds (Buffalo et al., 1999). Only the animals with perirhinal lesions, however, were impaired on the tactile DNMS task, suggesting a role of the perirhinal cortex in generalized memory.

Animals with adult lesions of TE have difficulty learning a computer version of the DNMS task (Buffalo, Ramus, Squire, & Zola, 2000) compared to animals with perirhinal lesions and control animals. After rule learning, animals with TE lesions perform worse than animals with perirhinal lesions and control animals at very short delays (1 second and 1 minute). At longer delays (15 seconds, 1 minute, 10 minutes, and 40 minutes), the TE and perirhinal groups perform worse than control animals but do not differ from each other (Buffalo et al., 1999, 2000). However, on a tactile version of the DNMS task, Buffalo and colleagues (1999) found that the perirhinal group was significantly impaired at rule learning and over delays, whereas the TE group did not differ from the control animals. Lesions to the rhinal cortex or mediodorsal thalamus (which receives projections from the rhinal cortex) also impair DMS performance, but only when a large stimulus set is used (as cited in Parker, Eacott, & Gaffan, 1997). Similar to the results from the VPC, successful performance on the DNMS involves the hippocampus formation, entorhinal cortex, perirhinal cortex, and area TE. The degree of involvement of each area is specific to the task requirements, the length of delay, and the age of the animal.

Adult animals with ablations of the inferior prefrontal convexity (IPC) show impairments on DNMS rule learning (Kowalska et al., 1991), and combined damage to area TE and the IPC prevents relearning of the task at intervals longer than 5 seconds (Weinstein, Saunders, & Mishkin, 1988, as cited by Malkova et al., 2000). In contrast, Malkova and colleagues (2000) found that animals with neonatal lesions to the IPC were able to learn the DNMS rule at 3 months of age in fewer trials than those with MTL lesions (amygdala, hippocampus, fusiform hippocampal gyrus, rostral and caudal entorhinal cortex, and caudal perirhinal cortex) and did not differ from control animals. At 2 years of age, the animals with IPC lesions performed better than the MTL group at relearning the DNMS rule but worse than controls. For the memory component, at 3 months and 2 years of age, MTL lesion animals performed worse than the IPC and control animals at delays longer than 10 seconds. These results suggest that there is some early functional plasticity in the IPC, but not when lesions are sustained during adulthood.

Suzuki and Clayton (2000) suggest that the DNMS task can be solved in two ways (see also Mandler, 2000). First, the subject can recall the stimulus, thought to be dependent on the hippocampus, or second, the subject can detect stimulus familiarity, thought to be dependent on the surrounding cortex. Thus, performance on DNMS tasks need not necessarily involve episodic recognition (Griffiths, Dickinson, & Clayton, 1999). Furthermore, animals must be trained to retrieve the food reward from under the stimulus, and thus training history of the animals as well as the variability in lesions may affect the circuitry used to perform the task.

Other Relational Memory Tasks

Transverse Patterning

One characteristic of both the DNMS and the VPC tasks is that the familiar item is tested in the context of a novel item; that is, the two items are paired at test. Given that one version of declarative memory is defined by relational representations (Eichenbaum et al., 1989), an additional task is of note: the transverse patterning task. In transverse patterning, the animal must learn that the correct or rewarded item depends on the context in which it is presented (A + B–; B + C–; C + A–). Thus, A is rewarded when paired with B but C is rewarded when paired with A. Performance on transverse patterning does not reach proficiency until 2 years of age in monkeys (Alvarado & Bachevalier, 2000; Killiany & Mahut, 1990) and not until 5 years of age in children (Rudy, Keith, & Georgen, 1993). Rudy and colleagues (1993) concluded that children younger than 4.5 years were not able to gain access to a configuration association system. Adult individuals with amnesia also fail at the transverse patterning task (Reed & Squire, 1999; Rickard & Grafman, 1998).

Animals with hippocampal lesions also show deficits on acquisition and performance of transverse patterning. Specifically, the animals were impaired on the transfer phase (C + A–) of the experiment but not on the earlier learning phases (A + B–; B + C–; Alvarado & Bachevalier, 2005). Monkeys with neonatal damage to the hippocampus and parahippocampal region were not able to learn transverse patterning but were able to learn a simpler association task (A + B–; B + C–; C + X–; Alvarado, Wright, & Bachevalier, 2002).

Eichenbaum and colleagues suggest that, as demonstrated by the transverse patterning task, the hippocampus is involved in learning the relations between stimuli, allowing for inferential responses (Eichenbaum, Dudchenko, Wood, Shapiro, & Tanila, 1999). The formation of unique relations between stimuli may not only be involved in the formation of episodic memories but may also play a role in semantic, recognition, and associative memory (Suzuki & Clayton, 2000).

Deferred Imitation

In the deferred imitation paradigm, an infant or toddler is shown a sequence of events that involves actions on objects. In a one-step imitation event, an experimenter might turn on a lighted display by touching it with his forehead (Meltzoff, 1988); in a two-step event, the child might place a car onto a covered track, then push a wooden plunger, such that the car moves to the end of the track (Bauer et al., 2006). Sequences may also differ in whether or not the steps are temporally constrained (i.e., step 1 must occur before step 2 can occur) or unconstrained (i.e., each step is independent of the other) or combined (i.e., partially constrained). For example, in the two-step sequence above, pushing the wooden plunger before putting the car on the track would not result in the car moving; thus, the sequence is temporally constrained. In both one- and two-step paradigms, either immediately or after a delay, the infant/toddler is given the items and "asked" to reproduce the sequence of events. Imitation tasks are thought to tap into declarative memory because they rely on representational capacities (Piaget, 1952), which are accessible to language (once language is developed; Bauer, Wenner, & Kroupina, 2002), rely on the MTL, and are thought to be nonverbal analogues to verbal report (e.g., Bauer, 2002; Mandler, 1990; Meltzoff, 1990). Interestingly, individuals with amnesia fail to reproduce the correct action sequence after a delay in deferred imitation tasks (McDonough, Mandler, McKee, & Squire, 1995).

Human infants are able to recall imitation events after 24 hours at 6 months of age, after 1 month at 9 months of age, after 3 months at 10 months of age, and after 12 months by 20 months of age (Bauer, Wenner, Dropik, & Wewerka, 2000; Carver & Bauer, 2001; Collie & Hayne, 1999). As children mature, sequences can be increased from one unique step to four steps, the number of imitation events can be increased, and the delay between the exposure to the imitation event (watching the experimenter perform the task) and the imitation event itself can be lengthened. Toddlers perform better earlier on action sequences that are temporally constrained compared to arbitrary, unconstrained sequences (e.g., Bauer & Hertsgaard, 1993; Bauer & Mandler, 1992). Memory expressed in deferred imitation experiments is context dependent at 6 months of age and object dependent until 12 months of age but becomes more flexibly expressed after the first year (Barnat et al., 1996; Hayne et al., 2000; see also Learmonth, Lamberth, & Rovee-Collier, 2004).

Bauer (2005) found that memory storage capacity may account for developmental improvements in the deferred imitation task during the second year of life (see also Howe & Courage, 1997; Howe & O'Sullivan, 1997). Bauer matched 13- and 16-month-old infants on immediate recall abilities (encoding abilities) and then compared their performance on 1-month and 3-month delay conditions. As expected, children performed more poorly as delay increased. However, younger children lost *more* information over time and were less able to make use of relearning cues.

Nonhuman primate species are able to imitate human actions; however, deferred imitation has only been shown in primates reared under human conditions (see Bering, 2004, for discussion). Enculturated but not mother-reared chimpanzees, orangutans, and bonobos are able to show deferred imitation (Bjorklund, Bering, & Ragan, 2000; Bjorklund, Yunger, Bering, & Ragan, 2002; Tomasello, Savage-Rumbaugh, & Kruger, 1993), but reports suggest that great apes develop deferred imitation later than human children (Parker, 1996).

Little is known about the specific neural systems underlying the deferred imitation paradigm. Adults with amnesia (adult onset; mixed etiology) perform fewer sequences than controls and patients with frontal lobe lesions (McDonough et al., 1995), but slight improvements between baseline and recall for the number of actions might reflect some residual declarative memory. Teenagers and adults with developmental amnesia are also impaired compared to controls at delayed recall of individual actions as well as action sequences (Adlam, Vargha-Khadem, Mishkin, & de Haan, 2005). However, these patients also performed more target actions after a 24-hour delay than at baseline, suggesting some preserved memory. Performance on the number of action pairs recalled was greater in the temporally constrained than unconstrained sequence type, but overall memory for number of actions recalled did not differ. All individuals had reduced hippocampal volumes (between 20 to 60% when known) and had sustained their injuries between 0 and 15 years of age.

Adult studies of imitation using fMRI have focused on observing, imitating, and generating hand movements, gestures, and other slight movements but have not focused on deferred imitation paradigms. Across these studies, it has been suggested that the system involved in imitation involves a distributed network that includes the premotor cortex (e.g., Buccino, Binkofski, & Riggio, 2004; Iacoboni et al., 2001; Koski et al., 2002; Muhlau et al., 2005), the superior temporal sulcus (e.g., Iacoboni et al., 2001), inferior frontal gyrus (e.g., Buccino et al., 2004; Iacoboni et al., 1999; Koski et al., 2002; Molnar-Szakacs, Iacoboni, Koski, & Mazziotta, 2005), superior parietal lobe (e.g., Iacoboni et al., 1999; Muhlau et al., 2005), inferior parietal cortex (Buccino et al., 2004; Chaminade, Meltzoff,

& Decety, 2005; Muhlau et al., 2005), lateral occipitotemporal junction (Chaminade et al., 2005; Muhlau et al., 2005), and cerebellum (Muhlau et al., 2005).

Summary

Results from nonhuman primates, lesion studies, and young children suggest that performance on the tasks typically referred to as "recognition" memory tasks have a complex developmental timeline. Tasks that rely on incidental learning or novelty preference develop relatively early; tasks that depend on discrimination and reward-based learning, recognition, and recall involve more complex circuitry but begin to make an appearance by the end of the first year of life; and tasks that involve relational learning or associations make their appearance during early childhood. Despite early success at some of these tasks, improvements in performance continue for many years. Bachevalier and Vargha-Khadem (2005) suggest that the progression in memory abilities is dependent on the maturation of the dentate gyrus, hippocampus, and the integration within MTL circuits (see also Tulving, 1985).

Although successful performance on the VPC, DNMS, and deferred imitation tasks can be demonstrated prior to the first year of life, differences in task requirements likely result in different structures being essential for function. Nemanic and colleagues (2004) argue that the VPC task involves passive exploration of two-dimensional stimuli and is best described as incidental learning. In passive learning, it is unclear what part of the event will become behaviorally relevant later. In contrast, the DNMS task involves active displacement of the sample (to achieve the reward) and has been proposed as intentional or purposeful encoding. The stimulus–reward link may emphasize which part of the event will become relevant. Furthermore, memories displayed within the VPC and deferred imitation tasks become more flexibly demonstrated after 1 year, suggesting additional modification in how the tasks are encoded, stored, and retrieved.

NOVELTY, FAMILIARITY, AND ERPs

In contrast to the approach discussed above, the recording of ERPs allows for the measurement of neural activity while a participant is performing a task. Furthermore, this approach allows for the collection of information during encoding or familiarization as well as during episodes of recall or test. Unlike behavioral tests that use few exposures, however, ERPs reflect averaged electrophysiological (EEG) responses. The ERP-evoked response is embedded within the background EEG activity. To increase the signal of the evoked activity relative to the background "noise," a large number of trials is needed. This methodological constraint requires that infants be exposed to numerous trials, usually of relatively short duration. Thus, a familiarization period during an ERP experiment might involve 50 trials with 500-millisecond (ms) exposure on each trial (total exposure = 25 seconds). Testing might involve altering presentation of the novel and familiar image for a total of 100 trials. Thus, ERP experiments of infant memory have different constraints than behavioral tests and require that attention be paid to the familiarity of the stimulus prior to familiarization and testing and to the repetition or frequency pattern of the stimulus.

To this end, we continue to discuss novelty and familiarity but within the context of ERP experiments (for an overview, see Table 6.2). As seen in the VPC experiment, young infants prefer novelty. To prefer novelty, however, an evaluative process must occur at some level that informs the system that one item is more novel or is more familiar than the other. Although it has been suggested that this process reflects pre-explicit processing (Nelson, 1994), it has also been suggested that familiarity-based memory is separate from episodic memory (e.g., Aggleton & Brown, 1999; Baddeley, Vargha-Khadem, & Mishkin 2001; O'Keefe & Nadel, 1978; Yonelinas et al., 2002). Whereas ERPs do not provide detailed source information, they can be used to differentiate processes related to familiarization and novelty in very young infants without the need for behavioral responses.

Repetition, Frequency, and Familiarity

Similar to habituation and paired-comparison methods, experiments that address the influence of repetition and frequency on familiarity often involve stimuli that are unfamiliar to the subject prior to the experimental manipulation. In order to understand how repetition and frequency influence familiarity, a standard oddball paradigm can be utilized. In such a paradigm, two novel stimuli are presented; one is presented frequently (~80% of trials) whereas the other is presented infrequently (~20% of trials). The relative probability of the stimulus presentation evokes a different "amount of processing" or facilitates the speed of processing. It is thought that the repeated frequent stimulus becomes more familiar than the repeated infrequent stimulus. ERP responses are the average response to these two categories of stimuli over the entire experiment.

TABLE 6.2. Summary of ERP Responses to Frequency and Familiarity

	Age	Middle (Nc)	Late (slow wave)	Other
		Visual oddball		
Courchesne et al. (1981)	4–7 months	Larger and later to infrequent		
Karrer and Ackles (1987a, 1988)	4–18 months	Larger to infrequent		
Nikkel and Karrer (1994)	6 months	Smaller with exposure to frequent stimulus		
Karrer and Monti (1995)	4–7 weeks	Faster to infrequent stimulus	More negative to infrequent	
Ackles and Cook (1998)	6 months	Larger to infrequent		
		Familiarization + test (ERP oddball)		
Nelson and Salapatek (1986)		Larger to habituation trials then novel test trials	Larger to novel than familiar trials at test	
Nelson and Collins (1991, 1992)	4, 6, 8 months; age-related differences	Smaller to frequent familiar test	Larger positive to infrequent familiar test; larger negative to infrequent novel test	
Nelson and deRegnier (1992)	12 months		Larger positive to infrequent novel test	
		Familiarization + test (behavioral and ERP)		
Snyder, Kuefner, et al. (2004)	6 months	Slower during familiarization in infants who showed familiarity preference at behavioral test		N700 slower to familiar at test
Snyder & Kuefner (2005)	6 months	Less amplitude during familiarization in infants who showed a novelty preference at behavioral test		
		A priori familiarity		
de Haan and Nelson (1997, 1999)	6 months	Greater to familiar		

Courchesne, Ganz, and Norcia (1981), using an 88%–12% design with two novel faces in 4- to 7-month-old infants, found that a negative component (Nc) was larger and peaked later for infrequent events. Using an 80%–20% paradigm also with 4- to 7-month-old infants, Karrer and Monti (1995) found that the Nc peaked earlier for the infrequent stimulus than the frequent stimulus and the slow wave was more negative for the infrequent than the frequent trials. For 6-, 12-, and 18-month-olds, the Nc was larger to the infrequent event (Karrer & Ackles, 1987a, 1988). The amplitude of the Nc in 6-month-old infants also decreases with exposure; smaller Nc amplitudes were found to the frequent stimulus (80%) during the last block of trials (Nickel & Karrer, 1994). Multiple probabilities— 90%–10%, 70%–30%, 60%–40%—also evoke a larger amplitude Nc to the infrequent stimulus (Ackles & Cook, 1998). Taken together, these studies suggest that infants can make use of frequency information by 1 month of age. ERP results suggest that infrequent stimuli are differentiated from frequent stimuli at the Nc component (negative midlatency component).

Similarly, using auditory ERPs, infrequent tones compared to frequent tones can produce a negative deflection at approximately 270–300 ms after stimulus presentation (called the mismatch negativity or MMN) in newborns (e.g., Alho, Sainio, Sajaniemi, Reinikainen, & Näätänen, 1990; Cheour et al., 2002). The MMN is thought to be a response to stimulus change, reflective of an automatic change detection process, and represents the sensory memory representation of the preceding auditory stimulus (see Näätänen, Jacobsen, & Winkler, 2005). It has also been proposed that the MMN reflects the outcome of a comparison process between the frequent and infrequent stimulus (Näätänen, 1999); this may be a preattentive process in that the MMN can be recorded without task requirements, in the absence of attention, and in individuals in a coma (see Näätänen, 2000, for a review).

The degree to which frequency detection reflects recognition memory per se is unclear. Similar to the VPC task, the memory trace developed during an oddball experiment is reflective of passive, incidental learning. If one is engaged in a perceptual analysis or a comparative process, then this might be reflective of an accessible conceptual knowledge system (Mandler, 1988). Similarly, the infant's response to novelty in both the visual and auditory oddball experiments may reflect differential processing of the "more" novel, infrequent stimulus and may thus be more similar to the conceptualization of pre-explicit memory proposed by Nelson (1996). Given that the MMN can be recorded in individuals who do not have conscious awareness due to coma, sedation, or during sleep, it is unclear if frequency detection fits under standard definitions of explicit, recognition, or declarative memory.

Familiarization and Frequency

In a set of studies from Nelson and colleagues that was designed to be similar to the classic behavioral tests of memory, ERPs were collected during familiarization and test. Because the focus of these experiments was to understand the processes invoked during testing conditions, the test images (novel, familiar) were presented based on different frequencies; this is referred to as a familiarization plus oddball design. Nelson and Salapatek (1986) used three designs to examine the influence of frequency on familiarity after familiarization. The first study familiarized the infants to a face (in which the face was presented with 100% probability) and then employed an 80% (familiarized face)–20% (novel face) test design. The second study familiarized the infants to a face and then employed a 50% (familiarized face)–50% (novel face) test design. The third study employed a 50% (novel face)–50% (novel face) design with no prior familiarization. The authors found two components that differed. First, the Nc (defined as the negative component at the midline central site between 550 and 700 ms) was greater (more negative) to the familiarization trials (100% probability) than the novel trials (novel face–20%, novel face–50%). Second, the later positive slow wave (850–1000 ms) at frontal and central midline sites was greater (more positive) to the test infrequent-novel (20% trials) than the test frequent-familiar (80% trials) stimuli for Experiment 1 but did not differ between the test familiar (50%) and test novel (50%) stimuli in Experiment 2.

Furthermore, Nelson and Collins (1991, 1992) familiarized 4-, 6-, and 8-month-old infants to two stimuli (two faces) for 10 trials each (alternating presentation). During the test ERP phase, one face was presented on 60% of trials (frequent-familiar) and the other on 20% of trials (infrequent-familiar). On the other 20% of trials, a set of 12 novel faces was presented (unfamiliar-infrequent). For the 4-month-olds, there were no significant differences in the ERP waveform for the frequent-familiar, infrequent-familiar, and infrequent-unfamiliar stimuli at test. For the 6-month-old infants, the early Nc (at ~400 ms) for the test frequent-familiar stimulus returned to baseline; for the test infrequent-familiar face, a late positive slow wave followed this negative deflection; and for the test infrequent novel faces, a sustained negative slow wave followed the early Nc. At 8 months of age, the frequent-familiar and infrequent-familiar stimuli were not differentiated in the ERP waveform, whereas the infrequent-unfamiliar stimulus evoked a negative slow wave similar to the 6-month-olds' response. The authors concluded that the early Nc did not differentiate between the types of stimulus events. However the later positive and negative slow waves did differ and were interpreted as indexing memory updating (positive slow wave) and novelty detection (negative slow wave).

Because the two familiar stimuli were encoded to the same degree, the resulting difference in the ERP components at 6 months to the frequent-familiar and infrequent-familiar stimuli may have been related to the infant's need to update the memory trace in the infrequent case. By 8 months of age, the responses to the two familiar events did not differ, suggesting that the memory trace was more stable, more established, did not need to be updated, and was not influenced by presentation frequency. In a follow-up study using the same paradigm with 12-month-olds, Nelson and deRegnier (1992) found that the infrequent-unfamiliar stimuli elicited a positive slow wave. The authors suggested that the 12-month-old infants might have been updating or abstracting a template of "novelty" from brief presentations. From these findings Nelson and Collins concluded that sometime after the first half year of life, infants could, in fact, dissociate a novel stimulus from a stimulus that had simply been seen infrequently. These studies suggest that the response to the familiar stimulus and the influence of frequency on familiarity changes across the first year.

It can be concluded that early responses to familiarity and frequency are critically linked in the first 6 months of life. Thus, in these paradigms, familiarity is influenced and maintained by frequency. Given that we do not know the state of encoding at the end of the habituation/familiarization period, and we do not know if infants would have shown a novelty preference if there were a test, how familiar the stimulus was to the infants at the beginning of the ERP experiment is unknown. It is possible that the responses during testing conditions reflect continued familiarization, such that the frequent-familiar becomes a fully familiarized stimulus whereas the infrequent-familiar is only partially encoded.

Nelson and Collins (1991, 1992) concluded that familiarity could be thought of as becoming independent of frequency in the second half of the first year. This conclusion assumes that the stimulus reaches a critical level of exposure, becomes familiar, and then does not need to be maintained or updated within this testing window. To fully test this view, one would need a way of determining if the infant became familiar with the stimuli, possibly using a familiarization time or criterion that is known to produce novelty preferences. If frequency does not alter the neural response to the familiar item, then it is likely that the two are independent. Frequent presentations of the familiar item may work to reactivate the memory trace and change attention or preference.

Familiarization and Novelty Preference

In order to further understand the neural processes involved when infants are performing a VPC task, Snyder and colleagues collected ERP data during encoding of the VPC (to the familiarized stimulus), behavioral data at test (to familiar or novel), and a posttest ERP experiment (to familiar and novel stimuli from the VPC test and an unexposed novel stimulus). Infants were grouped based on their performance on the VPC behavioral test as showing a novelty preference ($\geq 55\%$ time looking toward the novel stimulus at test), null preference (45–55% looking toward the novel stimulus at test), or a familiarity preference ($\leq 45\%$ time looking toward the novel stimulus at test). There was no difference in ERP activity during familiarization as a function of performance at VPC behavioral test (Snyder, 2003; Snyder, Blank, Cheek, Kuefner, & Marsolek, 2004; Snyder & Kuefner, 2005). During the posttest VPC oddball ERP experiment, the N700 peaked later in response to the familiar object compared to two novel objects, but did not differ in latency for the two novel objects. This difference in familiar and novel processing occurred even in those infants who demonstrated no preference at VPC test. These results suggest that differential processing of the novel and familiar item at test can be seen when using ERPs, despite a lack of difference when measured by behavioral performance. In addition, null or familiarity preferences can be differentiated from each other using ERPs. These results support the interpretation of the VPC task as reflecting a "flow of attentional preference" (Bahrick & Pickens, 1995; also see Courage & Howe, 1998). Bahrick and Pickens (1995) propose a four-stage model of infant attention that represents shifts in the flow of attentional preference, from novelty to null to familiarity preference, and reflects the accessibility of the representation over retention time.

Snyder, Stolarova, and Nelson (2005, as cited in Snyder, in press) tested 6-month-olds' brain activity during familiarization and then exposed the infants to the familiarized image and a novel image. However, unlike the behavioral VPC task described above, at test, the familiar and novel stimuli were presented serially, and the infant was allowed one continuous look at each stimulus. Again, infants were divided into groups based on their behavior at test. Infants who demonstrated a preference for the novel face at test showed a reduction in the amplitude of the ERP over temporal scalp regions during the familiarization phase, whereas a preference for the novel object was associated with a reduction in the amplitude over occipitotemporal scalp regions. Snyder (in press) has suggested a reinterpretation of the VPC and novelty preference data based on these findings. The reduction in activity with repetition was similar to that seen during repetition suppression in the visual processing pathway. Repetition suppression reflects a reduction of neuronal responses in the inferior temporal cortex as stimuli are repeated (see Desimone, 1996, for a discussion) and has been suggested to reflect a form of implicit memory. Furthermore, computational evidence shows that repetition of a specific visual pattern results in changes in the efficiency by which the pattern is processed, such that the number of units required to process the stimulus is reduced (McClelland & Rumelhart, 1985).

A Priori Familiarity and Novelty

The ERP studies reviewed above utilized stimuli that were unfamiliar to the subject prior to experimental exposure. An alternate way of examining familiarity and its neural signature is to use stimuli with which the young infant has extensive familiarity. In the auditory domain, this can be done through the use of a familiar voice and in the visual domain, through the use of a picture of a familiar person (mother's face) or a familiar item (favorite toy). A number of studies have investigated early processing of familiarity in the auditory modality. Newborns tested at 40 weeks postconception age and 10 days postnatal showed a larger and faster P2 to their mother's voice saying a familiar word (*baby*) than to an unfamiliar voice saying the same word; the unfamiliar voice elicited a greater late negative slow wave (deRegnier, Nelson, Thomas, Wewerka, & Georgieff, 2000). To test the effect of postnatal experience, healthy premature newborns (born 35–38 weeks) were tested within 7 days postbirth and compared to full-term infants. For the premature newborns, there was no difference between the mother's and the unfamiliar voice. For the full-term infants, the response was greater to the maternal voice than the unfamiliar voice at the negative slow wave. There were no group differences in the response to the unfamiliar voice (deRegnier, Wewerka, Georgieff, Mattia, & Nelson, 2002). At 4 months of age, infants demonstrated a greater negative response at 350 ms to their mother's voice as compared to an unfamiliar voice (Purhonen, Kilpelainen-Lees, Valkonen-Korhonen, Karhu, & Lehtonen, 2004).

Nelson and colleagues have published extensively on a visual memory paradigm that compares ERP signals to a highly familiar stimulus (mother's face) and a novel/unfamiliar stimulus (stranger's face). The stimuli are presented 50%–50%. Thus, the ERP can be compared between an item that is being retrieved from memory (mother's face) and an item that is concurrently being encoded into memory as the task is unfolding (unfamiliar face). In the original report by de Haan and Nelson (1997), the researchers found that the ERP response to the familiar face differed from the ERP response to the novel face, whereas the ERPs for two novel faces did not differ; larger peak Nc amplitudes were seen for the familiar face compared to a dissimilar looking unfamiliar face (Figure 6.1). The Nc effects for the familiar face were greater over the midline (Cz) and the right anterior temporal electrode (T4) sites. When familiar and unfamiliar objects were compared in a similar manner (de Haan & Nelson, 1999), the Nc was also

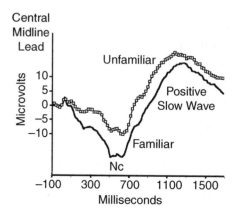

FIGURE 6.1. Graphical depiction of the pattern of ERP responses recorded from 4- and 6-month-olds to familiar and unfamiliar faces. Data from Webb, Long, and Nelson (2005).

greatest to the familiar object, but the distribution of responses differed slightly, with greater bilateral activation extending across posterior temporal electrodes. The authors concluded that the ERP differences reflected recognition of the familiar stimulus.

In addition, the authors demonstrated that the ERP to the familiar stimulus depended on the context in which the stimulus was viewed. Both the morphology and topography of infants' brain activity that differentiated a familiar stimulus from a novel stimulus depended on the degree of perceptual similarity between the stimuli. Specifically, the Nc was found to be larger (i.e., more negative) for the familiar face when the familiar and novel faces were dissimilar in appearance, but larger to the novel face when the two faces were similar in appearance. Likewise, the slow wave was found to differentiate familiar from unfamiliar faces both when the familiar face and the unfamiliar face were similar in appearance (de Haan & Nelson, 1997) and when they were dissimilar in appearance (Nelson et al., 2000). Such differences suggest that the degree of perceptual match between the two stimuli may alter the pattern of neural activation.

The relation between familiar and unfamiliar undergoes complex development over the first few years of life. In a longitudinal study of the response to familiar and unfamiliar faces, Webb, Long, and Nelson (2005) found that the Nc response as well as the slow wave shifted across the first year of life. For example, the Nc was greater to the familiar than unfamiliar face at 4 months but greater to the unfamiliar than familiar face at 12 months (Figure 6.2). Further reports suggest that the response shifts such that at 18–24 months, the Nc is greater to the familiar than unfamiliar, and

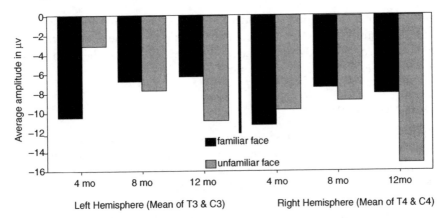

FIGURE 6.2. Mean amplitude of the Nc at 4, 8, and 12 months of age at right and left hemisphere sensors to familiar and unfamiliar faces. Data from Webb, Long, and Nelson (2005).

between 24 and 54 months the response is greater to the unfamiliar (Carver et al., 2003). Webb and colleagues note that behavioral preference (looking time) for the mother's face also shifts across the first year of life and may reflect the importance of attending to a familiar or a novel stimulus. As the Nc component is thought to reflect an obligatory attentional process, these results further highlight the possibility that this component may not be indexing memory per se.

In a reanalysis of data from Nelson's group, Snyder, Webb, and Nelson (2002) found that the Nc and slow wave dissociated cognitive processes associated with familiarity from processes associated with stimulus repetition: The Nc was modulated by familiarity alone. Individual differences in the number of trials an infant completed in an ERP session were observed to be associated with differences in the amplitude and latency of the Nc, possibly reflecting individual differences in both the magnitude and speed of stimulus processing. Furthermore, individual differences in the number of trials an infant completed also appeared to reflect differences in the extent to which the familiar and novel faces were encoded.

In addition, the slow wave component was modulated by repetition (Snyder et al., 2002). Specifically, the amplitude of the slow wave decreased with greater exposure to the stimulus. The slow wave component could be interpreted as a form of habituation to the stimulus. Whether this habituation reflects encoding per se or some other process is a matter of debate. Interestingly, however, the effect of repetition on the slow wave component did not appear to be influenced by the familiarity of the stimulus. Snyder (in press) has suggested two possible interpretations: The processes of encoding and recognition are independent (i.e., encoding does not cease once recognition occurs), or the effect of repetition on the slow wave component reflects the updating of the *specific* stimulus versus the updating of a more general representation of the familiar face.

Deferred Imitation

ERPs can also be used to assess memory status using the deferred imitation paradigm. Infants are exposed to the action sequences in the same manner as in the behavioral version of this task. The infant, after a "short" delay, is then shown pictures of the exposed imitation steps (familiar events) and imitation steps to which the infant was not exposed (unfamiliar events). After a delay, the infant is then tested, behaviorally, on the learned versus novel imitation events. Carver, Bauer, and Nelson (2000) found that ERP responses 1 week after exposure differed to the familiar as compared to the unfamiliar events, but only for those infants who recalled the imitation actions at 1 month after exposure. In order to better understand encoding and storage over the delay, another group of infants underwent ERP testing immediately after encoding and 1 week later (during storage); these infants were also tested behaviorally 1 month after the second ERP session. Bauer, Wiebe, Carver, Waters, and Nelson (2003) found that infants who were able to reproduce one or more of the familiar sequences and those who produced no ordered action pairs showed evidence of encoding at the first ERP session: The Nc was greater to the unfamiliar than familiar sequence pictures. At 1 week postencoding, during the second ERP session, infants who later recalled the action sequences demonstrated a faster NC response to the unfamiliar as compared to the familiar sequences. The authors interpreted these results to suggest that infants were able to encode the sequences but that performance after a 1-month delay was a function of memory storage. Thus, the Nc response 1 week after encoding predicted successful performance 1 month later.

Summary

Results from ERP experiments with young infants suggest that there are early neural differences in the response to familiarity, repetition, and novelty. The degree to which these are specific to *a* memory process versus reflecting general response properties is unknown. For example, the Nc is known to vary based on a priori familiarity (de Haan & Nelson, 1997, 1999; Snyder et al., 2002), frequency (Ackles & Cook, 1998; Courchesne et al., 1981; Karrer & Ackles, 1987a, 1988; Karrer & Monti, 1995; Nikkel

& Karrer, 1994), and repetition (Webb & Nelson, 2001). Although theoretical definitions would suggest that responses based on frequency and repetition should involve different neural systems than those based on familiarity (Nelson & Webb, 2003), it is unclear how modular these processes are. Further research examining the relation between ERP components and specific memory behaviors is needed.

OTHER INFLUENCES ON MEMORY

Task Specificity

Evidence from neuroimaging studies suggests that visual recognition memory may involve different neural processes depending on the type of stimulus involved in the memory task. For example, a number of studies with adults suggest that faces are perceived and represented by separate processes as compared to other types of objects. Using fMRI, it has been shown that areas within the posterior fusiform gyrus respond preferentially to faces (Clark et al., 1996; Kanwisher, McDermott, & Chun, 1997; Puce, Allison, Asgari, Gore, & McCarthy, 1996; Puce, Allison, Gore, & McCarthy, 1995) or to other stimuli that subjects have become experts at recognizing (e.g., Gauthier, Behrmann, & Tarr, 1999). In contrast, the lateral occipital complex (lateral bank of the fusiform gyrus) responds strongly to common objects (Grill-Spector, Kourtzi, & Kanwisher, 2001). In addition, the amygdala (e.g., Dubois et al., 1999) and temporofrontal cortex (e.g., Leveroni et al., 2000) have been found to be preferentially activated in processing of unknown faces in comparison to known faces.

The type of stimulus used in preference and recognition tasks also influences the circuitry of the memory system in infants. For example, by 4 months of age, infants begin to show a right-hemispheric advantage in learning to recognize new faces (Deruelle & de Schonen, 1991). De Haan and Nelson (1997, 1999) have also found that ERPs recorded from the right hemisphere differentiate an a priori familiar face (i.e., the mother's face) from an unfamiliar face (i.e., stranger's face); importantly, these responses are bilaterally distributed for objects. Behavioral memory paradigms using face stimuli also demonstrate novelty preferences over longer delays than those using object stimuli (Diamond, 1995; Fagan, 1972). This interaction between memory and stimulus type continues through the lifespan; dissociations have been found in paradigms that use familiar famous faces, unfamiliar faces, scrambled faces, words, nonwords, and objects with adult participants (e.g., Bentin & Moscovitch, 1988; see Nelson, 2001, for general discussion).

Developmental Disruptions

There are numerous conditions of early infancy that have known effects on memory or the MTL, such as iron deficiency, prematurity, hypoxic or ischemic events, epilepsy, and traumatic brain injury. Early tests of recognition memory and longitudinal studies of later memory abilities in special populations are important measures of the functioning of the recognition memory system and later impact on more complex behaviors. For example, Rose, Feldman, and Jankowski (2001) found that preterm infants compared to full-term infants had lower novelty scores, slower shift rates, more off-task behavior, and longer look durations—all suggestive of worse recognition memory. Visual recognition memory in the first year of life has also been found to be associated with cognitive abilities and IQ at 3 years of age in typical infants (Thompson, Fagan, & Fulker, 1991) and 6 years of age in typical and preterm infants (Rose, Feldman, & Wallace, 1992). Environmental factors also may impact later memory abilities. The cumulative quality of the early childrearing environment, particularly the family environment, is related to later attention and memory (National Institute of Child Health and Human Development, 2006).

Studies of patients with amnesia may be a less than optimal model for specifying the neuroanatomy underlying the development of recognition memory, but they provide important evidence for the role of plasticity in developing systems. Children with developmental amnesia show relatively spared item recognition (semantic memory) but impairments in delayed recall (Gadian et al., 2000; Isaacs et al., 2003), despite a 27–56% reduction in the volume of the hippocampus (Isaacs et al., 2003). In contrast, adult-onset amnesia cases show impairments in both semantic and episodic memory (Kitchener, Hodges, & McCarthy, 1998; Verfaellie, Koseff, & Alexander, 2000). In a further dissociation, individuals with isolated bilateral hippocampal damage have spared factual knowledge but disrupted event memory (Maguire & Cipolotti, 1998; Vargha-Khadem et al., 1997). These results highlight developmental compensatory mechanisms and further emphasize the likelihood of developmental transitions, both behaviorally and in terms of contributing neural systems, in memory.

CONCLUSIONS

Performance on tasks that have been defined as assessing recognition memory shows significant changes during the first years of life. In order to demonstrate "memory" for an item, the infant must first encode the stimulus, then store the stimulus in an accessible system, retrieve the item from storage, and finally, respond in a way that demonstrates memory. Given the limitations of the young child's behavioral and linguistic abilities, how recognition memories are demonstrated differs significantly from the tests used to define adult (mature) memory states. So, how do we characterize the memory abilities of preverbal children? Theoretically, the definitions are varied. Nelson (1994; Nelson & Webb, 2003) has defined pre-explicit memories as those that involve the hippocampus and are reflected in novelty preference. In contrast, Mandler (1988) suggests that early recall memory is defined by conceptual knowledge and reflects a comparative process between stimulus and representation. These two theories reflect very different conceptualizations of memory. Although they are not incompatible, they highlight different ways of defining the recognition memory system and have different implications for testing the development of recognition memory.

Reflecting on the specific tests that have been defined under the heading of recognition memory, there is significant evidence that novelty preferences in VPC experiments involve the MTL. However, the degree to which the hippocampus is critical to performance is unclear (see Table 6.1). Novelty preferences have been demonstrated in both early and late lesions of the hippocampus in nonhuman primate models. These neuroanatomical models suggest that the hippocampus is not necessary in order to demonstrate a novelty preference. This finding does not negate the possibility, however, that the hippocampus contributes to certain aspects of performance, such as performance over longer delays or contextual encoding. Furthermore, the hippocampal formation has been identified as playing a role in motivational behaviors (e.g., Tracy, Jarrard, & Davidson, 2001), spatial processing and memory (e.g., Iaria, Petrides, Dagher, Pike, & Bohbot, 2003; Maguire, Frackowiak, & Frith, 1996), relational memory (e.g., Astur & Constable, 2004; Davachi & Wagner, 2002; Eichenbaum & Cohen, 2001), episodic memory (e.g., Aggleton & Brown, 1999; Baddeley et al., 2001; O'Keefe & Nadel, 1978; Yonelinas et al., 2002), familiarity-based recognition memory and semantic memory (e.g., Squire & Zola-Morgan, 1991), and cross-modal associations (e.g., Alvarez & Squire, 1994; Rolls, 1996). Eichenbaum (2000) argues that the hippocampus is but one component of a larger memory system that interacts with cortical areas and, on its own, does not mediate any specific form of memory. It will be important to specifically define the processes that the hippocampus "controls" because these processes may form the structure for a number of different behaviors related to memory.

This review and others point to the complex dynamics of memory and memory development. The same regions may be involved in different circuitry, and different regions may interact to reflect common functions

(Bright & Kopelman, 2001). Memory is also dynamic; retrieval events trigger new encoding, and new encoding events may further engage the hippocampal system (Nadel & Bohbot, 2001). In addition, the use of memory tasks that involve reward, such as in the DNMS paradigm, may encourage or engage the development of alternate strategies (Nemanic et al., 2004). The behavioral responses on the VPC, DNMS, and deferred imitation tasks and the ERPs to frequency, familiarity, and novelty demonstrate the emergent capabilities of the infant memory system. Each of these measures has its own developmental trajectory and likely taps into different aspects of the system. One could argue that memory is the cornerstone of cognition and the foundation of development. The young infant, although limited in his or her behavioral repertoire, is surrounded with new items and events. How these events influence behavior has important implications for a lifetime of learning.

ACKNOWLEDGMENTS

The writing of this chapter was supported by Cure Autism Now. Additional support was provided by the National Institute of Mental Health Studies to Advance Autism Research and Treatment (No. U54 MH66399). I gratefully acknowledge Kelly Snyder for theoretical contributions and Donna Coch for contributions during the editing process.

REFERENCES

Ackles, P. K., & Cook, K. G. (1998). Stimulus probability and event-related potentials of the brain in 6-month-old human infants: A parametric study. *International Journal of Psychophysiology, 29*(2), 115–143.

Adlam A. L., Vargha-Khadem, F., Mishkin, M., & de Haan, M. (2005). Deferred imitation of action sequences in developmental amnesia. *Journal of Cognitive Neuroscience, 17*(2), 240–248.

Aggleton, J. P., & Brown, M. W. (1999). Episodic memory, amnesia and the hippocampal–anterior thalamic axis. *Behavioural and Brain Sciences, 22,* 425–498.

Alho, K., Sainio, K., Sajaniemi, N., Reinikainen, K., & Naatanen, R. (1990). Event-related brain potential of human newborns to pitch change of an acoustic stimulus. *Electroencephalography and Clinical Neurophysiology, 77*(2), 151–155.

Alvarado, M. C., & Bachevalier, J. (2000). Revisiting the development of medial temporal lobe memory functions in primates. *Learning and Memory, 7,* 244–256.

Alvarado, M. C., & Bachevalier J. (2005). Selective neurotoxic damage to the hippocampal formation impairs performance of the transverse patterning and location memory tasks in rhesus macaques. *Hippocampus, 15*(1), 118–131.

Alvarado, M. C., Wright, A. A., & Bachevalier J. (2002). Object and spatial relational memory in adult rhesus monkeys is impaired by neonatal lesions of the hippocampal formation but not the amygdaloid complex. *Hippocampus, 12*(4), 421–33.

Alvarez, P., & Squire, L. R. (1994). Memory consolidation and the medial temporal lobe: A simple network model. *Proceedings of the National Academy of Sciences, 91*(15), 7041–7045.

Astur, R. S., & Constable, R. T. (2004). Hippocampal dampening during a relational memory task. *Behavioral Neuroscience, 8*(4), 667–675.

Atkinson, R. C., & Shiffrin, R. M. (1968). Human memory: A proposed system and its control processes. In K. W. Spence & J. T. Spence (Eds.), *The psychology of learning and motivation* (pp. 89–195). New York: Academic Press.

Bachevalier, J. (1990). Ontogenetic development of habit and memory formation in primates. *Annals of the New York Academy of Sciences, 608,* 457–484.

Bachevalier, J., Beauregard, M., & Alvarado, M. C. (1999). Long-term effects of neonatal damage to the hippocampal formation and amygdaloid complex on object discrimination and object recognition in rhesus monkeys (*Macaca mulatta*). *Behavioral Neuroscience, 113*(6), 1127–1151.

Bachevalier, J., Brickson, M., & Hagger, C. (1993). Limbic-dependent recognition memory in monkeys develops early in infancy. *NeuroReport, 4*(1), 77–80.

Bachevalier, J., & Mishkin, M. (1992). Ontogenetic development and decline of memory functions in nonhuman primates. In I. Kostovic & S. Knezevic (Eds.), *Neurodevelopment, aging and cognition* (pp. 37–59). Cambridge, MA: Birkhauser.

Bachevalier, J., & Mishkin, M. (1994). Effects of selective neonatal temporal lobe lesions on visual recognition memory in rhesus monkeys. *Journal of Neuroscience, 14*(4), 2128–2139.

Bachevalier, J., & Vargha-Khadem, F. (2005). The primate hippocampus, ontogeny, early insult and memory. *Current Opinion in Neurobiology, 15*(2), 168–174.

Baddeley, A., Vargha-Khadem, F., & Mishkin, M. (2001). Preserved recognition in a case of developmental amnesia: Implications for the acquisition of semantic memory? *Journal of Cognitive Neuroscience, 13*(3), 357–369.

Bahrick, L. E., & Pickens, J. N. (1995). Infant memory for object motion across a period of three months: Implications for a four-phase attention function. *Journal of Experimental Child Psychology, 59*(3), 343–371.

Barnat, S. B., Klein, P. J., & Meltzoff, A. N. (1996). Deferred imitation across changes in context and object, memory and generalization in 14-month-old infants. *Infant Behavior and Development, 19,* 241–251.

Bauer, P. (2002). Long-term recall memory: Behavioral and neuro-developmental changes in the first 2 years of life. *Current Directions in Psychological Science, 11,* 137.

Bauer, P. J. (2005). Developments in declarative memory. *Psychological Science, 16*(1), 41–47.

Bauer, P. J., & Hertsgaard, L. A. (1993). Increasing steps in recall of events, factors facilitating immediate and long-term memory in 13.5- and 16.5-month-old children. *Child Development, 64*(4), 1204–1223.

Bauer, P. J., & Mandler, J. (1992). Putting the horse before the cart: The use of temporal order in recall of events by one year old children. *Developmental Psychology, 28,* 441–452.

Bauer, P. J., Wenner, J. A., Dropik, P. L., & Wewerka, S. S. (2000). Parameters of remembering and forgetting in the transition from infancy to early childhood. *Monographs of the Society for Research in Child Development, 65*(4), i–vi, 1–204.

Bauer, P. J., Wenner, J., & Kroupina, M. (2002). Making the past present: Later verbal accessibility of early memories. *Journal of Cognition and Development, 3*(1), 21–47.

Bauer, P. J., Wiebe, S., Carver, L., Lukowski, A., Haight, J., Waters, J., et al. (2006). Electrophysiological indexes of encoding and behavioral indexes of recall: Examining relations and developmental change late in the first life. *Developmental Neuropsychology, 29,* 293–320.

Bauer, P. J., Wiebe, S. A., Carver, L. J., Waters, J. M., & Nelson, C. A. (2003). Developments in long-term explicit memory late in the first year of life: Behavioral and electrophysiological indices. *Psychological Science, 14*(6), 629–635.

Bentin, S., & Moscovitch, M. (1988). The time course of repetition effects for words and unfamiliar faces. *Journal of Experimental Psychology: General, 117*(2), 148–160.

Bering, J. M. (2004). A critical review of the "enculturation hypothesis": The effects of human rearing on great ape social cognition. *Animal Cognition, 7*(4), 201–212.

Bjorklund, D. F., Bering, J. M., & Ragan, P. (2000). A two-year longitudinal study of deferred imitation of object manipulation in a juvenile chimpanzee (*Pan troglodytes*) and orangutan (*Pongo pygmaeus*). *Developmental Psychobiology, 37*(4), 229–237.

Bjorklund, D. F., Yunger, J. L., Bering, J. M., & Ragan, P. (2002). The generalization of deferred imitation in enculturated chimpanzees (*Pan troglodytes*). *Animal Cognition, 5*(1), 49–58.

Bright, P., & Kopelman, M. D. (2001). Learning and memory: Recent findings. *Current Opinion in Neurology, 14*(4), 449–455.

Brown, M. W., Wilson, F. A., & Riches, I. P. (1987). Neuronal evidence that inferomedial temporal cortex is more important than hippocampus in certain processes underlying recognition memory. *Brain Research, 409,* 158–162.

Buccino, G., Binkofski, F., & Riggio, L. (2004). The mirror neuron system and action recognition. *Brain and Language, 89*(2), 370–376.

Buffalo, E. A., Ramus, S. J., Clark, R. E., Teng, E., Squire, L. R., & Zola, S. M. (1999). Dissociation between the effects of damage to perirhinal cortex and area TE. *Learning and Memory, 6*(6), 572–599.

Buffalo, E. A., Ramus, S. J., Squire, L. R., & Zola, S. M. (2000). Perception and recognition memory in monkeys following lesions of area TE and perirhinal cortex. *Learning and Memory, 7*(6), 375–382.

Carver, L. J., & Bauer, P. J. (2001). The dawning of a past: The emergence of long-term explicit memory in infancy. *Journal of Experimental Psychology: General, 130*(4), 726–745.

Carver, L. J., Bauer, P. J., & Nelson, C. A. (2000). Associations between infant brain activity and recall memory. *Developmental Science, 3,* 234–246.

Carver, L. J., Dawson, G., Panagiotides, H., Meltzoff, A. N., McPartland, J., Gray, J., et al. (2003). Age-related differences in neural correlates of face recognition during the toddler and preschool years. *Developmental Psychobiology, 42*(2), 148–159.

Chaminade, T., Meltzoff, A. N., & Decety, J. (2005). An fMRI study of imitation, action representation and body schema. *Neuropsychologia, 43*(1), 115–127.

Cheour, M., Ceponiene, R., Leppanen, P., Alho, K., Kujala, T., Renlund, M., et al. (2002). The auditory sensory memory trace decays rapidly in newborns. *Scandinavian Journal of Psychology, 43,* 33–39.

Clark, V. P., Keil, K., Maisog, J. M., Courtney, S., Ungerleider, L. G., & Haxby, J. V. (1996). Functional magnetic resonance imaging of human visual cortex during face matching: A comparison with positron emission tomography. *NeuroImage, 4*(1), 1–15.

Cohen, L., & Gelber, E. R. (1975). Infant visual memory. In L. Cohen & Salapatek (Eds.), *Infant perception: From sensation to cognition* (Vol. 1, pp. 347–403). New York: Academic Press.

Cohen, N. J., & Eichenbaum, H. (1991). The theory that wouldn't die: A critical look at the spatial mapping theory of hippocampal function. *Hippocampus, 1*(3), 265–268.

Cohen, N. J., & Squire, L. R. (1980). Preserved learning and retention of pattern-analyzing skill in amnesia: Dissociation of knowing how and knowing that. *Science, 210,* 207–210.

Collie, R., & Hayne, H. (1999). Deferred imitation by 6- and 9-month-old infants: More evidence for declarative memory. *Developmental Psychobiology, 35*(2), 83–90.

Courage, M. L., & Howe, M. L. (1998). The ebb and flow of infant attentional preferences: Evidence for long-term recognition memory in 3-month-olds. *Journal of Experimental Child Psychology, 70*(1), 26–53.

Courchesne, E., Ganz, L., & Norcia, A. (1981). Event-related potentials to human faces in infants. *Child Development, 52,* 104–109.

Davachi, L., & Wagner, A. D. (2002). Hippocampal contributions to episodic encoding: Insights from relational and item-based learning. *Journal of Neurophysiology, 88*(2), 982–990.

Dawson, G., Meltzoff, A. N., Osterling, J., & Rinaldi, J. (1998). Neuropsychological correlates of early symptoms of autism. *Child Development, 69*(5), 1276–1285.

deBoer, T., Scott, L., & Nelson, C. A. (2005). Event-related potentials in developmental populations. In T. C. Handy (Ed.), *Event-related potentials: A methods handbook* (pp. 263–298). Cambridge, MA: MIT Press.

de Haan, M., & Nelson, C. (1997). Recognition of the mother's face by six-month-old infants: A neurobehavioral study. *Child Development, 68,* 187–210.

de Haan, M., & Nelson, C. (1999). Brain activity differentiates faces and object processing in 6- month old infants. *Developmental Psychology, 35,* 1113–1121.

deRegnier, R. A., Nelson, C. A., Thomas, K. M., Wewerka, S., & Georgieff, M. K. (2000). Neurophysiologic evaluation of auditory recognition memory in healthy newborn infants and infants of diabetic mothers. *Journal of Pediatrics, 137*(6), 777–784.

deRegnier, R. A., Wewerka, S., Georgieff, M. K., Mattia, F., & Nelson, C. A. (2002). Influences of postconceptional age and postnatal experience on the development of auditory recognition memory in the newborn infant. *Developmental Psychobiology, 41*(3), 216–225.

Deruelle, C., & de Schonen, S. (1991). Hemispheric asymmetries in visual pattern processing in infancy. *Brain and Cognition, 16*(2), 151–179.

Desimone, R. (1996). Neural mechanisms for visual memory and their role in attention. *Proceedings of the National Academy of Sciences USA, 93,* 13494–13499.

Diamond, A. (1990). Rate of maturation of the hippocampus and the developmental progression of children's performance on the delayed non-matching to sample and visual paired comparison tasks. *Annals of the New York Academy of Sciences, 608,* 394–433.

Diamond, A. (1995). Evidence of robust recognition memory early in life even when assessed by reaching behavior. *Journal of Experimental Child Psychology, 59*(3), 419–456.

Dolan, R. J., & Fletcher, P. C. (1997). Dissociating prefrontal and hippocampal function in episodic memory encoding. *Nature, 388,* 582–585.

Dubois, S., Rossion, B., Schiltz, C., Bodart, J. M., Michel, C., Bruyer, R., et al. (1999). Effect of familiarity on the processing of human faces. *NeuroImage, 9*(3), 278–289.

Ebbinghaus, H. (1885). *Memory: A contribution to experimental psychology.* New York: Teachers College.

Eichenbaum, H. (2000). A cortical-hippocampal system for declarative memory. *Nature Reviews Neuroscience, 1,* 41.

Eichenbaum, H., & Cohen, N. J. (2001). *From conditioning to conscious recollection: Memory systems of the brain.* New York: Oxford University Press.

Eichenbaum, H., Dudchenko, P., Wood, E., Shapiro, M., & Tanila, H. (1999). The hippocampus, memory, and place cells: Is it spatial memory or a memory space? *Neuron, 23*(2), 209–226.

Eichenbaum, H., Mathews, P., & Cohen, N. J. (1989). Further studies of hippocampal representation during odor discrimination learning. *Behavioral Neuroscience, 103*(6), 1207–1216.

Eichenbaum, H., Schoenbaum, G., Young, B., & Bunsey, M. (1996). Functional organization of the hippocampal memory system. *Proceedings of the National Academy of Sciences USA, 93,* 13500–13507.

Fagan, J. F. (1972). Infants' recognition memory for faces. *Journal of Experimental Child Psychology, 14*(3), 453–476.

Fahy, F. L., Riches, I. P., & Brown, M. W. (1993a). Neuronal signals of importance to the performance of visual recognition memory tasks: Evidence from recordings of single neurones in the medial thalamus of primates. *Progress in Brain Research*, *95*, 401–416.

Fahy, F. L., Riches, I. P., & Brown, M. W. (1993b). Neuronal activity related to visual recognition memory: Long-term memory and the encoding of recency and familiarity information in the primate anterior and medial inferior temporal and rhinal cortex. *Experimental Brain Research*, *96*(3), 457–472.

Gadian, D. G., Aicardi, J., Watkins, K. E., Porter, D. A., Mishkin, M., & Vargha-Khadem, F. (2000). Developmental amnesia associated with early hypoxic-ischaemic injury. *Brain*, *123*(3), 499–507.

Gauthier, I., Behrmann, M., & Tarr, M. J. (1999). Can face recognition really be dissociated from object recognition? *Journal of Cognitive Neuroscience*, *11*(4), 349–370.

Griffiths, D., Dickinson, A., & Clayton, N. (1999). Episodic memory: What can animals remember about their past? *Trends in Cognitive Science*, *3*(2), 74–80.

Grill-Spector, K., Kourtzi, Z., & Kanwisher, N. (2001). The lateral occipital complex and its role in object recognition. *Vision Research*, *41*(10–11), 1409–1422.

Haaf, R. A., Lundy, B. L., & Codren, J. T. (1996). Attention, recognition, and the effects of stimulus context in 6-month old infants. *Infant Behavior and Development*, *19*, 93–106.

Hayne, H., Boniface, J., & Barr, R. (2000). The development of declarative memory in human infants: Age-related changes in deferred imitation. *Behavioral Neuroscience*, *114*(1), 77–83.

Hayne, H., & Richmond, J. (2002, April). *Novelty detection: A measure of explicit memory?* Paper presented at the International Conference of Infant Studies, Toronto, Ontario, Canada.

Howe, M. L., & Courage, M. L. (1997). Independent paths in the development of infant learning and forgetting. *Journal of Experimental Child Psychology*, *67*(2), 131–163.

Howe, M. L., & O'Sullivan, J. T. (1997). What children's memories tell us about recalling our childhoods: A review of storage and retrieval processes in the development of long-term retention. *Developmental Review*, *7*(2), 148–204.

Iacoboni, M., Koski, L., Brass, M., Bekkering, H., Woods, R., Dubeau, M. C., et al. (2001). Re-afferent copies of imitated actions in the right superior temporal cortex. *Proceedings of the National Academy of Sciences*, *98*, 13995–13999.

Iacoboni, M., Woods, R., Brass, M., Bekkering, H., Mazziotta, J. C., & Rizzolatti, G. (1999). Cortical mechanisms of human imitation. *Science*, *286*, 2526–2528.

Iaria, G., Petrides, M., Dagher, A., Pike, B., & Bohbot, V. D. (2003). Cognitive strategies dependent on the hippocampus and caudate nucleus in human navigation: Variability and change with practice. *Journal of Neuroscience*, *23*(13), 5945–5952.

Isaacs, E., Vargha-Khadem, F., Watkins, K., Lucas, A., Mishkin, M., & Gadian, D. (2003). Developmental amnesia and its relationship to degree of hippocampal atrophy. *Proceedings of the National Academy of Sciences, 100,* 13060–13063.

Kanwisher, N., McDermott, J., & Chun, M. (1997). The fusiform face area: A module in human extrastriate cortex specialized for the perception of faces. *Journal of Neuroscience, 17,* 4302–4311.

Karrer, R., & Ackles, P. (1987a). Visual event-related potentials of infants during a modified oddball procedure. *Electroencephalography and Clinical Neurophysiology, 40*(Suppl.), 603–608.

Karrer, R., & Ackles, P. (1987b). Visual event-related potentials of infants during a modified oddball procedure. In R. Johnson, J. Rohrbaugh, & R. Parasuraman (Eds.), *Current trends in event related potential research* (pp. 603–608). Amsterdam: Elsevier.

Karrer, R., & Ackles, P. (1988). Brain organization and perceptual cognitive development in normal and Down syndrome infants: A research program. In P. Vietze & H. G. Vaughan, Jr. (Eds.), *The early identification of infants with developmental disabilities* (pp. 210–234). Philadelphia: Grune & Stratton.

Karrer, R., & Monti, L. A. (1995). Event-related potentials of 4-7-week-old infants in a visual recognition memory task. *Electroencephalography and Clinical Neurophysiology, 94*(6), 414–424.

Killiany, R., & Mahut, H. (1990). Hippocampectomy in infant monkeys facilitates object–reward association learning but not for conditional object–object associations. *Society for Neuroscience Abstracts, 16,* 847.

Kitchener, E. G., Hodges, J. R., & McCarthy, R. (1998). Acquisition of post-morbid vocabulary and semantic facts in the absence of episodic memory. *Brain, 121,* 1313–1327.

Koski, L., Wohlschläger, A., Bekkering, H., Woods, R. P., Dubeau, M. C., Mazziotta, J. C., et al. (2002). Modulation of motor and premotor activity during imitation of target-directed actions. *Cerebral Cortex, 12,* 847–855.

Kowalska, D. M., Bachevalier, J., & Mishkin, M. (1991). The role of the inferior prefrontal convexity in performance of delayed nonmatching-to-sample. *Neuropsychologia, 29,* 583–600.

Learmonth, A. E., Lamberth, R., & Rovee-Collier, C. (2004). Generalization of deferred imitation during the first year of life. *Journal of Experimental Child Psychology, 88*(4), 297–318.

Leveroni, C. L., Seidenberg, M., Mayer, A. R., Mead, L. A., Binder, J. R., & Rao, S. M. (2000). Neural systems underlying the recognition of familiar and newly learned faces. *Journal of Neuroscience, 20*(2), 878–886.

Liston, C., & Kagan, J. (2002). Brain development: Memory enhancement in early childhood. *Nature, 419,* 896.

Maguire, E. A., & Cipolotti, L. (1998). Selective sparing of topographical memory. *Journal of Neurology, Neurosurgery and Psychiatry, 65*(6), 903–909.

Maguire, E. A., Frackowiak, R. S., & Frith, C. D. (1996). Learning to find your way: A role for the human hippocampal formation. *Proceedings Biological Sciences, 263,* 1745–1750.

Malkova, L., Bachevalier, J., Webster, M., & Mishkin, M. (2000). Effects of neonatal inferior prefrontal and medial temporal lesions on learning the rule for delayed nonmatching-to-sample. *Developmental Neuropsychology, 18*(3), 399–421.

Malkova, L., Mishkin, M., & Bachevalier, J. (1995). Long-term effects of selective neonatal temporal lobe lesions on learning and memory in monkeys. *Behavioral Neuroscience, 109*(2), 212–226.

Mandler, J. M. (1988). How to build a baby: On the development of an accessible representational system. *Cognitive Development, 3*(2), 113–136.

Mandler, J. M. (1990). Recall of events by preverbal children. *Annals of the New York Academy of Sciences, 608,* 485–516.

Mandler, J. M. (1992). How to build a baby: II. Conceptual primitives. *Psychological Review, 99*(4), 587–604.

Mandler, J. (2000). Perceptual and conceptual processes in infancy. *Journal of Cognition and Development, 1,* 3–36.

Manns, J. R., Stark, C. E., & Squire, L. R. (2000). The visual paired-comparison task as a measure of declarative memory. *Proceedings of the National Academy of Sciences USA, 97,* 12375–12379.

McClelland, J., & Rumelhart, D. E. (1985). Distributed memory and the representation of general and specific information. *Journal of Experimental Psychology: General, 114*(2), 159–188.

McDonough, L., Mandler, J. M., McKee, R. D., & Squire, L. R. (1995). The deferred imitation task as a nonverbal measure of declarative memory. *Proceedings of the National Academy of Sciences, 92*(16), 7580–7584.

McKee, R. D., & Squire, L. R. (1993). On the development of declarative memory. *Journal of Experimental Psychology: Learning, Memory, and Cognition, 19*(2), 397–404.

Meltzoff, A. N. (1988). Infant imitation and memory: Nine month olds in immediate and deferred tests. *Child Development, 59,* 217–225.

Meltzoff, A. N. (1990). Towards a developmental cognitive science: The implications of cross-modal matching and imitation for the development of representation and memory in infancy. *Annals of the New York Academy of Sciences, 608,* 1–37.

Meltzoff, A. N., & Moore, C. (1999). A new foundation for cognitive development: The birth of the representational infant. In E. K. Scholnick (Ed.), *Conceptual development: Piaget's legacy. The Jean Piaget Symposium Series.* Mahwah, NJ: Erlbaum.

Mishkin, M. (1978). Memory in monkeys severely impaired by combined but not by separate removal of amygdala and hippocampus. *Nature, 273,* 297–298.

Mishkin, M., & Appenzeller, T. (1987). The anatomy of memory. *Scientific American, 256*(6), 80–89.

Molnar-Szakacs, I., Iacoboni, M., Koski, L., & Mazziotta, J. C. (2005). Functional segregation within pars opercularis of the inferior frontal gyrus: Evidence from fMRI studies of imitation and action observation. *Cerebral Cortex, 15*(7), 986–994.

Muhlau, M., Hermsdorfer, J., Goldenberg, G., Wohlschlager, A. M., Castrop, F., Stahl, R., et al. (2005). Left inferior parietal dominance in gesture imitation: An fMRI study. *Neuropsychologia, 43*(7), 1086–1098.

Näätänen, R. (1999). Phoneme representations of the human brain as reflected by event-related potentials. *Electroencephalography and Clinical Neurophysiology, 49*(Suppl.), 170–173.

Näätänen, R. (2000). Mismatch negativity (MMN): Perspectives for application. *International Journal of Psychophysiology, 37*, 3–10.

Näätänen, R., Jacobsen, T., & Winkler, I. (2005). Memory-based or afferent processes in mismatch negativity (MMN): A review of the evidence. *Psychophysiology, 42*, 25–32.

Nadel, L. (1994). Multiple memory systems: What and why, an update. In D. L. Schacter & E. Tulving (Eds.), *Memory systems* (pp. 39–63). Cambridge, MA: MIT Press.

Nadel, L., & Bohbot, V. (2001). Consolidation of memory. *Hippocampus, 11*(1), 56–60.

Nadel, L., & O'Keefe, J. (1974). The hippocampus in pieces and patches: An essay on the modes of explanation in physiological psychology. In R. Bellairs & E. G. Gray (Eds.), *Essays on the nervous system: A festchrift for Professor JZ Young*. Oxford, UK: Clarendon Press.

National Institute of Child Health and Human Development. (2006). *The NICHD Study of Early Child Care and Youth Development: Findings for children up to age 4 1/2 years*. (NIH Pub. No 05-4318). Washington, DC: U.S. Government Printing Office.

Nelson, C. A. (1996). Electrophysiological correlates of early memory development. In H. W. Reese & M. D. Franzen (Eds.), *Thirteenth West Virginia University conference on life span developmental psychology: Biological and neuropsychological mechanisms* (pp. 95–131). NJ: Erlbaum.

Nelson, C. A. (2001). The development and neural bases of face recognition. *Infant and Child Development, 10*, 3–18.

Nelson, C. A., & Collins P. (1991). An event-related potential and looking time analysis of infants' response to familiar and novel events: Implications for visual recognition memory. *Developmental Psychology, 27*, 50–58.

Nelson, C. A., & Collins, P. (1992). Neural and behavioral correlates of recognition memory in 4 and 8 month old infants. *Brain and Cognition, 19*, 105–121.

Nelson, C. A., & deRegnier, R. A. (1992). Neural correlates of attention and memory in the first year of life. *Developmental Neuropsychology, 8*(2–3), 119–134.

Nelson, C. A., & Salapatek, P. (1986). Electrophysiological correlates of infant recognition memory. *Child Development, 57*, 1483–1497.

Nelson, C. A., & Webb, S. J. (2003). A cognitive neuroscience perspective on early memory development. In M. Johnson & M. de Haan (Eds.), *The cognitive neuroscience of development: Studies in developmental psychology* (pp. 99–119). New York: Psychology Press.

Nelson, C. A., Wewerka, S., Thomas, K., Tribby-Walbridge, S., deRegnier, R., & Georgieff, M. (2000). Neurocognitive sequelae of infants of diabetic mothers. *Behavioral Neuroscience, 114*, 950–956.

Nemanic, S., Alvarado, M. C., & Bachevalier, J. (2004). The hippocampal/parahippocampal regions and recognition memory: Insights from visual paired comparison versus object-delayed nonmatching in monkeys. *Journal of Neuroscience, 24*(8), 2013–2026.

Nikkel, L., & Karrer, R. (1994). Differential effects of experience on the ERP and behavior of 6-month olds infants: trends during repeated stimulus presentations. *Developmental Neuropsychology, 10*, 1–11.

O'Keefe, J., & Nadel, L. (1978). *The hippocampus as a cognitive map.* Oxford, UK: Clarendon Press.

Overman, W. H. (1990). Performance on traditional matching to sample, non-matching to sample, and object discrimination tasks by 12- to 32-month-old children. A developmental progression. *Annals of the New York Academy of Sciences, 608*, 365–393.

Overman, W. H., Bachevalier, J., Turner, M., & Peuster, A. (1992). Object recognition versus object discrimination: Comparison between human infants and infant monkeys. *Behavioral Neuroscience, 106*(1), 15–29.

Parker, A., Eacott, M. J., & Gaffan, D. (1997). The recognition memory deficit caused by mediodorsal thalamic lesion in non-human primates: A comparison with rhinal cortex lesion. *European Journal of Neuroscience, 9*(11), 2423–2431.

Parker, S. T. (1996). Using cladistic analysis of comparative data to reconstruct the evolution of cognitive development in humans. In E. P. Martins (Ed.), *Phylogenies and the comparative method in animal behavior.* New York: Oxford University Press.

Pascalis, O., & Bachevalier, J. (1999). Neonatal aspiration lesions of the hippocampal formation impair visual recognition memory when assessed by paired-comparison task but not by delayed nonmatching-to-sample task. *Hippocampus, 9*(6), 609–616.

Pascalis, O., de Haan, M., Nelson, C. A., & de Schonen, S. (1998). Long-term recognition memory for faces assessed by visual paired comparison in 3- and 6-month-old infants. *Journal of Experimental Psychology: Learning, Memory, and Cognition, 24*(1), 249–260.

Pascalis, O., & de Schonen, S. (1994). Recognition memory in 3- to 4-day-old human neonates. *NeuroReport, 5*(14), 1721–1724.

Pascalis, O., de Schonen, S., Morton, J., & Deruelle, C. (1995). Mother's face recognition by neonates: A replication and extension. *Infant Behavior and Development, 18*, 79–95.

Piaget, J. (1952). *The origins of intelligence in children.* New York: International Universities Press.

Puce, A., Allison, T., Asgari, M., Gore, J. C., & McCarthy, G. (1996). Differential sensitivity of human visual cortex to faces, letter strings, and textures: A functional magnetic resonance imaging study. *Journal of Neuroscience, 16*(16), 5205–5215.

Puce, A., Allison, T., Gore, J. C., & McCarthy, G. (1995). Face-sensitive regions in human extrastriate cortex studied by functional MRI. *Journal of Neurophysiology, 74*(3), 1192–1199.

Purhonen, M., Kilpelainen-Lees, R., Valkonen-Korhonen, M., Karhu, J., & Lehtonen, J. (2004). Cerebral processing of mother's voice compared to unfamiliar voice in 4-month-old infants. *International Journal of Psychophysiology, 52*(3), 257–266.

Reed, J. M., & Squire, L. R. (1999). Impaired transverse patterning in human amnesia is a special case of impaired memory for two-choice discrimination tasks. *Behavioral Neuroscience, 113*(1), 3–9.

Resende, M., Chalan-Fourney, J., & Bachevalier, J. (2002). Neonatal neurotoxic lesions of the hippocampal formation do not impair recognition memory in infant macaques. *Society for Neuroscience Abstracts, 28*, 1832.

Richmond, J., Sowerby, P., Colombo, M., & Hayne, H. (2004). The effect of familiarization time, retention interval, and context change on adults' performance in the visual paired-comparison task. *Developmental Psychobiology, 44*(2), 146–155.

Rickard, T. C., & Grafman J. (1998). Losing their configural mind: Amnesic patients fail on transverse patterning. *Journal of Cognitive Neuroscience, 10*(4), 509–524.

Robinson, A. J., & Pascalis, O. (2004). Development of flexible visual recognition memory in human infants. *Developmental Science, 7*(5), 527–533.

Rolls, E. T. (1996). The orbitofrontal cortex. *Philosophical Transactions of the Royal Society of London B: Biological Sciences, 351*, 1433–1444.

Rolls, E. T., Cahusac, P. M., Feigenbaum, J. D., & Miyashita, Y. (1993). Responses of single neurons in the hippocampus of the macaque related to recognition memory. *Experimental Brain Research, 93*(2), 299–306.

Rose, S. A. (1983). Differential rates of visual information processing in full-term and preterm infants. *Child Development, 54*(5), 1189–1198.

Rose, S. A., Feldman, J. F., & Jankowski, J. J. (2001). Visual short-term memory in the first year of life: Capacity and recency effects. *Developmental Psychology, 37*(4), 539–549.

Rose, S. A., Feldman, J. F., & Wallace, I. F. (1992). Infant information processing in relation to six-year cognitive outcomes. *Child Development, 63*(5), 1126–1141.

Rovee-Collier, C. (1997). Dissociations in infant memory: Rethinking the development of implicit and explicit memory. *Psychological Review, 104*(3), 467–498.

Rovee-Collier, C. (2001). Information pick-up by infants: What is it, and how can we tell? *Journal of Experimental Child Psychology, 78*(1), 35–106.

Rudy, J. W., Keith, J. R., & Georgen, K. (1993). The effect of age on children's learning of problems that require a configural association solution. *Developmental Psychobiology, 26*(3), 171–184.

Schacter, D. L. (1987). Implicit expressions of memory in organic amnesia: Learning of new facts and associations. *Human Neurobiology, 6*(2), 107–118.

Schacter, D. L. (1992). Understanding implicit memory: A cognitive neuroscience approach. *American Psychologist, 47*(4), 559–569.

Schacter, D. L. (1994). Implicit knowledge: New perspectives on unconscious processes. *International Review of Neurobiology, 37*, 271–288.

Schacter, D. L., & Tulving, E. (1994). *Memory systems.* London: MIT Press.

Serres, L. (2001). Morphological changes of the human hippocampal formation from midgestation to early childhood. In C. A. Nelson & M. Luciana (Eds.), *Handbook of developmental cognitive neuroscience* (pp. 45–58). Cambridge, MA: MIT Press.

Snyder, K.A. (2003). *Neural mechanisms underlying novelty preferences.* Unpublished doctoral dissertation, University of Minnesota.

Snyder, K. A. (in press). Neural mechanisms underlying memory and attention in preferential-looking tasks. In L. M. Oakes & P. J. Bauer (Eds.), *Short- and long-term memory in infancy and early childhood: Taking the first steps toward remembering.* Oxford, UK: Oxford University Press.

Snyder, K. A., Blank, M. P., Cheek, D., Kuefner, D., & Marsolek, C. (2004, April). *Converging evidence for a dissociation between preferential-looking in the visual paired-comparison task and recognition memory.* Poster presented at the annual meeting of the Cognitive Neuroscience Society, San Francisco.

Snyder, K. A., & Kuefner, D. (2005, April). *Infant ERPs during encoding predict performance on the visual paired-comparison task.* Poster presented at the annual meeting of the Cognitive Neuroscience Society, New York.

Snyder, K. A., Kuefner, D., Schunk, E., Blank, M., Cheek, D., & Marsolek, C. (2004, June). Rethinking the relation between preferential-looking in the visual paired-comparison task and recognition memory. *Proceedings of the International Society for Infant Studies,* Chicago.

Snyder, K. A., Webb, S. J. & Nelson, C. A. (2002). Theoretical and methodological implications of variability in infant brain response during a recognition memory paradigm. *Infant Behavior and Development, 25*(4), 466–494.

Squire, L. R. (1987). The organization and neural substrates of human memory. *International Journal of Neurology, 21–22,* 218–222.

Squire, L. R. (1994). Declarative and nondeclarative memory: Multiple brain systems supporting learning and memory. In D. L. Schacter & E. Tulving (Eds.), *Memory systems* (pp. 203–231). London: MIT Press.

Squire, L. R., Knowlton, B., & Musen, G. (1993). The structure and organization of memory. *Annual Review of Psychology, 44,* 453–495.

Squire, L. R., & Zola-Morgan, S. (1991). The medial temporal lobe memory system. *Science, 253,* 1380–1386.

Suzuki, W. A., & Clayton, N. S. (2000). The hippocampus and memory: A comparative and ethological perspective. *Current Opinion in Neurobiology, 10*(6), 768–773.

Thompson, L. A., Fagan, J. F., & Fulker, D. W. (1991). Longitudinal prediction of specific cognitive abilities from infant novelty reference. *Child Development, 62*(3), 530–538.

Tomasello, M., Savage-Rumbaugh, S., & Kruger, A. C. (1993). Imitative learning of actions on objects by children, chimpanzees, and enculturated chimpanzees. *Child Development, 64*(6), 1688–1705.

Tracy, A. L., Jarrard, L. E., & Davidson, T. L. (2001). The hippocampus and motivation revisited: Appetite and activity. *Behavioral Brain Research, 127*(1–2), 13–23.

Tulving, E. (1985). Memory and consciousness. *Canadian Psychology, 26,* 1–12.

Tulving, E., & Markowitsch, H. J. (1997). Memory beyond the hippocampus. *Current Opinion in Neurobiology, 7*(2), 209–216.

Tulving, E., Markowitsch, H. J., Kapur, S., Habib, R., & Houle, S. (1994). Novelty encoding networks in the human brain: Positron emission tomography data. *NeuroReport, 5,* 2525–2528.

Tulving, E., & Schacter, D. (1990). Priming and human memory systems. *Science, 247,* 301–305.

Vargha-Khadem, F., Gadian, D. G., Watkins, K. E., Connelly, A., Van Paesschen, W., & Mishkin, M. (1997). Differential effects of early hippocampal pathology on episodic and semantic memory. *Science, 277,* 376–380. Erratum in *277,* 1117.

Verfaellie, M., Koseff, P., & Alexander, M. P. (2000). Acquisition of novel semantic information in amnesia: Effects of lesion localization. *Neuropsychologia, 38,* 484–492.

Webb, S. J., Long, J. D., & Nelson, C. A. (2005). The longitudinal development of visual event-related potentials across the first year of life. *Developmental Science, 8,* 605–616.

Webb, S. J., & Nelson, C. A. (2001). Perceptual priming for upright and inverted faces in infants and adults. *Journal of Experimental Child Psychology, 79,* 1–22.

Webster, M. J., Bachevalier, J., & Ungerleider, L. G. (1995). Transient subcortical connections of inferior temporal areas TE and TEO in infant macaque monkeys. *Journal of Comparative Neurology, 352,* 213–226.

Webster, M. J., Ungerleider, L. G., & Bachevalier, J. (1991). Connections of inferior temporal areas TE and TEO with medial temporal-lobe structures in infant and adult monkeys. *Journal of Neuroscience, 11*(4), 1095–1116.

Weinstein, J., Saunders, R., & Mishkin, M. (1988). Temporo-prefrontal interactions in rule learning by macaques. *Society for Neuroscience Abstracts, 14,* 1230.

Williams, G. V., Rolls, E. T., Leonard, C. M., & Stern, C. (1993). Neuronal responses in the ventral striatum of the behaving macaque. *Behavioural Brain Research, 55,* 243–252.

Wilson, F., & Rolls, E. (1993). The effects of stimulus novelty and familiarity on neuronal activity in the amygdala of monkeys performing recognition memory tasks. *Experimental Brain Research, 93,* 367–382.

Yonelinas, A. P., Kroll, N. E., Quamme, J. R., Lazzara, M. M., Sauve, M. J., Widaman, K. F., et al. (2002). Effects of extensive temporal lobe damage or mild hypoxia on recollection and familiarity. *Nature Neuroscience, 11,* 1236–1241.

Zola, S. M., Squire, L. R., Teng, E., Stefanacci, L., Buffalo, E. A., & Clark, R. E. (2000). Impaired recognition memory in monkeys after damage limited to the hippocampal region. *Journal of Neuroscience, 20*(1), 451–463.

CHAPTER 7

Experience and Developmental Changes in the Organization of Language-Relevant Brain Activity

Debra L. Mills
Elizabeth A. Sheehan

How the adult brain becomes specialized for language and other cognitive functions is a central question in the field of cognitive neuroscience (Elman et al., 1996; Johnson, 2005). Recent developmental studies suggest that experience plays an important role in shaping the organization of the brain for a variety of sensory and cognitive processes such as music, face recognition, speech perception, and language development (see Johnson, 2005; Muller, 1996; Nelson & Luciana, 2001, for reviews). Greenough and colleagues have shown that in rats an enriched environment leads to experience-dependent modifications in synaptic connections that occur through the process of learning (Greenough, Black, & Wallace, 2002). Because the environment is external to the animal, it cannot induce changes in the brain without learning. It is the act of learning a new skill that triggers an increase in the number of synapses per neuron rather than passive exposure to the environment (Kleim et al., 1998). The process of establishing new synapses through learning in conjunction with eliminating unused connections through a series of subtractive neural events, some of which are also influenced by experience, shapes the organization of the brain

183

for different cognitive processes (Greenough, Black, Klintsova, Bates, & Weiler, 1999). To some extent this view implies that structural changes in postnatal brain development are the result of increasing functional specialization (Johnson, 2001; see also Johnson, Chapter 5, this volume). The important role of experiential factors in brain development is good news from an educational perspective. By understanding how different types of experience affect brain development, scientists and educators can develop and assess more effective teaching strategies for typically developing children and treatments for children with learning impairments.

This chapter reviews a series of studies using the event-related potential (ERP) technique to examine changes in brain activity linked to increasing age and proficiency during the course of language development. The first section describes developmental trajectories for lateralization of brain activity to spoken words observed across the lifespan. The second section examines the functional significance of these patterns of lateralization and the role of experience in setting up these specializations. We then turn to other language-specific and domain-general processes that contribute to vocabulary development, such as prosody, phonology, working memory, and semantic processing of gestures. Finally, we address the implications of this line of research from an educational perspective.

THE ERP TECHNIQUE

Large populations of cortical neurons aligned in parallel and firing simultaneously generate electrical fields that can be recorded from electrodes placed on the scalp; this is the basis for electroencephalographic (EEG) recordings. In ERP research, this activity is sampled every few milliseconds as the participant watches or listens to experimental stimuli. ERPs are averages of epochs of this brain activity time-locked to specific stimuli, such as spoken words, and reflect changes in neural activity on a millisecond-by-millisecond basis. ERPs are typically depicted as waves of activity at several locations across the scalp by plotting voltage in microvolts along the Y-axis and latency in milliseconds along the X-axis. They are characterized by a series of positive and negative fluctuations in voltage, called components. ERP components are named both for their polarity, *P* for positive and *N* for negative, and either their latency—the time at which they reach maximum amplitude—or their position in the waveform. For example, a positive component that reached maximum amplitude at 100 milliseconds (ms) after the onset of the stimulus would be called a P100, or a P1 if it were the first positive peak. The latencies, amplitudes, and distributions of these components respectively reflect the timing, amount, and (to some extent)

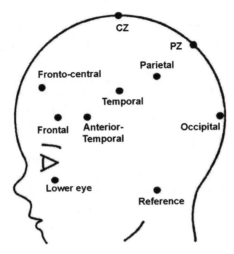

FIGURE 7.1. Electrode placements for 10–20 and nonstandard sites in our typical ERP studies with young infants and children.

location of the underlying brain activity. The functional significance of ERP components is determined by comparing the relative latencies, amplitudes, and distributions of the components to the stimuli across different experimental conditions. ERPs are safe, noninvasive, and the most practical brain imaging technique currently available for studying the development of cerebral specializations. This technique has the added benefits that it does not require an overt response (the children are not asked to do anything except sit still), and the same paradigm can be used to study development across several age groups. Figure 7.1 illustrates the placement of electrodes used in the majority of ERP studies with young children. In our most recent work we have recorded from twice the number of electrodes shown in the figure. Note that in all of the figures in this chapter, negative voltage is plotted in the upward direction.

LIFESPAN DEVELOPMENTAL CHANGES IN THE ORGANIZATION OF BRAIN ACTIVITY FOR AUDITORY WORDS

It is widely accepted that for the majority of both left- and right-handed typical adults, the left hemisphere has a privileged status for most aspects of language processing. The extent to which lateralization for language *develops* has been a topic of considerable interest and controversy for several decades. Lenneberg (1967) proposed that at birth the two hemispheres are equipotential for developing language skills. According to his theory, lateralization for language occurs progressively as a function of increasing age, stabilizing in the left hemisphere only after puberty. This position fell out of favor in the 1970s due to a series of studies showing both anatomical (Witelson & Pallie, 1973) and functional left-hemispheric asymmetries for language in infants using both behavioral (Entus, 1977; Kinsbourne, 1975) and electrophysiological (Molfese, 1973; Molfese, Freeman, & Palermo, 1975) techniques, as well as evidence from cases of hemispherectomized children suggesting early lateralization (Dennis & Whitaker, 1976; Kohn & Dennis, 1974). With recent innovations in brain imaging techniques, the debate has been revived with evidence on both sides. Consistent with Lenneberg's position, recent studies of children with focal brain injury have found that infants and children do not show the same degree or specific patterns of impairments as adults with the same lesions (for a review, see Bates & Roe, 2001). That is, children show a greater degree of brain plasticity than adults. A large number of neuroimaging (fMRI, PET, and ERP) studies also suggest that children show less specialization or a different pattern of specialization compared with adults engaged in similar tasks (Durston et al., 2002; Moses & Stiles, 2002; Passarotti et al., 2003; Stiles, Bates, Thal, Trauner, & Reilly, 2002; Stiles et al., 2003; Tamm, Menon, & Reiss, 2002). Other recent neuroimaging studies (Dehaene-Lambertz & Baillet, 1998; Dehaene-Lambertz & Dehaene, 1994; Dehaene-Lambertz, Dehaene, & Hertz-Pannier, 2002; Dehaene-Lambertz & Pena, 2001; Pena et al., 2003) suggest that there are left-hemispheric asymmetries or biases for processing language stimuli present in very young infants and even at birth. These early asymmetries are often assumed to be immutable and have been interpreted as evidence for an innate left-hemispheric specialization for language. Yet very few studies on either side of the debate have examined developmental trajectories for the early left-hemispheric asymmetries.

In this section we examine changes in the timing, morphology, and distributions of ERPs to auditory words from infancy through adulthood. If ERP asymmetries in young infants reflect an innate left-hemispheric bias for processing speech, then left-greater-than-right asymmetries elicited to auditory words should be present throughout development. In contrast, developmental changes in ERP distributions from bilateral to left-lateralized with increasing age would be consistent with a progressive lateralization position. Fluctuations in the distribution of components across the lifespan that vary with proficiency rather than chronological age would not support either position, but would be consistent with the interpretation that brain activity is dynamic and depends on a variety of factors other than brain maturation or innate specialization.

Figure 7.2 shows ERPs recorded over the left temporal region to familiar auditory words using a cross-sectional sample of 307 participants from 3 months to 75 years of age. Approximately half of the participants at each age group were female. These data have been described in other papers examining shorter periods of development (i.e., 3–10 months: Addy & Mills, 2005; 13–20 months: Mills, Coffey-Corina, & Neville, 1997; 28–36 months: Mills & Neville, 1997, and St. George & Mills, 2001; childhood: Holcomb, Coffey, & Neville, 1992; and elderly adults: de Ochoa, Mills, & Kutas, 2007). To control for developmental changes in ERP amplitudes, the original data were converted into standard scores (described below) and reanalyzed to examine age-related consistencies and differences in distribution. Age groups showing the same patterns in anterior–posterior or lateral distributions are collapsed in the illustrations. The ERPs shown in Figure 7.2 were recorded to familiar words for all age groups. For infants ages 3–42 months the stimuli were presented as a series of single auditory words (object names), approximately one word every 2 seconds. For infants 3–11 months of age, these were words heard several times per day or week, according to parental report. If the child had started to understand words, the words were those his or her parent rated as comprehended on a parental rating scale. If the child had started talking, the stimuli were words the child both said and understood. For children ages 5 years to adults, the words were presented in sentence format: for example, "The sun is shining and the birds are singing." Only open class words (nouns, verbs, and adjectives) from the middle of the sentence (i.e., excluding the first and last words) were used in the ERP averages shown in the figure.

Marked developmental changes were observed in the morphology of the ERP components elicited by auditory words, particularly during the first 3 years of life (refer to Figure 7.2). Developmental ERP studies employing a variety of cognitive and sensory stimuli have shown that the latencies and amplitudes of components tend to decrease with increasing age (Coch, Grossi, Skendzel, & Neville, 2005; Coch, Maron, Wolf, & Holcomb, 2002; Fuchigami, Okubo, Fujita, & Okuni, 1993; Holcomb et al., 1992; Little, Thomas, & Letterman, 1999). Decreasing latencies most likely reflect changes in speed of processing and may be related to maturational changes in myelination as well as increasing proficiencies in processing different types of information. Developmental changes in ERP amplitudes likely reflect several factors, including changes in the amount of neural activity generated, head size, skull thickness, resistance at the scalp, and closing of the fontenelles around 18 months of age.

Charting developmental changes in ERPs across the lifespan is challenging because very few components have direct correlates across infant and adult populations (Nelson & Luciana, 2001). The approach taken here was to compare the latencies, amplitudes, and lateral and anterior–

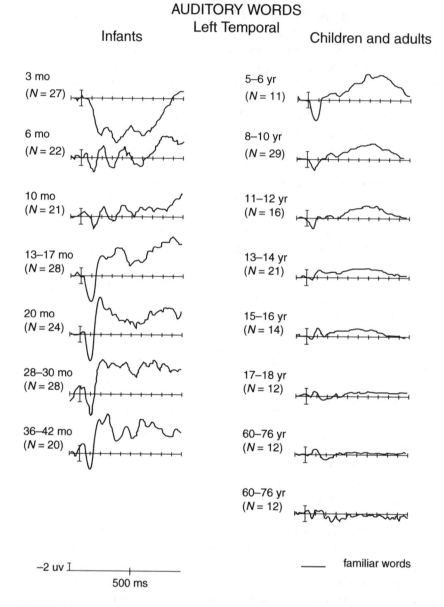

FIGURE 7.2. ERPs to familiar auditory words across different age groups, from infants 3 months of age to elderly adults.

posterior distributions of the first positive (P1) and first negative (N1) components at each age range. These early components are more likely to reflect similar processes in infants and adults and are within the latency windows of the components reflecting asymmetries in earlier studies.

First Positive Component, P1

The P1 indexes auditory sensory processing and has been localized to the primary auditory cortex within the superior temporal gyrus (Huotilainen et al., 1998; Toma et al., 2003). The amplitude of the P1 is influenced by both exogenous and endogenous factors and increases with increased stimulus intensity and attention (Hillyard, Mangun, Woldorff, & Luck, 1995). In the present study the P1 was defined as the most positive-going peak between 0 and 175 ms. A clear and discrete P1 peak was observed at all ages except 3 months. Consistent with previous studies (Coch et al., 2002; Key, Dove, & McGuire, 2005; Mills, Coffey, & Neville, 1993), both the latency and the amplitude of the P1 decreased with increasing age. The latency of the first positivity peaked at 160 ms at 3 months, at 100 ms from 6 to 30 months, and at 50 ms in young adults, and showed a slight increase to 65 ms in the elderly population.

Developmental changes in the anterior–posterior and lateral distributions of the P1 are illustrated as standardized scores in the left and right side of Figure 7.3, respectively. Standard scores were calculated by computing the mean of the peak amplitudes for a given component across all electrode locations at each age; standard scores are expressed as standard deviations from that mean. A score of zero reflects the mean of the peak amplitudes for a given age group. A positive score of 1 reflects one standard deviation from that mean in the direction of positive polarity, whereas a score of –1 reflects one standard deviation in the direction of negative polarity.

For all age groups, the P1 was larger over anterior (frontal, anterior temporal, and temporal regions) than posterior (parietal and occipital) regions (refer to the left side of Figure 7.3). The standard scores were averaged across all age groups because there were no developmental changes in the anterior–posterior distribution of the P1 component across time. Similarity across age groups in the anterior–posterior distribution of the P1 is consistent with the position that this component is generated in the primary auditory cortex across development, that is, in infants, children, and adults. In contrast, the lateral distribution of the P1 varied with age (refer to the right side of Figure 7.3). The P1 was larger over the left than the right hemisphere for children from 3 months to 3 years of age, was symmetrical in children 6–12 years of age, and was larger over the right than the left

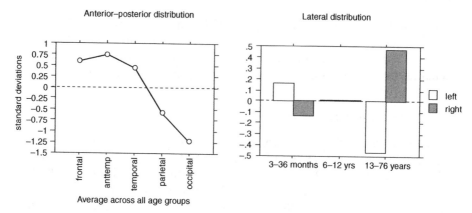

FIGURE 7.3. Standard scores for P1 amplitudes. The left side of the figure shows the anterior–posterior distribution of the P1, which was remarkably similar across all age groups. The right side of the figure shows changes in the lateral distribution of the P1 as a function of development. The P1 was larger over the left than the right hemisphere from 3 to 36 months, was symmetrical from 6 to 12 years, and was larger over the right than the left hemisphere from 13 to 76 years.

hemisphere in children 13 years of age and adults. Thus, the lifespan ERP results show that the asymmetries observed early in development are not immutable and do vary with age.

First Negative Component, N1

In adults the amplitude of the N1, like the P1, is modulated by stimulus intensity and attention. Source localization studies suggest that the auditory N1 in adults is most likely generated in the temporal lobe in the auditory cortex (Scherg, Vajsar, & Picton, 1989; Vaughn & Rigger, 1970). Fractionation studies suggest that there are several subcomponents in the N1 with multiple sources within different regions of the temporal lobe (Alcaini, Giard, Echallier, & Pernier, 1994; Woldorff, 1993; for reviews, see Key et al., 2005; Naatanen & Picton, 1987). In infants the first negative component has been linked to phonological processing (Dehane-Lambertz & Baillet, 1998; Molfese, Burger-Judisch, & Hans, 1991), and its amplitude is modulated by word familiarity and comprehension (Mills, Conboy, & Paton, 2005). As reported for adults, it is likely that multiple overlapping sources contribute to the first negative component in infants.

The developmental trajectories observed for the first negative-going component also tell a story of change across the lifespan (refer to Figure 7.2). Like the P1, the amplitude and latency of the N1 decrease with increasing age. The first negative component peaked at around 225 ms from 3 to 17 months, 200 ms from 20 months to 3 years of age, and 150 ms at 5–6 years, decreasing gradually to 100 ms at 17 years of age. For the elderly adults, the N1 latency, like the P1 latency, increased slightly relative to the young adults, peaking at 140 ms. The anterior–posterior distribution showed two developmental patterns (refer to the left side of Figure 7.4 and note that negative voltage is plotted down; hence, increasing N1 is shown below the baseline). From 3 months through 17 months of age, the first negative peak was larger from posterior than anterior regions. From 20 months through 76 years of age, the N1 amplitude was largest over temporal and parietal regions relative to frontal, anterior temporal, and occipital regions. The two developmental patterns overlap for anterior temporal, temporal, and parietal regions. This overlap is consistent with the areas closest to the putative generators of the N1 in the auditory cortex. The primary differences in the two patterns are in the frontal and occipital regions. These differences could reflect maturational changes in the auditory system linked to redundant connections to frontal and occipital regions early in development (Neville & Bavelier, 2002).

The lateral distribution of the N1 also varied with increasing age (refer to the right side of Figure 7.4). The first negative component was larger over the right than the left hemisphere from 3 to 17 months; was symmetri-

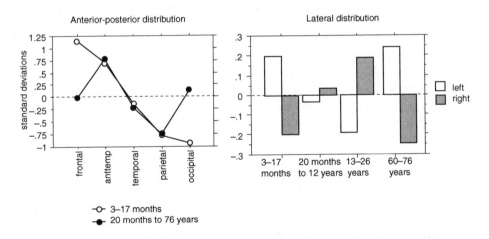

FIGURE 7.4. Standard scores for N1 amplitudes. The left side of the figure shows the anterior–posterior distribution averaged across two age groups. From 3 to 17 months the N1 was larger over posterior than anterior regions. From 20 months through adulthood, the N1 was largest over temporal and parietal regions. The right side of the figure shows developmental changes in the lateral distribution of the N1. Like the P1, the lateral distribution of the N1 varied with age.

cal from 20 months to 12 years of age; and was larger over the left than the right hemisphere from 13 to 26 years. A left-greater-than-right asymmetry for the auditory N1 to words in adults and adolescents has been reported in several papers and is thought to reflect the mature and stable pattern (Neville & Bavelier, 2002). In elderly adults, the N1 asymmetry reversed again and was larger over the right than the left hemisphere.

Although the first positive and first negative components are thought to be generated in the auditory cortex and are sensitive to sensory and attentional processes, the P1 and N1 differed from each other in their anterior–posterior and lateral distributions and the ages at which they showed changes in these distributions. These differences suggest that the two components index activity from nonidentical neural systems, have different developmental time courses, and reflect somewhat different aspects of auditory language processing. The complex pattern of changing lateral asymmetries suggests that the functional organizations of the brain systems indexed by these ERP components show a dynamic and protracted course of development. Moreover, these data highlight the need for establishing lifespan developmental trajectories. Selecting a restricted age range, even one that spans several years, can lead to completely different conclusions. For example, if one looked only at the P1 data from 3 months to 3 years, it might be interpreted as reflecting an immutable left-hemispheric bias for processing speech. In contrast, examining only changes from 6 years through old age could be interpreted as consistent with a progressive lateralization hypothesis from symmetrical to right-lateralized. Additionally, before one can make claims about ERP or other asymmetries, the functional significance of those asymmetries must be determined. Language is not a single entity. There are many aspects of language processing, including acoustic, phonological, prosodic, semantic, syntactic, and discourse processing. An asymmetry reflected by any single ERP component, or in response to any single type of stimulus, should not be taken as evidence for lateralization for "language" or any other complex cognitive function.

Although these data show that ERP asymmetries do *develop*, the extent to which maturational versus experiential factors influence that development is still a question of general interest. Also of interest is whether functional asymmetries are linked to better language skills. Abnormalities in both structural and functional asymmetries have been noted in a variety of atypical populations, such as children with autism, dyslexia, language impairment, schizophrenia, and Williams syndrome (Bellugi, Lichtenberger, Mills, Galaburda, & Korenberg, 1999; Dawson, Finley, Phillips, & Lewy, 1989; De Fosse et al., 2004; Herbert et al., 2002, 2005; Mills et al., 2000; Saugstad, 1998). It has been suggested that slow brain maturation and the failure to develop lateral asymmetries may underlie linguistic deficits in these atypical populations (Saugstad, 1998). Rather than assume a causal link from abnormal brain development to abnormal function, we make the opposite suggestion: that slow and effortful processing may be an underlying factor associated with the absence of lateral asymmetries in some atypically developing populations.

In the next section we review a series of studies examining the relation between vocabulary size and ERP differences to comprehended and unknown words, suggesting that the rate of word learning, rather than absolute vocabulary size or chronological age, influences the development of ERP asymmetries (Conboy & Mills, 2006; Mills et al., 1997; Mills & Neville, 1997; Mills, Plunkett, Pratt, & Schafer, 2005; Mills et al., 2004).

LANGUAGE EXPERIENCE AND ERP ASYMMETRIES TO KNOWN AND UNKNOWN WORDS

At the beginning of the chapter, we discussed the role of learning in shaping the organization of the brain. Applying this work to child language acquisition, we are working from the assumption that when a child learns a word, new synapses are formed. In turn, these new connections interact in a dynamic manner with other developmental changes and sculpt the organization of the brain for language. The word *experience* is used here to refer to the dynamic process of learning new words. In this section, we examine the functional significance of the first positive and negative ERP components to auditory words in more detail and show how experiential factors, as indexed by proficiency with different aspects of language processing, affect the lateral asymmetry of these components. In the studies reviewed below, the infant's absolute vocabulary size was taken as an index of relative amount of language experience as measured by the MacArthur–Bates Communicative Development Inventory (CDI; Fenson et al., 1994). A picture-pointing task and an additional 4-point Likert-type parental rating scale were used to identify words the child understood and/or produced. In these studies, single auditory words were presented serially in random order at the rate of one every 2–3 seconds.

To establish the functional significance of the first negative and positive components, ERP latencies and amplitudes were compared for familiar, unknown, and backward words in infants from 3 to 36 months old (Addy & Mills, 2005; Mills, Coffey-Corina, & Neville, 1993; Mills et al., 1997; Neville & Mills, 1997). For infants the first positive component peaked at approximately 100 ms and the first negative component peaked at approximately 200 ms, hereafter called the P100 and N200, respectively.

ERPs to backward words differed from ERPs to forward words by 150 ms after word onset (Neville & Mills, 1997), did not reveal developmental trends that varied with vocabulary size, and are not addressed further here.

The remainder of the chapter focuses primarily on ERPs in children between 13 and 20 months of age. This period of development is particularly interesting because of rapid changes in several aspects of language development. Typically infants start saying their first words soon after their first birthdays. They make slow progress until accumulating a vocabulary of about 50–100 words, and then show a rapid increase in vocabulary size in a very short time (Thal, Bates, Goodman, & Jahn-Samilo, 1997). This phenomenon, called the vocabulary burst, has led researchers to postulate several different hypotheses that suggest a reorganization of cognitive processes in order to explain the marked acceleration in vocabulary size. These hypotheses include changes in representational capacity for symbolic functioning (McCune, 1995; McCune-Nicolich, 1981; Nazzi & Bertoncini, 2003; Werner & Kaplan, 1963), the insight that objects do or should have names (Baldwin & Markman, 1989; Dore, 1974; McShane, 1979), changes in categorization abilities (Gopnik & Meltzoff, 1987), and changes in social pragmatics such as joint attention (Baldwin & Moses, 2001; Tomasello, 2001). In this section we review a series of cross-sectional studies designed to examine how changes in age and vocabulary size vary with changes in the timing and lateral distribution of the first positive (P100) and negative (N200) components to known and unknown words around the time of the vocabulary burst (Conboy & Mills, 2006; Mills, Coffey-Corina, & Neville, 1993, 1997; Mills et al., 2004; Mills, Plunkett, Prat, & Schafer, 2005).

Infant P100 Lateral Asymmetries and Vocabulary Size

As noted earlier, the first positive component, P100, in infants is probably the functional equivalent of the P50 in adults and is linked to auditory sensory processing. In adults, P1 amplitudes and latencies are modulated by variations in the physical or acoustic properties of stimuli. Therefore, we controlled for a variety of acoustic differences across conditions such as volume, duration, and number of syllables. Additionally, different types of consonants, such as stops, fricatives, or liquids, are characterized by differences in the shape and spectral frequencies of formant transitions at the onset of the consonant. In order to control for systematic differences in acoustic attributes at the beginnings of familiar and unfamiliar words, the phonological characteristics of the known and unknown words were designed to be similar. Across the studies employing these controlled auditory stimuli, the P100 amplitude did not differ between known and unknown words, with one exception (Mills et al., 2004). In that study, 20-month-olds, but not 14-month-olds, showed P100 amplitude differences when the unknown words consisted of nonsense words that differed from the known words by a minimal contrast in the initial phoneme (e.g., *milk* vs. *nilk*). Because the amplitude of the P100 is modulated by attention in both adults and children (Luck & Hillyard, 2000; Richards & Hunter, 2002), the interpretation of the P100 amplitude difference in this paradigm was that inclusion of the phonemic contrast words increased attention to sensory and perceptual detail. In a study of bilingual toddlers (Conboy & Mills, 2006), although the amplitude of the P100 did not differ for known as compared to unknown words in either language, the latency of the P100 was later for Spanish than English. One possible explanation is that phonological differences between Spanish and English modulated these P100 latency differences. In summary, our findings examining P100 latencies and amplitudes to familiar, unknown, and backward words are consistent with the position that the P100 indexes acoustic and phonological processing and may be modulated by increased attention to acoustic information.

Deficits in acoustic processing are hypothesized to underlie or contribute to some aspects of language disorders (Neville, Coffey, Holcomb, & Tallal, 1993; Tallal, 1978). In very young infants ERP sensitivity to different speech contrasts has been shown to be predictive of later language abilities (Molfese, Molfese, & Espy, 1999). To examine a possible link between auditory sensory processing and early language abilities, the distribution of the P100 was compared across three groups of children who were matched on chronological age but varied in vocabulary size. Infants from 13 to 17 months, 20 months, and 28 to 30 months of age were divided into two categories of "high" and "low" producers, based on the size of their productive vocabularies relative to the MacArthur–Bates CDI norm for their age group. High producers were defined as children who scored above the 50th percentile for their age, whereas low producers scored below the 30th percentile (Mills & Neville, 1997). Figure 7.5 shows that for the high producers in each age group, the P100 was larger over left than right temporoparietal regions. In contrast, the P100 was symmetrical for the low producers in each age group. Note that the left-greater-than-right asymmetry was not linked to any particular vocabulary size or language milestone. This finding was determined by comparing children at different ages who were matched on vocabulary size. For example, the 13- to 17-month-old high producers and the 20-month-old low producers both had a mean of 44 words produced, and the 20-month-old high producers and 28- to 30-month-old low producers both had a mean of approximately 196 words. But only the high producers, that is, the younger children, showed the left-

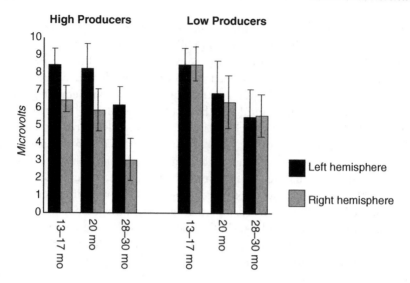

FIGURE 7.5. P100 amplitudes over temporoparietal regions of the left and right hemispheres for 13- to 17-, 20-, and 28- to 30-month-old high and low producers. The P1 is larger over the left than the right hemisphere for the high producers and symmetrical for the low producers.

greater-than-right P100 asymmetry in each case. Thus the left-greater-than-right P100 asymmetry appears to be linked to percentile rankings rather than absolute vocabulary size.

We hypothesized that the lateral asymmetry of the P100 is linked to faster rates of learning, whereas the lack of this asymmetry is associated with slower and more effortful processing (Mills, Conboy, & Paton, 2005). According to this hypothesis, slow and effortful processing requires more cortical tissue to perform the word learning task. In contrast, more experienced word learners can afford to use more specialized systems when processing known words or learning new ones. This perspective suggests that it is the process and rate of learning that differentially shape the organization of the brain. An alternate explanation is that an initial preparedness to process language stimuli in the left hemisphere will result in better language skills. This explanation implies that the presence or absence of an innate bias for the two hemispheres to process speech and nonspeech sounds influences language development. Saugstad (1998) suggested that slower brain development results in a lack of hemispheric asymmetries. This maturational hypothesis implies that slower brain maturation or the lack of a left-hemispheric asymmetry would result in slower learning. That is, it is possible that the low producers showed a bilateral distribution for the P100 because they had more slowly maturing brains. More specifically, they were late talkers because their brains did not show a left-hemispheric predisposition for language.

In a recent study of 20-month-olds learning Spanish and English simultaneously (Conboy & Mills, 2006), we observed a similar pattern of a left-greater-than-right P100 asymmetry to known words in the children who had a large total conceptual vocabulary across both languages. Children with smaller total vocabularies showed a symmetrical P100 to known words. We also examined P100 differences for the dominant as compared to the nondominant language. Language dominance was determined by the vocabulary size for each individual language. For the high-vocabulary children, the P100 was left-lateralized only for their dominant language and was symmetrical for the nondominant language. For the children with smaller vocabularies the P100 was symmetrical for both the dominant and nondominant language. We suggested that this asymmetrical processing for known words in the dominant language of high-vocabulary children was related to a more efficient, faster, and automatic processing system for that language. The asymmetry cannot be due to faster rates of brain maturation or an innate preparedness to process speech stimuli in the left hemisphere because both patterns were found in the same developing brains.

In summary, although the lateral distribution of the first positive component changes with increasing age across the lifespan (refer to Figure 7.3), these changes are not exclusively due to brain maturation; other neurocognitive mechanisms are involved in driving these changes. The findings from 13- to 30-month-old monolingual children show that the presence of the left-greater-than-right asymmetry is linked to language proficiency rather than chronological age. The findings from 20-month-old bilingual toddlers show that this asymmetry is linked to proficiency in one language relative to the other and must be due to the effects of different experience rather than genetic or maturational factors.

Infant N200 Asymmetries and Vocabulary Size

Unlike the P100, the amplitude of the first negative component observed in the known/unknown/backward word paradigm, N200, *did* differ for known as compared to unknown words. From 200 to 400 ms after word onset, hereafter called the N200–400, ERP amplitudes were larger to known than unknown words in infants as young as 10 months of age whose parents reported that the infants understood the meanings of the words (Addy & Mills, 2005; Conboy & Mills, 2006; Mills et al., 1993, 1997, 2004; Mills, Coffey-Corina, & Neville, 1994; Mills, Plunkett, et al., 2005). Although the amplitude of the N200 can be modulated by phonological differences in certain paradigms (Connolly, Service, D'Arcy, Kujala, & Alho, 2001; D'Arcy, Connolly, Service, Hawco, & Houlihan, 2004; Dehaene-Lambertz, 2000; Dehaene-Lambertz & Gliga, 2004; Dehaene-Lambertz & Pena, 2001), we argue that in our studies the dominant factor modulating component amplitude is word meaning (see Mills, Conboy, et al., 2005, for a complete argument). Briefly, our argument that these differences are not due to phonological differences in word types is as follows. In two studies in which word types did differ in phonology (Conboy & Mills, 2006; Mills et al., 2004), N200–400 amplitude differences were not observed when the phonologically different types of words were both processed as known words. For example, in the study of bilingual toddlers (Conboy & Mills, 2006), although Spanish and English clearly differ in phonology, the N200–400 amplitude varied only as a function of whether the word was known or unknown, not whether the word was presented in Spanish or English. Additionally, in a word learning paradigm, pairing a novel word with an object increased the amplitude of the N200–400, whereas repeating the word the same number of times led to a decrease in N200–400 amplitude (Mills, Plunkett, et al., 2005). Because the stimuli were physically identical and counterbalanced across participants and conditions, the increased N200–400 amplitudes could not be explained by phonological differences. It was the association with a meaningful stimulus that modulated the amplitude of the N200–400 to the newly learned words.

The lateral distribution of the N200–400, like the P100, has been shown to vary as a function of vocabulary size across several studies. However, in these studies it is the distribution of the ERP effect—that is, the N200–400 amplitude difference between known as compared to unknown words—that changes with language experience. In an earlier edition of this book, we (Mills et al., 1994) described developmental changes in cerebral specialization for language comprehension, from bilateral to left-lateralized, in children from 13 to 20 months of age (see Figure 7.6). More specifically, at 13–17 months of age, the N200–400 was larger to known than unknown words over anterior and posterior regions of both the left and right hemispheres (Mills et al., 1997). In contrast, at 20 months of age—that is, after the vocabulary burst—these differences were more focally distributed and apparent only over temporal and parietal regions of the left hemisphere (Mills et al., 1993). For both age groups, when children were divided into two groups based on vocabulary size, the N200–400 difference was more focally distributed for children with a larger vocabulary size. We proposed that this shift in the distribution of N200–400 differences was tied to marked changes in vocabulary development such as the vocabulary burst.

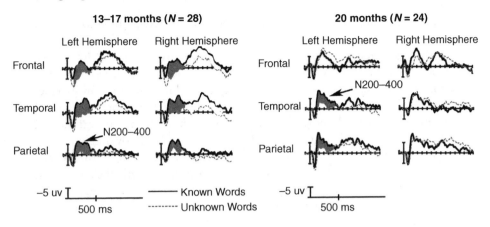

FIGURE 7.6. ERPs to known (solid lines) and unknown (dashed lines) words for 13- to 17- and 20-month-old typically developing infants. Shaded areas denote statistically reliable differences in ERPs to known and unknown words. Negative polarity in microvolts is plotted up. The N200–400 was larger to known than unknown words for both age groups. The distribution of this effect was broadly distributed over anterior and posterior regions of both hemispheres at 13–17 months, but was limited to temporal and parietal regions of the left hemisphere at 20 months.

Since these early studies, we have replicated this effect using other stimuli with 14- and 20-month-old typically developing infants (Mills et al., 2004) and 20- and 28- to 30-month-old late talkers—that is, older children who were matched for vocabulary size with the 13- to 17- and 20-month-old groups. In the latter study (Mills, Conboy, et al., 2005; Mills, Prat, Llamas, & Thal, 2007), 20-month-old late talkers, like the language-matched typically developing 13- to 17-month-olds, showed a bilateral distribution of the N200–400 differences to known as compared to unknown words. In contrast, the 28- to 30-month-old late talkers, like the language-matched 20-month-old typically developing children, showed a left-lateralized ERP effect. This study provided further evidence that the more focalized ERP response was linked to vocabulary size rather than chronological age. Similarly, in the study of 20-month-old bilingual toddlers (Conboy & Mills, 2006), the N200–400 amplitude difference to known as compared to unknown words was more focally distributed for children classified as high as compared to low on vocabulary size, and also more focally distributed for children's dominant language. Although there were some differences between monolingual and bilingual toddlers, these data show unequivocally that changes in the distribution of the N200–400 known/unknown word effect cannot be explained by group differences in brain maturation.

We interpreted the observed changes in the lateral organization of brain activity to known as compared to unknown words as linked to the vocabulary burst or absolute vocabulary size around 100–150 words. However, connectionist models suggest that increasing experience with "image–label" associations leads to a rapid nonlinear increase in productive performance in the network, similar to the vocabulary spurt observed in child language development (Plunkett, Sinha, Møller, & Strandsby, 1992). It is plausible that the 20-month-olds in our study might simply have had 7 more months of experience knowing a particular word than the 13-month-olds. Therefore, the amount of experience with the individual words, rather than absolute vocabulary size, may have accounted, at least in part, for changes in the distribution of the observed ERP effects in previous studies.

To test the contrasting hypotheses that absolute vocabulary size as opposed to experience with individual words is linked to the lateral distribution of ERP differences to known as compared to unknown words, we examined ERPs to newly learned words in 20-month-olds with small and large vocabularies (Mills, Plunkett, et al., 2005). The procedure was described earlier in this section. If the distribution of brain activity is linked to the amount of experience with individual words rather than vocabulary size, then we would expect a bilateral distribution in ERP differences to newly learned words versus not-trained (simply repeated) words, as displayed by the 13- to 17-month-old infants in the Mills and colleagues (1997) study to known and unknown words. In contrast, if the lateral distribution of these effects were determined by the vocabulary spurt or a productive vocabulary of over 100 words, then we would expect the distribution of the effect to vary with vocabulary size; that is, a bilateral distribution for the low producers and ERP effects limited to the left hemisphere for the high producers. The results showed that across vocabulary groups, the N200–400 was larger to newly learned than repeated words over anterior and posterior regions of both the left and right hemispheres. This finding supports the "word experience" hypothesis. When we examined the distribution of ERP effects according to vocabulary size, the 20-month-old high producers showed ERP effects that were significantly different over both hemispheres but were larger over the left than the right. These results suggest an interaction between vocabulary size and experience with the individual words. A similar pattern that showed effects of both vocabulary size and language experience was observed in the study of bilingual 20-month-olds (Conboy & Mills, 2006). In that study, the organization of brain activity varied according to vocabulary size for the high and low producers and by experience with individual words in the dominant as compared to nondominant language.

The results of these studies support the position that experience shapes the organization of lateral asymmetries in neural language processing. In normal language development, increasing proficiency is linked with increased cerebral specializations (more focally distributed ERPs). However, the change in lateralization does not appear to be linked to the attainment of an absolute number of words or to reaching the "vocabulary burst" milestone as originally proposed. Thus our original interpretation of the bilateral to left-lateralized "shift" in distribution described in an earlier edition of this volume (Mills et al., 1994) has been revised in light of these new findings. We now offer the following working hypothesis: As the strength of a word–object association increases, the amount of brain activity it takes to discriminate newly learned words from unfamiliar words decreases. That is, the brain activity needed to discriminate known from unknown words becomes more focally distributed as an emergent property of learning those specific words. In our training study, even the high producers did not show the same pattern of lateralization as shown by the 20-month-olds in either the Mills and colleagues 1997 or 2004 studies. It is likely that the novel trained word–object associations were weaker than those of the "known" words in the previous studies. More generally, we propose a trend from a broadly distributed to a more focalized pattern of neural activity during the course of learning that might not be specific to language. Slow and effortful processing, which is a hallmark of early word learning, leads to a broad distribution of brain activity. When an association or skill is well learned and more automatic, the pattern of brain activity elicited by that cognitive process becomes more focally distributed. The level of proficiency of the learner at a given time interacts with this process. For example, although the mechanism—from broad to more focal patterns of activity—may be the same in an adult and an infant, it will occur much faster in a skilled adult than in an unskilled infant learner. That is, these asymmetries emerge through the process of learning. It is our position that the observed functional asymmetries are not static attributes that develop in a linear manner as a function of maturation, but instead are dynamic and vary with task demands. Future studies manipulating levels of task difficulty in both infants and adults will test this hypothesis.

Given that the results do not support the position that a reorganization in brain activity leads to or explains the vocabulary burst, the question remains as to what other factors contribute to this apparent stage-like shift in language abilities. In the next several sections we examine the role of experience in shaping the organization of neural systems for other language-specific and domain-general processes that contribute to vocabulary development, such as prosody, phonological processing, working memory, and the processing of meaningful gestures.

PROSODY

It is well known that adults use prosodic modifications of speech, commonly called "baby talk" or "motherese," when they talk to infants. In infant research, this speech register is referred to as infant-directed speech (IDS) as opposed to adult-directed speech (ADS). IDS is characterized by a higher pitch, greater variability in prosodic changes, increased repetition, elongated vowels, and slower tempo as compared to ADS. Using behavioral measures of attention, such as looking time, prior research has consistently demonstrated that infants prefer IDS to ADS as early as the first few weeks after birth (Cooper & Aslin, 1990; Fernald, 1985; Papousek, Bornstein, Nuzzo, Papousek, & Symmes, 1990). This particular speech register is thought to capture the infants' attention and highlight certain aspects of the speech signal, which may aid in later word recognition (Bertoncini, 1998; Christophe, Dupoux, Bertoncini, & Mehler, 1994; Fernald, 2000; Hirsh-Pasek et al., 1987; Jusczyk et al., 1992).

In an extension of behavioral work in this area, Zangl and Mills (2007) examined patterns of brain activity to familiar and unfamiliar words presented in IDS and ADS. Six- and 13-month-old infants listened to words in four different conditions: familiar IDS, unfamiliar IDS, familiar ADS, and unfamiliar ADS. The ERP components of interest in this study were the N200–400 and a negative-going component peaking around 800 ms, N600–800.

In infants, a frontal negativity peaking around 800 ms, termed the Nc (Courchesne, 1978), has been linked to the allocation of attention such that a larger amplitude Nc is thought to be associated with a greater allocation of attentional resources (Nelson & Monk, 2001). Therefore, if IDS serves to increase attention to specific words, as suggested by behavioral research, we predicted that ERP amplitude to words presented in IDS would be larger than that to words presented in ADS, within the latency range of the Nc component. Furthermore, we hypothesized that if IDS serves to facilitate comprehension, the amplitude of the N200–400, which has been linked to word meaning in our previous studies (see above), would be greater for familiar words presented in IDS relative to ADS.

As predicted, at both 6 and 13 months, N600–800 was larger to words presented in IDS than ADS (see Figure 7.7). However, at 6 months this effect was observed only for familiar words, whereas at 13 months, the N600–800 was larger to IDS than ADS for both familiar and unfamiliar words. Also as predicted, for 13-month-olds, but not 6-month-olds, the N200–400 was larger to familiar words presented in IDS. In a continuation of this study, preliminary findings show that for 20-month-olds, IDS serves to increase neural activity relative to ADS but only for unfamiliar words.

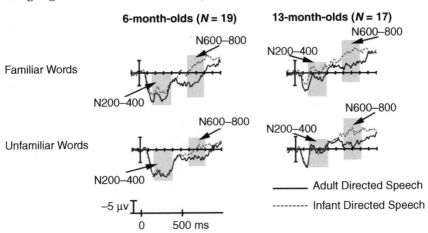

FIGURE 7.7. ERPs to known and unknown words presented in adult-directed speech (solid lines) and infant-directed speech (dashed lines) for 6- and 13-month-old infants. At 6 months IDS elicited larger negative amplitudes from 600 to 800 ms after word onset only for familiar words. At 13 months this effect was significant for both familiar and unfamiliar words.

The ERP differences found with age and word familiarity indicate a dynamic role for IDS over development and are consistent with behavioral studies showing a developmental change in preference for IDS (Cooper & Aslin, 1994; McRoberts, 2000). We propose that these differences reflect changes in both language development and domain-general cognitive development. For young infants, IDS draws attention to potentially meaningful words for which they may already have formed a phonological representation but not necessarily mapped word meaning; in this case, the words rated as familiar to the infant. For older infants, IDS highlights both familiar and unfamiliar words, interacts with increased attentional and working memory capacity, and may boost infants' ability to focus on and learn new individual words. For more experienced word learners such as 20-month-olds, IDS serves to focus attention on novel but potentially meaningful words.

To examine the effects of experience on the organization of neural activity to IDS, we tested 6-month-old infants with altered early experience with IDS: infants of depressed mothers (Huot et al., 2005). Depressed mothers tend to use less IDS than nondepressed mothers (Bettes, 1988; Kaplan, Bachorowski, Smoski, & Zinzer, 2001). If the boost in neural activity to IDS observed in the studies of typically developing infants is related to innate processes designed to take advantage of the special acoustic features of IDS, we should see the same ERP patterns in infants of depressed mothers as we did in the study described above. However, if experience plays a role in the functional significance of IDS, we predicted that infants of depressed mothers would not show the same pattern of activation to IDS. The results from 18 6-month-old infants of depressed mothers indicated that these infants did not show an increase in neural activity to IDS at any point in the waveform. We are following these children longitudinally, and continuing analyses will examine the relation between maternal parenting behaviors, the timing and length of maternal depression, and the use of medication during pregnancy on the ERP results. Analysis of cortisol levels taken across three time points showed that the two groups of infants did not differ in baseline levels or reactive levels of cortisol—an important control because cortisol levels have been shown to influence ERPs related to attentional processing (Gunnar & Nelson, 1994). Preliminary findings suggest that it is reduced experience with maternal IDS that is associated with the lack of ERP differences to IDS as compared to ADS in this group. Future studies will examine the possible beneficial effects of nondepressed fathers by examining patterns of ERP activity to male IDS.

PHONOLOGICAL PROCESSING

The ability to discriminate phonetically similar speech sounds is quite evident early in development. However, behavioral work in this area has demonstrated that children around 14 months of age have difficulty distinguishing phonetically similar words when they are also required to map those words onto meaning (Stager & Werker, 1997; Werker, Cohen, Lloyd, Casasole, & Stager, 1998; but see also Swingley & Aslin, 2000, 2002, for an alternative interpretation). Comparing ERPs to three types of words—known words (e.g., *bear*), phonetically similar nonsense words (e.g., *gare*), and phonetically dissimilar nonsense words (e.g., *kobe*)—Mills and colleagues (2004) examined neural activity for processing phonetic detail in the context of meaningful words. The ERP results supported the behavioral work showing that inexperienced word learners do not use information about minimal phonetic differences when processing word meaning. The 14-month-olds showed a larger amplitude response over the 200–400 ms window to known words as compared to phonetically dissimilar nonsense words (e.g., *bear* vs. *kobe*; see Figure 7.8). As predicted, ERPs to known words and phonetically similar words (e.g., *bear* and *gare*) did not differ. In contrast, more experienced word learners, 20-month-olds, showed a larger N200–400 response to known words (e.g., *bear*) when compared to both the phonetically similar and phonetically dissimilar non-

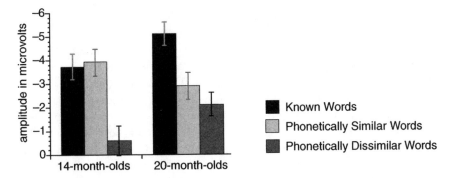

FIGURE 7.8. N200–400 amplitudes to known words (e.g., *bear*), nonsense words that were phonetically similar to the known words (e.g., *gare*), and nonsense words that were phonetically dissimilar to the known words (e.g., *kobe*). At 13 months known and phonetically similar nonsense words elicited similar ERPs. At 20 months, known words and phonetically similar nonsense words elicited distinct ERP patterns.

sense words (e.g., *gare* and *kobe*); indeed, the ERPs to both types of nonsense word were indistinguishable from each other in this group.

These results suggest that inexperienced word learners mistakenly interpret the phonetically similar word as a known word by disregarding the phonetic information in favor of the semantic information. In contrast, by 20 months of age, infants can utilize both phonetic and semantic information and therefore process the phonetically similar and nonsense words as the same. These findings provide evidence that novice word learners may accept a broader range of pronunciations of a word as acceptable. With increasing age and language experience, older infants have more accessible knowledge of phonological detail, narrowing their range of acceptable pronunciations and avoiding mistakes in word recognition.

WORKING MEMORY

Changes in the ability to access detailed phonetic information in word learning contexts, as well as other linguistic and cognitive correlates of the vocabulary burst, may be linked to changes in domain-general processes such as working memory. For example, Gershkoff-Stowe (2002) hypothesized that vocabulary differences between 13 and 20 months are due to differences in memory development.

Using ERPs, Mills, Conboy, and colleagues (2005) investigated the role of memory, specifically working memory, and vocabulary size in semantic processing. Adults and children at ages 13, 20, and 36 months were tested in two cross-modal paradigms designed to elicit an N400 response, with and without a working memory component. The N400 response is a negative component occurring 400 ms after the onset of a stimulus and is larger when a stimulus is incongruent with the preceding context (Kutas & Hillyard, 1980). In the first experiment, children viewed a picture and then 500 ms later heard a word while the picture was still on the screen (Mills, Conboy, et al., 2005). The word either named the object in the picture (match) or named an object in a different picture (mismatch). In both studies, the infants understood the meanings of the words, as assessed by a Likert-type parental rating scale and a picture-pointing task. If the infants did not see the picture, the EEG from that trial was not included in the ERP average. A significant N400 effect to the mismatched words was observed at all ages as early as 200 ms after the onset of the word (see Figure 7.9, left side). That is, there were no developmental changes and no differences in the N400 for high as compared to low comprehenders at each age group, suggesting that the neural mechanisms underlying the N400 response are similar to adults' even in early word learners. These results differ somewhat from those of Friederici and colleagues (Friedrich & Friederici, 2004, 2005) in the timing of the N400 response. However, the infants in those studies, especially the low comprehenders, did not understand the meanings of all of the words and in some instances did not see the picture.

In the second experiment, the word was presented first and a picture that either matched or mismatched with the preceding word was presented 500 ms later (Larson, Lewis, Horton, Addy, & Mills, 2005). This procedure introduced a working memory component by inserting a delay between the offset of the word and the onset of the picture. Adults, 36-, and 20-month-olds all showed an N400 response, but it differed in latency and distribution (see Figure 7.9, right side). The adults showed an increased negativity to the mismatched pictures (N400) from 200–600 ms after the onset of the picture. For the 20-month-olds, the N400 peaked later and was significant at medial and central sites. The 36-month-olds showed an N400 latency and distribution similar to the adults. As a group the 13-month-olds did not show a significant N400 response when the delay was introduced. However, if a larger vocabulary is associated with stronger word-association bonds and therefore decreases memory load, then vocabulary size should be correlated with the N400 effect in this paradigm. When divided into two groups for high as compared to low comprehension, 13-month-olds who had a receptive vocabulary over 100 words showed a significant N400 response that had a longer latency than that shown by 20-month-olds. Infants at 13 months who had receptive vocabularies under 100 words did not show an N400 response. These findings demonstrate the

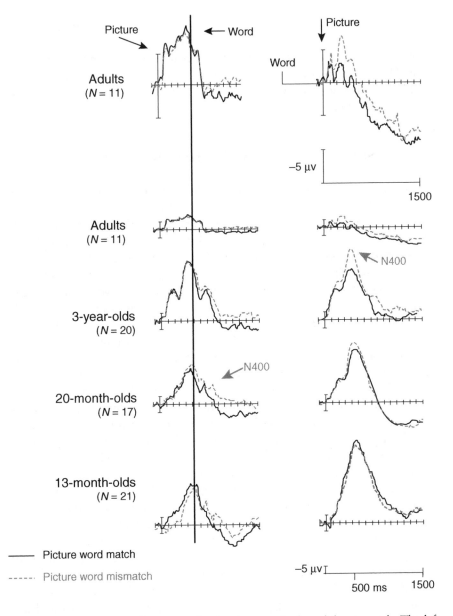

FIGURE 7.9. ERPs to picture–word pairs that matched or did not match. The left side of the figure represents ERPs to pictures followed by a word. All ages showed an N400 effect that was similar in timing and distribution. The onset of the N400 effect occurs after the onset of the word, as shown by the vertical black bar. The right side of the figure represents ERPs to a picture that followed a word. Marked developmental differences were apparent in the timing of the N400 when a working memory component was added. (Apparent amplitude differences in ERPs to the pictures in the two conditions for 13- and 20-month-olds were due to data collection in different ERP labs and different distances from the stimulus presentation monitor.)

important role of domain-general processes in children's semantic processing. The extent to which these neural processes are specific to language is explored in the next section, as we examine the organization of brain activity in processing meaning for words and gestures.

PROCESSING MEANINGFUL GESTURES

When learning to communicate with others, infants use a variety of both verbal and nonverbal techniques. By 12 months of age, infants use gestures and words similarly to identify objects, events, and their desires (Acredolo & Goodwyn, 1985, 1988; Bates, Bretherton, Snyder, Shore, & Volterra, 1980; Blake & Dolgoy, 1993; Iverson, Capirci, & Caselli, 1994). However, at approximately 20 months of age, infants begin to move toward the use of predominately verbal communication, and their use of "gestural naming" decreases (Acredolo & Goodwyn, 1988; Iverson, Capirci, & Caselli, 1994). At this point in development and continuing through adulthood, gestures tend to augment spoken language instead of replacing it.

One growing area of research is the study of representational or symbolic gestures. Representational gestures are used to stand for an object or event. Some of these gestures are iconic in that they depict inherent properties of the item or event they represent, such as the function or physical characteristics of an object. For example, an iconic gesture for *cup* could be displaying the motion of taking a drink. To compare the processing of words and gestures over development, we examined ERPs to iconic gestures (Sheehan, Namy, & Mills, in press).

Participants were presented with a video of the same model either producing an iconic gesture or speaking a word. Following each video, either a matched or mismatched picture was shown. An example of a matched trial is the gesture for phone (thumb and pinkie extended, to ear) followed by the picture of a phone. ERPs were time-locked to the presentation of the picture and examined for evidence of an N400 response. Adults showed a significantly larger and broadly distributed N400 on mismatched trials (as compared to matched trials) for both pictures following a word and pictures following a gesture (see Figure 7.10). The distribution of this effect was identical for pictures preceded by words and gestures. Twenty-six-month-olds showed an N400 response for the mismatched word–picture pairs at specific sites, but this effect was not significant for mismatched gesture–picture pairs at any electrode location. Surprisingly, 18-month-olds showed a pattern more similar to adults: an N400 mismatch effect for both the word–picture and gesture–picture pairs.

The differing N400 mismatch pattern for 18- and 26-month-olds is consistent with behavioral research in this area. Namy and Waxman

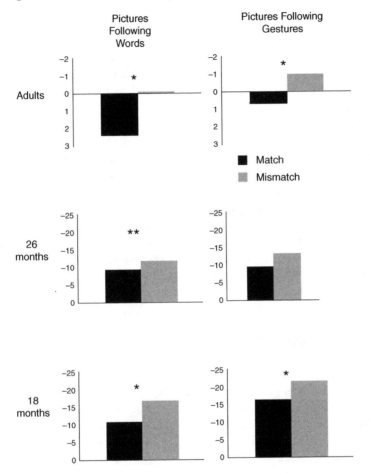

FIGURE 7.10. N400 amplitude differences to matched as compared to mismatched pictures that followed either a word or a gesture. * $p < .05$; ** only significant at specific electrode sites.

(1998) tested infants' developing symbolic ability by training infants to identify an arbitrary gesture or a novel word as an object name for object categories, such as *fruit* or *vehicle*. After a training period with a novel gesture or a novel word (both were arbitrary, but the context in which they were presented was held constant), the infants were tested using a forced-choice task. The authors found that infants at 18 months would accept a novel gesture or a novel word as a name for an object category. At 26 months there was a different pattern: The older infants readily accepted a novel word as an object name but would only accept a novel gesture as a name under a more limited set of conditions, such as increased exposure to the gesture or when the gesture was iconically related to the referent. These results were interpreted as showing that words gain priority over gestures as children gain more experience with language.

The ERPs from adults and 18-month-olds suggest that semantic processing of words and gestures is mediated by similar neural systems in both modalities, as evidenced by similarities in the distribution of the N400 mismatch effect between conditions. Whereas at 18 months infants showed an N400 mismatch effect for both words and gestures, at 26 months, infants showed an N400 mismatch effect only to the word–picture pairings. Thus, for 18-month-olds and adults who process gestures semantically, the neural systems involved in processing meaning, as indexed by the N400, are similar across modalities. In contrast, although the 26-month-olds appear to process words semantically, gestures did not activate the same neural systems. This lack of a mismatch effect for pictures preceded by gestures at 26 months is consistent with the hypothesis offered by Namy and Waxman (1998) that, with increasing language experience, children become more sensitive to the conventional use of symbols appropriate for conveying meaning.

SUMMARY AND CONCLUSIONS

Experience with language has been found to affect the organization of language-relevant brain activity across multiple studies employing different experimental paradigms and at different ages. Developmental changes in the lateral distribution of ERPs across the lifespan suggest that cerebral specializations for language occur along a protracted course of development. None of the findings reviewed support a strong nativist position that left-hemispheric asymmetries observed in very young infants are immutable and reflect an innate language acquisition device within the left hemisphere. In contrast, across all of the studies the findings are consistent with the position that *cerebral specialization for language emerges as a function of learning and to some extent depends on the rate of learning*. The findings from both phonological and gesture processing suggest that inexperienced word learners initially accept a broader range of symbols and sounds for communication, but with increasing experience become more discriminating in delineating acceptable forms for spoken language. A similar trend is observed in developmental changes in the organization of brain activity from broadly distributed patterns to more focal activity with increasing proficiency. We do not mean to suggest that these finding are consistent with a pattern of progressive lateralization that occurs as a function of brain maturation. Instead the studies suggest that functional specializations are dynamic, change as a function of the immediate task, and interact with a variety of language-specific and domain-general processes such as prosody, phonology, working memory, and nonverbal communication (e.g., gestures). Future studies will examine these hypotheses further by measuring the effect of task difficulty on patterns of brain activity.

From an educational perspective, this type of research can be applied at many levels. Both behavioral and electrophysiological studies contribute to our basic understanding of the processes involved in normal language development. The findings reviewed here suggest that a variety of domain-general cognitive functions such as attention and memory interact with more language-specific functions such as phonological processing and processing of prosodic information. Accurate assessment of these mediating factors can, in turn, provide information that can be used to help children with different types of language delay. Additionally, early observation of abnormal patterns of activity can be used to identify infants who might be at risk for language delay. This idea is not new; ERPs have been shown to be an effective tool in early detection of later language problems (Molfese et al., 1999). However, here we suggest that the observed abnormal patterns of activity may not be the cause but rather the result of language delay. The implications of this position suggest that if effective learning strategies are implemented, the patterns of brain activity can be changed as well. Finally, another practical application is the use of electrophysiological techniques to test the effectiveness of different educational programs, and the potential beneficial effects of preschool programs in terms of language experience, in the case of children with suboptimal home environments.

ACKNOWLEDGMENTS

The research reported here was supported by grants from the National Institute of Deafness and Communication Disorders (No. NIH 5 RO1-DC0048111), to Helen Neville, and the Emory University Research Committee, to Debra Mills. We thank Chantel Prat, Terra Llamas, Marie St. George, Molly Larson, Dede Addy, and Amy Hood for help in data collection and averaging. We are particularly indebted to the participants in the studies and their parents.

REFERENCES

Acredolo, L., & Goodwyn, S. (1985). Symbolic gesturing in language development: A case study. *Human Development, 28,* 40–49.

Acredolo, L., & Goodwyn, S. (1988). Symbolic gesturing in normal infants. *Child Development, 59,* 450–466.

Addy, D. A., & Mills, D. L. (2005, April). *Brain activity to familiar, unfamiliar, and backward words in infants 3- to 10-months of age.* Poster presented at the biennial meeting of the Society for Research in Child Development, Atlanta, GA.

Alcaini, M., Giard, M., Echallier, J., & Pernier, J. (1994). Selective auditory attention effects in tonotopically organized cortical areas: A topographic ERP study. *Human Brain Mapping, 2,* 159–169.

Baldwin, D. A., & Markman, E. M. (1989). Establishing word object relations: A first step. *Child Development, 60,* 381–398.

Baldwin, D. A, & Moses, L. J. (2001). Links between social understanding and early word learning: Challenges to current accounts. *Social Development, 10,* 309–329.

Bates, E., Bretherton, I., Snyder, L., Shore, C., & Volterra, V. (1980). Vocal and gestural symbols at 13 months. *Merrill–Palmer Quarterly, 26,* 407–423.

Bates, E., & Roe, C. (2001). Language development in children with focal brain injury. In C. Nelson & M. Luciana (Eds.), *Handbook of developmental cognitive neuroscience* (pp. 281–307). Cambridge, MA: MIT Press.

Bellugi, U., Lichtenberger, L., Mills, D., Galaburda, A., & Korenberg, J. (1999). Bridging cognition, brain and molecular genetics: Evidence from Williams syndrome. *Trends in Neuroscience, 22,* 193–236.

Bertoncini, J. (1998). Initial capacities for speech processing: Infant's attention to prosodic cues to segmentation. In F. Simion & G. Butterworth (Eds.), *The development of sensory, motor, and cognitive capacities in early infancy: From perception to cognition* (pp. 161–170). Hillsdale, NJ: Erlbaum.

Bettes, B. (1988). Maternal depression and motherese: Temporal and intonational features. *Child Development, 59,* 1089–1096.

Blake, J., & Dolgoy, S. (1993). Gestural development and its relation to cognition during the transition to language. *Journal of Nonverbal Behavior, 17*(2), 87–102.

Christophe, A., Dupoux, E., Bertoncini, J., & Mehler, J. (1994). Do infants perceive word boundaries? An empirical study of the bootstrapping of lexical acquisition. *Journal of the Acoustical Society of America, 95,* 1570–1580.

Coch, D., Grossi, G., Skendzel, W., & Neville, H. (2005). ERP nonword rhyming effects in children and adults. *Journal of Cognitive Neuroscience, 17,* 168–182.

Coch, D., Maron, L., Wolf, M., & Holcomb, P. J. (2002). Word and picture processing in children: An event-related potential study. *Developmental Neuropsychology, 22,* 373–406.

Conboy, B., & Mills, D. L. (2006). Two languages, one developing brain: Event-related potentials to words in bilingual toddlers. *Developmental Science, 9,* F1–F12.

Connolly, J. F., Service, E., D'Arcy, R. C. N., Kujala, A., & Alho, K. (2001). Phonological aspects of word recognition as revealed by high-resolution spatio-temporal brain mapping. *NeuroReport, 12,* 237–243.

Cooper, R. P., & Aslin, R. N. (1990). Preference of infant-directed speech in the first month after birth. *Child Development, 61,* 1584–1595.

Cooper, R. P., & Aslin, R. N. (1994). Developmental differences in infant attention to the spectral properties of infant-directed speech. *Child Development, 65,* 1663–1677.

Courchesne, E. (1978). Neurophysiological correlates of cognitive development: Changes in long-latency event-related potentials from childhood to adulthood. *Electroencephalography and Clinical Neurophysiology, 45,* 468–482.

D'Arcy, R. C. N., Connolly, J. F., Service, E., Hawco, C. S., & Houlihan, M. E. (2004). Separating phonological and semantic processing in auditory sentence processing: A high-resolution event-related brain potential study. *Human Brain Mapping, 22,* 40–51.

Dawson, G., Finley, C., Phillips, S., & Lewy, A. (1989). A comparison of hemispheric asymmetries in speech-related brain potentials of autistic and dysphasic children. *Brain and Language, 37,* 26–41.

De Fosse, L., Hodge, S. M., Makris, N., Kennedy, D. N., Caviness, V. S, Jr., McGrath, L., et al. (2004). Language-association cortex asymmetry in autism and Specific Language Impairment. *Annals of Neurology, 56,* 757–766.

Dehaene-Lambertz, G. (2000). Cerebral specialization for speech and non-speech stimuli in infants. *Journal of Cognitive Neuroscience, 12,* 449–460.

Dehaene-Lambertz, G., & Baillet, S. (1998). A phonological representation in the infant brain. *NeuroReport, 9,* 1885–1888.

Dehaene-Lambertz, G., & Dehaene, S. (1994). Speed and cerebral correlates of syllable discrimination in infants. *Nature, 370,* 292–295.

Dehaene-Lambertz, G., Dehaene, S., & Hertz-Pannier, L. (2002). Functional neuroimaging of speech perception in infants. *Science, 298,* 2013–2015.

Dehaene-Lambertz, G., & Gliga, T. (2004). Common neural basis for phoneme processing in infants and adults. *Journal of Cognitive Neuroscience, 16,* 1375–1387.

Dehaene-Lambertz, G., & Pena, M. (2001). Electrophysiological evidence for automatic phonetic processing in neonates. *NeuroReport, 12,* 3155–3158.

Dennis, M., & Whitaker, H. A. (1976). Hemispheric equipotentiality and language acquisition. In S. J. Segalowitz & F. A. Gruber (Eds.), *Language development and neurological theory* (pp. 93–105). New York: Academic Press.

de Ochoa, E., Mills, D. L., & Kutas, M. (2007). [Brain activity to semantic and word order violations in auditory sentences with elderly adults]. Unpublished raw data.

Dore, J. (1974). A pragmatic description of early language development. *Journal of Psycholinguistic Research, 4,* 423–430.

Durston, S., Thomas, K., Yang, Y., Ulug, A. M., Zimmerman, R. D., & Casey, B. J. (2002). A neural basis for the development of inhibitory control. *Developmental Science, 5,* 9–16.

Elman, J. L., Bates, E. A., Johnson, M. H., Karmiloff-Smith, A., Parisi, D., & Plunkett, K. (1996). *Rethinking innateness: A connectionist perspective on development.* Cambridge, MA: MIT Press.

Entus, A. (1977). Hemispheric asymmetry in processing of dichotically presented speech and nonspeech stimuli by infants. In S. Segalowitz & F. Gruber (Eds.), *Language development and neurological theory* (pp. 63–73). New York: Academic Press.

Fenson, L., Dale, P. S., Reznick, J. S., Bates, E., Thal, D. J., & Pethick, S. J. (1994). Variability in early communicative development. *Monographs of the Society for Research in Child Development, 59*, 1–173.

Fernald, A. (1985). Four-month-old infants prefer to listen to motherese. *Infant Behavior and Development, 8*, 181–195.

Fernald, A. (2000). Speech to infants as hyperspeech: Knowledge-driven processes in early word recognition. *Phonetica, 57*, 242–254.

Friedrich, M., & Friederici, A. D. (2004). N400-like semantic incongruity effect in 19-month-olds: Processing known words in picture contexts. *Journal of Cognitive Neuroscience, 16*, 1465–1477.

Friedrich, M., & Friederici, A. D. (2005). Lexical priming and semantic integration selected in the event-related potential of 14-month-olds. *NeuroReport, 16*, 653–656.

Fuchigami, T., Okubo, O., Fujita, Y., & Okuni, M. (1993). Auditory event-related potentials and reaction time in children: Evaluation of cognitive development. *Developmental Medicine and Child Neurology, 35*, 230–237.

Gershkoff-Stowe, L. (2002). Object naming, vocabulary growth, and the development of word retrieval abilities. *Journal of Memory and Language, 46*, 665–687.

Gopnik, A., & Meltzoff, A. (1987). The development of categorization in the second year and its relation to the other cognitive and linguistic developments. *Child Development, 58*, 1523–1531.

Greenough, W. T., Black, J. E., Klintsova, A., Bates, K. E., & Weiler, I. J. (1999). Experience and plasticity in brain structure: Possible implications of basic research findings for developmental disorders. In S. Broman & J. Fletcher (Eds.), *The changing nervous system: Neurobehavioral consequences of early brain disorders* (pp. 51–70). New York: Oxford University Press.

Gunnar, M., & Nelson, C. S. (1994). Event-related potentials in year-old infants predict negative emotionality and hormonal responses to separation. *Child Development, 65*, 80–94.

Herbert, M. R., Harris, G. J., Adrien, K.T., Ziegler, D. A., Makris, N., Kennedy, D. N., et al. (2002). Abnormal asymmetry in language association cortex in autism. *Annals of Neurology, 52*, 588–596.

Herbert, M. R., Ziegler, D. A., Deutsch, C. K., O'Brien, L. M., Kennedy, D. N., Filipek, P. A., et al. (2005). Brain asymmetries in autism and developmental language disorder: A nested whole-brain analysis. *Brain, 128*, 213–226.

Hillyard, S. A., Mangun, G. R., Woldorff, M. G., & Luck, S. (1995). Neural systems mediating selective attention. In M. S. Gazzaniga (Ed.), *The cognitive neurosciences* (pp. 665–681). Cambridge, MA: MIT Press.

Hirsh-Pasek, K., Kemler Nelson, D., Jusczyk, P., Cassidy, K., Druss, B., & Kennedy, L. (1987). Clauses are perceptual units for young infants. *Cognition, 26*, 269–286.

Holcomb, P. J., Coffey, S. A., & Neville, H. J. (1992). Visual and auditory sentence processing: A developmental analysis using event-related brain potentials. *Developmental Neuropsychology, 8*, 203–241.

Huot, R., Larson, M., Addy, D., Stowe, Z., Walker, E., & Mills, D. L. (2005,

April). *Maternal depression alters brain activity of offspring in response to infant-directed speech.* Poster presented at biennial meeting of the Society for Research in Child Development, Atlanta, GA.

Huotilainen, M., Winkler, I., Alho, K., Escera, C., Virtanen, J., & Ilmoniemi, R. L. (1998) Combined mapping of human auditory EEG and MEG responses. *Electroencephalography and Clinical Neurophysiology, 108,* 370–379.

Iverson, J., Capirci, O., & Caselli, M. (1994). From communication to language in two modalities. *Cognitive Development, 9,* 23–43.

Johnson, M. H. (2001). Functional brain development in humans. *Nature Reviews Neuroscience, 2,* 475–483.

Johnson, M. H. (2005). *Developmental cognitive neuroscience.* Malden, MA: Blackwell.

Jusczyk, P., Hirsh-Pasek, K., Kemler Nelson, D., Kennedy, L., Woodward, A., & Piwoz, J. (1992). Perception of acoustic correlates of major phrasal units by young infants. *Cognitive Psychology, 24,* 252–293.

Kaplan, P. S., Bachorowski, J. A., Smoski, M. J., & Zinzer, M. C. (2001). Role of clinical diagnosis in effects of maternal depression on infant-directed speech. *Infancy, 2,* 533–544.

Key, A. P. J., Dove, G. O., & Maguire, M. (2005). Linking brainwaves to the brain: An ERP primer. *Developmental Neuropsychology, 27,* 183–215.

Kinsbourne, M. (1975). The ontogeny of cerebral dominance. *Annals of the New York Academy of Sciences, 263,* 244–250.

Kohn, B., & Dennis, M. (1974). Patterns of hemispheric specialization after hemidecortication for infantile hemiplegia. In M. Kinsbourne & W. L. Smith (Eds.), *Hemispheric disconnection and cerebral function* (pp. 34–47). Springfield, IL: Thomas.

Kutas, M., & Hillyard, S. A. (1980). Reading senseless sentences: Brain potentials reflect semantic incongruity. *Science, 207,* 203–220.

Larson, M., Lewis, E., Horton, C., Addy, D., & Mills, D. (2005, March). *Working memory and early language development.* Poster at biennial meeting of the Society for Research in Child Development, Atlanta, GA.

Lenneberg, E. (1967). *Biological foundations of language.* New York: Wiley.

Little, V. M., Thomas, D. G., & Letterman, M. R. (1999). Single-trial analyses of developmental trends in infant auditory event-related potentials. *Developmental Neuropsychology, 16,* 455–478.

Luck, S. J., & Hillyard, S. A. (2000). The operation of selective attention at multiple stages of processing: Evidence from human and monkey electrophysiology. In M. S. Gazzaniga (Ed.), *The new cognitive neurosciences* (pp. 687–700). Cambridge, MA: MIT Press.

McCune, L. (1995). A normative study of representational play in the transition to language. *Developmental Psychology, 31,* 198–206.

McCune-Nicolich, L. (1981). The cognitive bases of relational words in the single word period. *Journal of Child Language, 8,* 15–34.

McRoberts, G. W. (2000, July). *The role of infant age and age-of-addressee in ID speech preferences.* Paper presented at the international conference of Infant Studies, Brighton, UK.

McShane, J. (1979). The development of naming. *Linguistics, 17*, 879–905.

Mills, D. L., Alvarez, T. D., St. George, M., Appelbaum, L. G., Neville, H., & Bellugi, U. (2000). Electrophysiological studies of face recognition in Williams syndrome. *Journal of Cognitive Neuroscience, 12*(Suppl.), 47–64.

Mills, D. L., Coffey-Corina, S. A., & Neville, H. (1993). Language acquisition and cerebral specialization in 20-month-old infants. *Journal of Cognitive Neuroscience, 5*, 317–334.

Mills, D. L., Coffey-Corina, S. A., & Neville, H. H. (1994). Variability in cerebral organization during primary language acquisition. In G. Dawson & K. Fischer (Eds.), *Human behavior and the developing brain* (pp. 427–455). New York: Guilford Press.

Mills, D. L., Coffey-Corina, S. A., & Neville, H. J. (1997). Language comprehension and cerebral specialization from 13 to 20 months. *Developmental Neuropsychology, 13*, 397–445.

Mills, D. L., Conboy, B., & Paton, C. (2005). Do changes in brain organization reflect shifts in symbolic functioning? In L. Namy (Ed.), *Symbol use and symbolic representation* (pp. 123–153). Mahwah, NJ: Erlbaum.

Mills, D. L., & Neville, H. J. (1997). Electrophysiological studies of language and language impairment. *Seminars in Pediatric Neurology, 4*, 125–134.

Mills, D., Plunkett, K., Prat, C., & Schafer, G. (2005). Watching the infant brain learn words: Effects of language and experience. *Cognitive Development, 20*, 19–31.

Mills, D. L., Prat, C., Llamas, T., & Thal, D. (2007). *Cerebral specializations during early language development: Electrophysiological evidence from late talkers*. Manuscript in preparation.

Mills, D., Prat, C., Stager, C., Zangl, R., Neville, H., & Werker, J. (2004). Language experience and the organization of brain activity to phonetically similar words: ERP evidence from 14- and 20-month olds. *Journal of Cognitive Neuroscience, 16*, 1452–1464.

Molfese, D. L. (1973). Central asymmetry in infants, children and adults: Auditory evoked responses to speech and music. *Journal of the Acoustical Society of America, 53*, 363–373.

Molfese, D. L., Burger-Judisch, L. M., & Hans, L. L. (1991). Consonant discrimination by newborn infants: Electrophysiological differences. *Developmental Neuropsychology, 7*, 177–195.

Molfese, D., Freeman, R., & Palermo, D. S. (1975). The ontogeny of brain lateralization for speech and nonspeech stimuli. *Brain and Language, 2*, 356–368.

Molfese, D. L., Molfese, V. J., & Espy, K. A. (1999). The predictive use of event-related potentials in language development and the treatment of language disorders. *Developmental Neuropsychology, 16*, 373–377.

Moses, P., & Stiles, J. (2002). The lesion methodology: Contrasting views from adult and child studies. *Developmental Psychobiology, 40*, 266–277.

Muller, R. A. (1996). Innateness, autonomy, universality?: Neurobiological approaches to language. *Behavioral and Brain Sciences, 19*, 611–675.

Naatanen, R., & Picton, T. (1987). The N1 wave of the human electric and magnetic response to sound: A review and analysis of the component structure. *Psychophysiology, 24,* 375–425.

Namy, L., & Waxman, S. (1998). Words and gestures: Infants' interpretations of different forms of symbolic reference. *Child Development, 69,* 295–308.

Nazzi, T., & Bertoncini, J. (2003). Before and after the vocabulary spurt: Two modes of word acquisition? *Developmental Science, 6,* 136–142.

Nelson, C. A., & Luciana, M. (2001). *Handbook of developmental cognitive neuroscience.* Cambridge, MA: MIT Press.

Nelson, C. A., & Monk, C. S. (2001). The use of event-related potentials in the study of cognitive development. In C. Nelson & M. Luciana (Eds.), *Handbook of developmental cognitive neuroscience* (pp. 125–136). Cambridge, MA: MIT Press.

Neville, H. J., & Bavelier, D. (2002). Specificity and plasticity in neurocognitive development in humans. In M. Johnson & Y. Munakata (Eds.), *Brain development and cognition: A reader* (2nd ed., pp. 251–271). Malden, MA: Blackwell.

Neville, H. J., Coffey, S. A., Holcomb, P. J., & Tallal, P. (1993). The neurobiology of sensory and language processing in language impaired children. *Journal of Cognitive Neuroscience, 5,* 235–334.

Neville, H. J., & Mills, D. L. (1997). Epigenesis of language. *Mental Retardation and Developmental Disabilities Research Reviews, 3,* 282–292.

Papousek, M., Bornstein, M., Nuzzo, C., Papousek, H., & Symmes, D. (1990). Infant responses to prototypical melodic contours in parental speech. *Infant Behavior and Development, 13,* 539–545.

Passarotti, A. M., Paul, B. M., Bussiere, J. R., Buxton, R. B., Wong, E. C., & Stiles, J. (2003). The development of face and location processing: An fMRI study. *Developmental Science, 6,* 100–117.

Pena, M., Maki, A., Kovacic, D., Dehaene-Lambertz, G., Koizumi, H., Bouquet, F., et al. (2003). Sounds and silence: An optical topography study of language recognition at birth. *Proceedings of the National Academy of Science, 100,* 11702–11705.

Plunkett, K., Sinha, C., Møller, M. F., & Strandsby, O. (1992). Symbol grounding or the emergence of symbols?: Vocabulary growth in children and a connectionist net. *Connection Science, 4,* 293–312.

Richards, J. E., & Hunter, S. K. (2002). Testing neural models of the development of infant visual attention. *Developmental Psychobiology, 40,* 226–236.

Saugstad, L. F. (1998). Cerebral lateralisation and rate of maturation. *International Journal of Psychophysiology, 28,* 37–62.

Scherg, M., Vajsar, J., & Picton, T. (1989). A sourced analysis of the late human auditory evoked potentials. *Journal of Cognitive Neuroscience, 1,* 336–355.

Sheehan, E., Namy, L., & Mills, D. L. (in press). Developmental changes in neural activity to familiar words and gestures. *Brain and Language.*

Stager, C., & Werker, J. (1997). Infants listen for more phonetic detail in speech perception than in word-learning tasks. *Nature, 388,* 381–382.

St. George, M., & Mills, D. L. (2001). Electrophysiological studies of language development. In J. Weissenborn & B. Hoehle (Eds.), *Language acquisition and language disorders* (pp. 247–259). Amsterdam: Benjamins.

Stiles, J., Bates, E. A., Thal, D., Trauner, D. A., & Reilly, J. (2002). Linguistic and spatial cognitive development in children with pre- and perinatal focal brain injury: A ten-year overview from the San Diego longitudinal project. In M. Johnson & Y. Munakata (Eds.), *Brain development and cognition: A reader* (2nd ed., pp. 272–291). Malden, MA: Blackwell.

Stiles, J., Moses, P., Roe, K., Akshoomoff, N. A., Trauner, D., Hesselink, J., et al. (2003). Alternative brain organization after prenatal cerebral injury: Convergent fMRI and cognitive data. *Journal of the International Neuropsychological Society, 9,* 604–622.

Swingley, D., & Aslin, R. N. (2000). Spoken word recognition and lexical representation in very young children. *Cognition, 76,* 147–166.

Swingley, D., & Aslin, R. N. (2002). Lexical neighborhoods and the word-form representations of 14-month-olds. *Psychological Science, 13,* 480–484.

Tallal, P. (1978). An experimental investigation of the role of auditory temporal processing in normal and disordered language development. In A. Caramazza & D. Zurif (Eds.), *Language acquisition and language breakdown: Parallels and divergences* (pp. 25–61). Baltimore: Johns Hopkins University Press.

Tamm, L., Menon, V., & Reiss, A. L. (2002). Maturation of brain function associated with response inhibition. *Journal of the American Academy of Child and Adolescent Psychiatry, 41,* 1231–1238.

Thal, D. J., Bates, E., Goodman, J., & Jahn-Samilo, J. (1997). Continuity of language abilities: An exploratory study of late- and early-talking toddlers. *Developmental Neuropsychology, 13,* 239–273.

Toma, R. J., Hanlon, F. M., Moses, S. N., Edgar, J. C., Huang, M., & Weisend, M. P. (2003). Lateralization of auditory sensory gating and neurophysiological dysfunction in schizophrenia. *American Journal of Psychiatry, 160,* 1595–1605.

Tomasello, M. (2001). Perceiving intentions and learning words in the second year of life. In M. Tomasello & E. Bates (Eds.), *Language development: The essential readings* (pp. 111–128). Malden, MA: Blackwell.

Vaughn, H. G., Jr., & Rigger, W. (1970). The sources of auditory evoked responses recorded from the human scalp. *Electroencephalography and Clinical Neurophysiology, 28,* 360–367.

Werker, J., Cohen, L., Lloyd, V., Casasole, M., & Stager, C. (1998). Acquisition of word–object associations by 14-month-old infants. *Developmental Psychology, 34,* 1289–1309.

Werner, H., & Kaplan, B. (1963). *Symbol formation.* New York: Wiley.

Witelson, S. F., & Pallie, W. (1973). Left hemisphere specialization for language in the newborn: Neuroanatomical evidence of asymmetry. *Brain, 96,* 641–647.

Woldorff, M. G. (1993). Distortion of ERP averages due to overlap from temporally adjacent ERPs: Analysis and correction. *Psychophysiology, 30,* 98–119.

Zangl, R., & Mills, D. L. (2007). Brain activity to infant versus adult directed speech in 6- and 13-month-olds. *Infancy, 11*(1), 31–62.

CHAPTER 8

Temperament and Biology

Jerome Kagan
Nancy Snidman

It is always more fruitful in immature scientific disciplines to focus on the phenomena to be explained rather than on how to operationalize a concept believed to apply to a set of phenomena. Hence, this chapter on the concept *temperament* begins with a description of the observations that motivated the invention of the term. Infants and young children vary in behaviors, acute emotions, and moods that are influenced by their biology and are preserved over time, albeit modestly. The implicit model for human temperaments is the psychological variation noted among strains or subspecies of animals. Dog breeds vary in timidity following encounter with novelty (Scott & Fuller, 1965), and quail chicks vary in the duration of body immobility when placed on their back and restricted by a human hand (Williamson et al., 2003).

Although there is general consensus on the sense meaning of a temperamental bias, there is far less agreement on the number and types of temperaments and their measurement. Readers can consult books that present diverse views on this issue, especially Kohnstamm, Bates, and Rothbart (1989), Strelau and Angleitner (1991), Bates and Wachs (1994), and Plomin and McClearn (1993).

Although political tension created by European immigration exiled temperamental constructs during the first half of the 20th century, the research of Thomas and Chess (1977) was an important reason for their return. These two psychiatrists inferred nine temperamental dimensions, along with three abstract categories, from lengthy interviews with well-educated parents and observations of their infants. The most prevalent of the three temperamental categories was the "easy child," about 40% of the sample, who was regular in bodily activity and approached unfamiliar objects with an engaging mood. A second category, about 15% of the sample, was called "slow-to-warm-up" because these children reacted to unfamiliarity with withdrawal. The smallest group, about 10% of the sample, was labeled "difficult" because they were labile, irritable, avoided novelty, and seemed poorly adapted to their homes.

NEUROCHEMISTRY AND TEMPERAMENT

We believe that the biological bases for most, but probably not all, temperamental biases are heritable neurochemical profiles, a hypothesis anticipated earlier (McDougall, 1929; Rich, 1928). Research on voles provides an illustration. Prairie and montane voles, two closely related strains, differ in the tendency to pair bond following several hours of mating. Prairie voles pair bond but montane voles do not. Variation in the promoter region of the genes that influence the distribution of receptors for vasopressin in males and oxytocin in females contributes to the dramatic behavioral difference. This genetic difference between the two strains determines where in the brain the receptors for vasopressin or oxytocin will be activated. The receptors in limbic sites believed to mediate states of pleasure are, for genetic reasons, more active in prairie voles than in montane voles (Insel, Wang, & Ferris, 1994).

Because there is heritable variation in the concentration, density, and location of receptors for more than 150 different molecules that can affect brain function, a very large number of neurochemical profiles could potentially influence behaviors and moods. Even if a majority of these profiles had little relevance for temperament, the very large number of possible profiles suggests that human populations contain a great many temperaments, each one influenced by a neurochemistry that affects the usual psychological reaction to particular classes of events. Some molecules are excitatory and others inhibitory, and a balance between these two processes determines the brain state evoked by an event. For example, the balance between opioids and corticotropin releasing hormone in the locus coeruleus contributes to an animal's reaction to a stressor (van Bockstaele, Bajic, Proudfit, & Valentino, 2001). Variation in the density of receptors for a molecule is often independent of the concentration of the molecule. Some mice strains show high levels of tyrosine hydroxylase in the cortex (an enzyme involved in the synthesis of dopamine and norepinephrine) but a low density of receptors for norepinephrine, whereas other strains are high or low on both of these properties (Dyaglo & Shishkina, 2000). If we assume that the concentration of a particular molecule, as well as the density of its varied receptors, can be low, moderate, or high, there will be nine possible profiles for each molecule. If there were 150 molecules, then at least 1,400 neurochemical profiles, reciprocally influencing each other, could form the biological bases of human temperaments.

Contemporary research nominates a number of relevant molecules. These include norepinephrine, dopamine, serotonin, acetycholine, gamma-aminobutyric acid (GABA), glutamate, opioids, corticotropin releasing hormone (CRH), vasopressin, prolactin, and oxytocin. Many of these molecules are found in varied brain sites. GABA, for example, is found in close to 40% of all synapses, although it has its greatest density in the basal ganglia and limbic system. Most molecules have more than one receptor. For example, dopamine has five types of receptors and serotonin, nine each with varying densities in different brain sites.

Scientists do not yet understand how this complex web of neurochemical events contributes to the brain's reaction to an incentive event because each of the different balances among many molecules is linked to a distinct brain state. But all psychologists have to work with are the behavioral outcomes and some biological correlates. However, speculative arguments are possible. Consider the fact that GABA-ergic and serotonergic circuits usually inhibit neuronal activity. Hence, infants born with a compromise in either of these transmitter systems should be less effective in modulating extreme excitement or distress. This implication finds support in the fact that very irritable 2-year-olds, compared with relaxed children, inherit the shorter form of an allele located in the promoter region for the serotonin transporter gene (Auerbach et al., 1999). Japanese differ from Europeans in the prevalence of the short or long forms of this allele, and Japanese infants are less irritable than European infants (Kumakiri et al., 1999). In addition, adults with the shorter allele show greater amygdalar activity in response to fear-provoking stimuli, compared with adults with the longer form (Hariri et al., 2002). However, nature is not consistently compliant; very shy Israeli children inherit the longer, rather than the shorter, form of this allele (Arbelle et al., 2003).

A second hypothetical cascade involves a molecule called gastrin-releasing peptide, which acts on the receptors of interneurons to release GABA that, in turn, inhibits neural activity. Mice lacking the gene for this class of receptor fail to release GABA in the amygdalar neurons and, as a consequence, preserve traces of the association between a conditioned stimulus and electric shock for a longer period of time (Shumyatsky et al., 2002). It is possible, therefore, that children who possess an allele of the gene for this peptide associated with compromised GABA activity in the amygdala would preserve a fearful posture over longer periods of time (Maren, Yap, & Goosens, 2001; Sanders, 2001).

Variation in dopamine release and in the density of its varied receptors regulates cortical excitability, intensity of sensory pleasure, and reactions to novel events. The moment a rat places its paws in an unfamiliar environment, dopamine is released in the nucleus accumbens and can remain there for as long as 8 seconds (Rebec, Christianson, Guevra, & Bardo, 1997). In addition, higher levels of cortical dopamine suppress neuronal activity in the corpus striatum, resulting in fewer volleys from striatum to cortex, and, as a result, lower cortical excitability. Greater dopamine activity in the cortex also implies that a new event will produce a proportionally smaller rise in dopamine. These facts imply that children or adults with greater cortical dopamine activity might have a lower preference for novel experiences than those with less dopamine activity. It is relevant that females have more dopamine receptors in the brain than males (Kaasinen, Nagren, Hietala, Farde, & Rinne, 2001) and that females are less likely than males to seek novel, high-risk experiences (Hyde, 2005).

Variation in norepinephrine and its receptors modulates preferred reactions to novelty, alertness, sustained attention in the face of distracting stimuli, and thresholds for detecting subtle changes in sensory input. Wistar rats that explore unfamiliar areas have greater norepinephrine activity in the nucleus accumbens than other animals from this strain; as a result, projections from the amygdala are enhanced when they arrive at the nucleus accumbens (Roozendaal & Cools, 1994). Release of norepinephrine in the amygdala is potentiated by epinephrine acting on norepinephrine receptors in the basolateral nucleus (McGaugh & Cahill, 2003). Hence, variation in the density of receptors for norepinephrine in the amygdala, together with the sensitivity of the basolateral receptors to epinephrine, should affect behaviors that are classified as temperamental (Cecchi, Khoshbouei, Javors, & Morilak, 2002).

The varied classes of opioids monitor the intensity of visceral afferent feedback from the body to the nucleus tractus solitarius in the medulla. Less opioid activity means more intense volleys from the medulla to the amygdala. As a consequence, the orbitofrontal prefrontal cortex, which receives projections from the amygdala, will be vulnerable to greater activation. One possible consequence of this cascade is a more intense state of worry, tension, or dysphoria, or greater difficulty extinguishing a conditioned fear (McNally & Westbrook, 2003). By contrast, individuals with greater opioid activity in the medulla should enjoy more frequent moments of serenity (Miyawki, Goodchild, & Pilowsky, 2002; Wang & Wessendorf, 2002). Some variation in opioid activity can originate in prenatal events rather than in heredity. Female mice embryos lying between two males or next to a male, when compared with those lying between two females, are affected by the surge in testosterone the male embryo secretes. One consequence of their prenatal position is an increase in mu-opioid receptors in the midbrain that, postnatally, is accompanied by a higher pain threshold (Morley-Fletcher, Palanza, Parolaro, Vigano, & Laviola, 2003).

CRH, secreted by the hypothalamus, influences a great many systems but especially the hypthalamic–pituitary–adrenal axis. One consequence is the secretion of cortisol. Capuchin monkeys with high cortisol levels are more avoidant of novelty than animals with lower cortisol levels (Byrne & Suomi, 2002). In humans, there is a relation between an allele at a CRH locus and avoidant behavior in children, especially among children who have a parent with panic disorder (Smoller et al., 2004).

High doses of glucocorticoids injected into the central nucleus of the amygdala potentiate the release of CRH as well as the startle (Lee, Schulkin, & Davis, 1994) and prolonged freezing (Takahashi & Rubin, 1994) responses in rats. CRH stimulates the secretion of cortisol, and monkeys that avoid novel objects and situations and, in addition, have high cortisol levels are likely to show right rather than left frontal activation in the EEG (Kalin, Larson, Shelton, & Davidson, 1998). Monkeys with an extreme degree of right frontal activation had higher levels of CRH across the interval from 4 to 52 months of age (Kalin, Shelton, & Davidson, 2000).

Despite this list of interesting facts, there is no simple or linear relation between cortisol levels and reactions to aversive events or self-reported moods. For example, adults given either 20 or 40 mg of cortisol, compared with a placebo, were asked to rate unpleasant and neutral words and pictures and, in addition, to describe their changing moods. Although the subjects who received cortisol showed a rise in circulating hormone, there was no relation between their cortisol level and reports of their feelings or their ratings of the emotionality of the words and pictures (Abercrombie, Kalin, Thurow, Rosenkranz, & Davidson, 2003). Gunnar (1994) has argued that high levels of cortisol do not determine any particular behavior across persons and situations. Cortisol levels are subject to too many temporary states to be used as a sensitive sign of any temperament. Bold, extraverted, preschool children are more active than shy ones early in the school year and show, on a few occasions, very high cortisol levels. However, several months later, after the shy children have become accustomed to a school setting and have begun to socialize with their peers, they, too, show occasional days with high cortisol levels. Thus, the variation in the number of spikes in cortisol is related to a child's temporary state and level of activity. We found no significant relation between early morning salivary cortisol levels in 87 5- and 7-month-old infants and either their reactivity to stimuli, frequency of smiling, or fearfulness (Kagan, 1994). It is unlikely that any single biological variable will define a temperamental bias—there are no silver bullets.

The immaturity of current knowledge relating neurochemistry to temperamental qualities frustrates any attempt to posit a specific relation between a chemical profile and a temperament. Because genetic variation accounts for less than 10% of the variation in most complex behaviors, it is unlikely that a particular allele affecting a brain molecule or receptor distribution determines any specific temperamental type. Hence, at the present time, a human temperament cannot be defined by a specific neurobiology. One reason for this skepticism is that the number of possible neurochemical profiles that can influence behavior is much larger than the number of ways a child can display a class of behavior. Furthermore, each measure of bodily activity is subject to local influences unrelated to the central brain mechanisms that are believed to be the primary foundation of a temperament. Psychologists also appreciate the reciprocal relations between brain and body, on the one hand, and psychological states, on the other.

Finally, it is important to appreciate the extraordinary specificity of brain–mind relationships. The areas of the brain that cause a rat to avoid a probe that delivers electric shock are not the same as those that cause a rat to bury woodchips following the same electric shock; the amygdala is necessary for the former, whereas the septum is necessary for the latter (Treit, Pesold, & Rotzinger, 1993a, 1993b). The circuit that mediates defensive aggression to a noxious stimulus does not require the amygdala, whereas the freezing response to an intruder does; by contrast, freezing does not require the hypothalamus, but the rise in heart rate in response to an intruder is likely to involve the amygdala and its projection to the lateral hypothalamus (Fanselow, 1994). In summary, the different responses that are often regarded as equivalent indexes of a fear state are mediated by distinct neural circuits and, therefore, probably create different states of fear.

AGREEMENTS AND CONTROVERSIES

Most investigators of temperament agree on a small number of issues. First, the major structures of the limbic system—parahippocampal region, hippocampus, cingulate, septum, hypothalamus, and amygdala, as well as their projections—participate in the variation regarded as temperamental. Second, the excitability of these structures is influenced by many genes. Third, the known biological correlates of a temperament have only modest associations with the behavioral components of the category (Bates & Wachs, 1994; Kagan, 1994).

This trio of agreements is set against three nodes of controversy. One tension is the difference between investigators who begin their research with a priori concepts and those who begin with phenomena. The former try to find measures for their theoretical conception of temperament. The latter, a smaller group, following Francis Bacon, allow the data to guide inferences of a temperamental concept.

A second controversy involves the idea of essences. Some investigators write about a temperamental type as if it had a fixed set of behavioral and psychological measures, resembling the way a disease is described. The less popular view maintains that each child begins life with a particular temperamental profile that undergoes change as a result of experience. As experiences are encountered and accommodated to, psychological and biological changes occur. Because there are dramatic behavioral changes over the first dozen years, the temperamental categories assigned to infants necessarily differ from the constructs used for adolescents or adults that are products of environments sculpting the initial temperaments. A drop of black ink in a container of glycerine soon becomes invisible when stirred. Although the ink cannot be seen, it has altered the composition of the glycerine. An infant's temperamental bias, like the drop of black ink, is not observable in older children or adults, even though it influences moods and behaviors. Scientists might one day discover the critical features that define each of the many temperaments.

SOURCES OF EVIDENCE

Another significant controversy involves the evidence used to measure a temperamental type or dimension. The validity of every inference is intimately tied to the origin of its observations. Estimates of the age of a species vary considerably if fossils rather than proteins are the basis for the judgment. The usual evidence in studies of temperament is a verbal report provided by a parent or, less often, by teachers or peers. A less frequent source is behavioral observations, usually in the laboratory, but occasionally at home or in a school setting. The least common source of evidence involves biology. Each source of information has a unique structure. Behavioral observations are not a valid proxy for parental descriptions or biology; biological measures are not a proxy for behavior or parent reports; and parental reports are not a valid proxy for behavioral observations, especially when emotions and reactions to emotionally salient situations are the dependent variables of interest. That does not mean that parental descriptions are of no value; to the contrary, they can reflect the parent's perception of the child and whether that perception is consistent or inconsistent with the parent's ego ideal.

Although adult descriptions of children on questionnaires have the advantage of sampling behaviors across settings and time, and can refer to events that cannot be observed in the laboratory (e.g., the reaction to serious injury or illness), these data have special problems. The most popular questionnaires are the Infant Characteristics Questionnaire (ICQ; Bates, 1989), the Infant Behavior Questionnaire (IBQ; Rothbart, 1981), the Child Behavior Questionnaire (CBQ; Rothbart, Ahadi, & Hershey, 1994), the Revised Infant Temperament Questionnaire (RITQ; Carey & McDevitt, 1978), and the Emotionality, Activity, Sociability Questionnaire (EAS; Buss & Plomin, 1984). The reasons for skepticism toward sole reliance on questionnaires can be stated succinctly. First, questionnaires cannot gather data about qualities that are not observable, especially biological variation. Second, psychologists can ask informants only about qualities the latter understand, using words that are part of a familiar vocabulary. A small group of infants are minimally irritable, smile frequently, have a low heart rate, low muscle tension, and greater activation of the EEG in the left frontal area. The psychologist who invented a novel temperamental name for this combination of qualities could not ask a parent to rate his or her child on this quality because the parent has no access to the child's biology.

Moreover, parents vary in the accuracy of their descriptions, where accuracy is defined by a filmed record of the child's behavior. Parents of infants did not agree in their ratings of fearfulness, smiling, or sociability because the fathers interpreted high activity in their children as reflecting a positive emotional mood, whereas the mothers regarded the same behavior as reflecting anger (Goldsmith & Campos, 1990). Languages are not rich enough to describe all the important feelings and behaviors that are components of a temperamental category. Finally, the social class and personality of parents influence their descriptions of children. Mothers who never attended college described their infants as less adaptive and less sociable than college-educated parents (Spiker, Klebanov, & Brooks-Gunn, 1992). An exhaustive review of the level of agreement among parents, teachers, and peers on the occurrence of a variety of behavioral and emotional problems in over 269 samples revealed poor agreement among the informants as to whether a child was fearful, aggressive, or impulsive (Achenbach, 1985; Klein, 1991).

In sum, even though parents and teachers have opportunities to observe children in a variety of natural situations over long periods of time, and laboratory observations are often artificial and of short duration, there are unique influences on adult descriptions that are absent when behaviors requiring minimal inference are recorded on film and coded by disinterested observers. Because future discoveries of significance are likely to come from behavioral observations combined with parental, teacher, or peer reports, rather than from either source of data alone, it is important that psychologists not treat conclusions derived from only one of these sources of information as being equivalent in meaning to the other. George von Bekesy, who received a Nobel Prize for his research on hearing, told a young scientist, "The method is everything." Each method, whether questionnaire, behavioral observation, or biology, provides different information, and each requires a distinct construct. Although questionnaire data should not be ignored, scientists who rely only on questionnaires must recognize that the validity of their inferences is restricted to that class of information. The same caveat applies, of course, to those who gather only behavioral observations. Future research will reveal that substantial progress will follow greater reliance on a combination of informant report and behavioral observations gathered across diverse settings.

Infant Temperaments

Developmental psychologists regard a small number of infant behaviors as temperamental, even though their foundation in biology remains uncertain. These include variation in irritability (usually defined by crying and fretting), smiling, activity, and profiles of attention. An extreme level of irritability is preserved, to a modest degree, through part or all of the first year (Birns, Barten, & Bridger, 1969), and newborn irritability to stimulation predicts a less sociable child 2 years later. However, the later consequences of infant irritability that is spontaneous or a reaction to stimulation are different from the consequences of crying produced by the restraint of holding the infant's hands or arms. Infants who cry to restraint have higher vagal tone than those who cry to stimulation (Fox, 1989).

Frequency of spontaneous smiling in infants is heritable (Freedman & Keller, 1963; Repucci, 1968), moderately stable from 3 months to the end of the first year, and predicts smiling following success on a cognitive challenge at 2 years of age (Kagan, 1971). A small number of 4-month-olds (10% of a large sample) who smiled frequently to stimulation had significantly lower diastolic blood pressures at 21 months and low baseline heart rates as preadolescents (Kagan & Snidman, 2004). Furthermore, 2-week-olds who showed high heart rate variability to stimulation were frequent smilers when they were 4 months old (Fish & Fish, 1995).

The concept *activity level* changes its referential meaning between infancy and the preschool years; hence, it is not surprising that there is little preservation of this construct from infancy to the toddler years (Feiring & Lewis, 1980; Matheny, 1983). Variation in activity in monozygotic and dizygotic twins, assessed at 14, 20, and 24 months, was moderately stable and heritable (Saudino & Cherny, 2001). However, a concept of general activity that does not stipulate the age, context of assessment, or time of day is probably not useful theoretically.

Rothbart, Derryberry, and Posner (1994) have described three categories of attention that might constitute temperamental biases. First, there is variation in the rapidity and consistency with which infants orient to a moving object or sound, and the posterior attention network (portions of the parietal cortex, thalamus, and superior colliculus, which are modulated by noradrenergic axons from the locus coeruleus) is involved in this disposition. Second, an anterior attentional network, involving the prefrontal cortex, anterior cingulate, and the supplementary motor area, participates more fully in inhibiting orientation to a distracting stimulus. It is believed that dopaminergic inputs from the ventral tegmental area and basal ganglia modulate this network. Finally, Posner and Peterson (1990) have posited a vigilance system, involving the right lateral midfrontal cortex and influenced by noradrenergic axons in the locus coeruleus, that mediates an alert state that is preserved over a longer period of time.

Temperaments in Older Children

Bates (1989) has nominated seven temperamental concepts in children older than 2 or 3 years of age: variation in distress, disobedience, reaction to unfamiliarity, reactivity to stimulation, activity level, attention regulation, and sociability. Eisenberg et al. (2003) add the ability to regulate emotion and its accompanying behaviors.

Reaction to Unfamiliarity

The child's reactions to unfamiliar people, objects, events, or contexts— whether affective restraint, caution, or avoidance, on the one hand, or spontaneous approach, on the other—have been the targets of the most extensive empirical inquiry. The behavioral reaction to an unfamiliar event depends on (1) whether the child perceives it as a threat, (2) the ease with which it is assimilated, and (3) the availability of an appropriate coping response. All 1-year-olds reach toward a new toy after playing with a different one because the novel object poses no threat, is assimilated at once, and a relevant response is available. However, not all 1-year-olds reach toward a stranger who has extended his or her hand because that event is not assimilated easily and the child may not know what response to display. Thus, children, like adults, live in a corridor bordered on one side by the appeal of the new and on the other by an avoidance of the unfamiliar.

We and our colleagues classify children who consistently display an avoidant or affectively subdued reaction to unfamiliar events that are not obviously dangerous *inhibited*, and children who show minimal avoidance to unfamiliarity as *uninhibited*. The heritability of these two categories, based on behavioral observations of a large sample of monozygotic and dizygotic twins observed at 14, 20, 24, and 36 months of age approached 0.5 (Kagan & Saudino, 2001). However, only 10% of the children were consistently inhibited at all four ages (Kagan & Saudino, 2001). Heritability estimates were higher when the analysis was restricted to children who were extremely inhibited or uninhibited in a play session consisting of four children (DiLalla, Kagan, & Reznick, 1994).

Longitudinal observations on New Zealand children revealed that 3-year-olds rated as shy and subdued, versus sociable and spontaneous, preserved these qualities, albeit modestly, through 18 years of age; the older adolescents described themselves as cautious and likely to avoid dangerous situations (Caspi & Silva, 1995). Of course, not all inhibited 2-year-olds become excessively shy adolescents because adults encourage children to be bold, and inhibited children often try to develop a more sociable profile. Rubin, Burgess, and Hastings (2002) found that 2-year-olds who were inhibited in the laboratory were most likely to preserve that persona if they had intrusive, hypercritical mothers and were likely to lose that style if their mothers discouraged withdrawal.

There is the possibility that degree of inhibition might be influenced by the season in which conception occurred. Preschool children who were members of the National Longitudinal Sample of Youth were rated for shyness on two different occasions in their homes, separated by 2 years. Fifteen percent of this large sample was rated as very shy on both occasions, and these children were more likely to have been conceived during the period from late July to late September. New Zealand children rated as shy were most likely to be conceived in the months of January and February. Because New Zealand is in the Southern Hemisphere, daylight begins to decrease during these months. Thus, both groups of fetuses that became shy children spent the opening months of their gestation at a time of decreasing daylight (Gortmaker, Kagan, Caspi, & Silva, 1997). The decrease in hours of daylight is accompanied by increased secretion of melatonin and decreased serotonin by the pregnant mother. These changes could affect embryos that were genetically disposed to developing a shy profile and enhance the probability of inhibited behavior during childhood or an affective disorder in the adult years (Pjerk et al., 2004).

Inhibited and Uninhibited Children

The concept of *inhibition to the unfamiliar* is defined by initial avoidance, distress, or subdued affect in response to unfamiliar people, events, objects, or situations in children older than 1 year (Kagan & Snidman, 2004). The child with an inhibited style can learn to control shyness with strangers but often retains an avoidant style to unfamiliar challenges or places. The complementary category, *uninhibited to the unfamiliar*, is defined by a sociable, affectively spontaneous reaction to unfamiliar events. Because some children can acquire a shy or a sociable demeanor as a result of experience alone, without a temperamental contribution, psychologists must differentiate between these two types. They should not treat *shy* behavior as a quality that is due to one cause or separable from the child's life history, physiology, and the context of observation.

The brain states created by (1) encounter with unfamiliarity, (2) a conditioned stimulus signaling an aversive unconditioned event, (3) a biologically significant stimulus, and (4) the anticipation of an undesirable event in the future are distinct states mediated by different neural circuits. For example, cessation of activity in a 2-year-old who sees a clown enter a room is mediated by a circuit involving the amygdala and the central gray, but a startle reaction to a sudden, unexpected loud sound need not involve the amygdala. Acquisition of a classically conditioned rise in heart rate requires the hypothalamus and the sympathetic chain, but not the central gray. Classically conditioned avoidance of tastes, but not odors, can be acquired by anesthetized rats, suggesting that the conditioned avoidance of tastes involves a different circuit than the one mediating acquired avoidance to novel visual events (Rattoni, Forthman, Sanchez, Perez, & Garcia, 1988).

High and Low Reactivity

Observations on a large number of healthy 4-month-old Caucasian infants exposed to unfamiliar visual, auditory, and olfactory stimuli reveal obvious variation in vigorous motor activity and crying. The infants who show high motor activity combined with crying are called *high-reactive*; those who show minimal motor activity and little or no crying are called *low-reactive*. This variation can be understood by assuming that infants vary in the threshold of excitability in the amygdala and its projections to the ventral striatum, hypothalamus, cingulate, frontal cortex, central gray, and medulla.

The amygdala consists of many neuronal collections, each with a distinct pattern of connectivity, neurochemistry, and functional consequences.

Each collection projects to at least 15 different sites and receives input from about the same number of regions, resulting in about 600 known amygdala connections (Stefanacci & Amaral, 2002). Although a simplification, most anatomists regard the amygdala as comprising four basic areas: the basolateral, cortical, medial, and central areas. The first two, which are phylogenetically younger, receive rich thalamic and cortical inputs from many sensory origins (including some from the viscera), establish associations between stimuli, and are more closely connected to the cortex, hippocampus, and basal ganglia. The behavioral reactions of flight or attack are mediated primarily by projections from the basolateral nucleus to the ventromedial striatum and the ventral pallidum (Fudge, Kunishio, Walsh, Richard, & Haber, 2002).

The medial nucleus receives primarily olfactory and taste information and projects to the hippocampus, thalamus, hypothalamus, and central nucleus. The central nucleus receives input from taste, vision, and the viscera but, most important, from the other three areas. The central area, which is relatively larger than the basolateral area in rats than in primates, is the origin of a large number of projections, especially to the bed nucleus, basal forebrain, hypothalamus, brainstem, and autonomic nervous system. These projections are responsible for automatic bodily changes that include hormone secretion, activation of the autonomic nervous system, and alterations in posture and muscle tone. The central nucleus is typically activated by discrete events to produce a transient reaction, whereas more continually stressful conditions activate the bed nucleus of the stria terminalis to create a more chronic emotional state. Level of CRH in the central nucleus is correlated with the degree of reactivity to a phasic event, whereas CRH levels in the bed nucleus are more highly correlated with reactivity to a chronic stressor (Walker, Toufexis, & Davis, 2003).

Fear or Surprise

Scientists debate whether the amygdala reacts primarily to imminently threatening events to produce varied states of fear or primarily to unexpected or unfamiliar events to produce varied states of surprise. Not all unfamiliar events are dangerous, and some dangerous events are not novel. Obviously, dangerous events should create different states in brain and mind than unfamiliar ones. We believe that the primary function of the amygdala is to react to unexpected or unfamiliar events. This view is based on research reporting that the behavioral reactions of monkeys, chimpanzees, and human infants to a snake are no different from their reactions to discrepant events that are harmless (Marks, 1987). Monkeys born and reared in a laboratory—and therefore protected from encounters with live snakes—showed a longer period of motor inhibition to the presentation of a snake, whether alive or an artifact, than to blue masking tape. However, the restraint only occurred on the first testing session; during later sessions the animals showed no more restraint to the snake than to the blue masking tape. Further, most animals did not show any difference in degree of withdrawal to the snake compared to the masking tape (Nelson, Shelton, & Kalin, 2003).

Select neurons in the amygdala, bed nucleus, hippocampus, and brainstem reliably respond to discrepant events whether or not they are harmful (Wilson & Rolls, 1993), and the reactivity of these neurons to a discrepant event habituates rapidly once the event becomes familiar (La Bar, Gatenby, Gore, LeDoux, & Phelps, 1998). Adults in an fMRI scanner, looking at faces with neutral expressions, showed greater amygdala activation to new, compared with familiar, faces, even though no face displayed a fearful or a threatening expression (Schwartz et al., 2003a), as did adults who were inhibited during childhood (Schwartz et al., 2003b). It is believed that high-reactive infants are born with a low threshold of excitability in the amygdala (projections from the amygdala can mediate motor activity and crying); conversely, low-reactive infants are born with a high threshold of excitability in this structure. Observations of high- and low-reactive infants when they were 14 and 21 months old revealed that the former displayed more avoidance and crying to unfamiliarity than the latter (Kagan, 1994).

The high-reactive children observed at 4 years of age talked and smiled less often than the low-reactive children during a 1-hour interview with an unfamiliar female examiner. Restraint on spontaneous conversation and smiling in unfamiliar social situations seem to be analogous to freezing to an unexpected event in animals. Experience influences the display of a subdued or avoidant profile, as evidenced by research indicating that placement in daycare mutes degree of inhibition displayed to unfamiliar peers; apparently the day care experience helps inhibited children learn how to cope with unfamiliarity (Fox, Henderson, Rubin, Calkins, & Schmidt, 2001). The mothers of inhibited children who were oversolicitous when their children cried were most likely to have children who were reticent when they played with unfamiliar peers (Rubin, Cheah, & Fox, 2001).

The high- and low-reactive children were evaluated again at 7 years of age. The 7-year-olds who had been labeled as high-reactive were more likely than the low-reactive children to display/report anxious symptoms, and about 18% of all high-reactive children were consistently inhibited at 14 months, 21 months, 4 years, and 7 years of age. Not one high-reactive infant was consistently uninhibited across all four assessments (Kagan & Snidman, 2004).

When these children were evaluated between 10 and 12 years of age, 40% of those labeled as high-reactive retained an inhibited profile from 4 to 11 years of age, whereas 70% of those labeled as low-reactive retained an uninhibited profile across the same 7-year interval. It is important to note that the 4-month temperamental category was a better predictor of social behavior with an unfamiliar examiner at age 11 than the level of fear displayed at 14 or 21 months.

Biological Assessments

Four biological variables gathered on the 11-year-olds are regarded as indirect signs of amygdalar activity, even though other brain sites participate in each biological reaction (Kagan & Snidman, 2004).

Hemispheric Asymmetry in the EEG

Fox (1991, 1994) and Davidson (2003a, 2003b) have reported that the cortical neurons of the left frontal lobe are more active than those on the right when individuals are relaxed and feeling in a happy mood, whereas the right frontal area is more active when individuals are in a state of uncertainty, fear, or tension. The measure of asymmetry of activation is the difference in the amount of desynchronization of alpha frequencies between the left and right frontal areas (see Davidson, Ekman, & Saron, 1990; Schmidt & Fox, 1994; Tomarken, Davidson, & Henriques, 1990). Because amygdalar activity is transmitted to the frontal lobe through the nucleus basalis, it is possible, though not proven, that greater desynchronization of alpha frequencies in the right frontal lobe could reflect greater activity in the right amygdala (Kapp, Supple, & Whelen, 1994; Lloyd & Kling, 1991). It is also possible that the distribution of receptors for CRH, or CRH level, contributes to the asymmetry of activation. Monkeys with stable and extreme right frontal activation across a 4-year interval had higher CRH levels (Kalin et al., 2000).

The 11-year-olds who had been high-reactive infants showed greater EEG activation over the right than the left hemisphere at parietal sites, and high-reactive children who also had been highly fearful in the second year were more likely than low-reactive children to show right-hemispheric activation over frontal sites as well (Kagan & Snidman, 2004). Furthermore, Fox's laboratory has reported that high-reactive infants who, at 4 and 7 years of age, were reticent when playing with unfamiliar children of the same sex were more likely than others to have shown right frontal activation when they were 9 months old (Polak, Fox, Henderson, & Rubin, 2005).

Wave 5

The biological measure that best separated high- from low-reactive children at age 11 was the magnitude of the brainstem evoked potential from the inferior colliculus. The waveform generated by the colliculus, called Wave 5, occurs between 5.5 and 6.0 milliseconds (ms) following the onset of sound and reflects the neuronal activity generated by termination of the fibers of the lateral lemniscus on the inferior colliculus (Chiappa, 1983). The important fact is that the amygdala projects, indirectly through projections to the locus coeruleus and central gray, to the colliculus and therefore can enhance the excitability of this structure. These facts mean that children who possess a more excitable amygdala should have a larger Wave 5 to auditory stimulation. The data confirmed this expectation: High-reactive children had larger Wave 5 values than low-reactive children to a series of click sounds (Kagan & Snidman, 2004). It is relevant that adults displayed a larger Wave 5 when they thought they might receive an electric shock than when they were certain no shock would be delivered (Baas, Milstein, Donlevy, & Grillon, 2006).

Event-Related Potentials

A third variable that separated high- and low-reactive children was the magnitude of the event-related potential to unfamiliar visual scenes. The amygdala sends projections to the locus coeruleus, ventral tegmentum, and basal nucleus of Meynert, which in turn project to the cortical pyramidal neurons that mediate the magnitude of the event-related potential. These facts suggest that children with a more excitable amygdala might show larger P300 or N400 waveforms to unfamiliar events. The high-reactive children displayed larger N400 waveforms to ecologically invalid scenes (e.g., a child's head on an animal's body) than low-reactive children, and high-reactive children who had very large waveforms to the discrepant scenes possessed more intense symptoms of anxiety or depression 4 years later when they were 15-year-olds. Furthermore, during the last assessment at 15 years of age, high-reactive children showed shallower habituation of the N1 and N4 waveforms across three blocks of discrepant pictures (20 pictures in each block) than low-reactive children who did show steep habituation of both waveforms. This result implies that high-reactive children possess a neurochemistry that is more responsive to unfamiliarity (Kagan, Snidman, Kahn, & Towsley, 2007).

Sympathetic Activity

The amygdala projects to the sympathetic nervous system. A Fourier analysis of supine heart rate revealed that more high- than low-reactive children had more power in the low-frequency band of the spectrum (0.5–.15 Hz), reflecting both sympathetic and parasympathetic activity, and less power in the high-frequency band (0.2 Hz), which reflects vagal tone. The combination of greater power in the lower-frequency band, together with a high resting heart rate, characterized one of every three high-reactive children, but only one of five low-reactive children. More 11-year-olds with high vagal tone smiled frequently during the second year, and, at age 11, described themselves as usually happy. A longitudinal study of 31 pregnant mothers and their fetuses revealed that fetuses with high heart rates less often displayed smiling and laughter at 6 months of age (Di Pietro, 1995) and high heart rate variability, which is associated with greater vagal tone and is correlated with a tendency to approach unfamiliarity (Richards & Cameron, 1989) and unfamiliar people (Fox, 1989), as well as with smiling and laughter (Stifter, Fox, & Porges, 1989). In addition, inhibited children observed at 5 and 7 years of age showed greater pupillary dilation, greater cardiac acceleration, and larger changes in blood pressure to cognitive stressors than uninhibited children (Kagan, 1994). Finally, children classified as socially reticent showed higher sympathetic tone than children who played alone or who were sociable (Henderson, Marshall, Fox, & Rubin, 2004).

About one of every four high-reactive children and one of every three low-reactive children preserved their expected behavioral and biological profiles to age 11 years. By contrast, only 1 of 20 children classified as high- or low-reactive developed a combination of behavior and biology characteristic of the complementary group. These results are similar to those reported by Fox and colleagues.

It is important to note that none of the biological variables has the same meaning or significance across all individuals. The meaning of left frontal activation in the EEG profiles of the 11-year-olds provides an example. The low-reactive children who were described by their mothers as extremely sociable, who smiled frequently at the examiner, and who had low levels of cortical arousal showed extreme left frontal activation. But high-reactive children described as shy and timid, who smiled infrequently and had high cortical arousal were equally likely to show extreme degrees of left frontal activation. Thus, left frontal activation does not have the same meaning in youth with different temperaments. Left or right frontal activation in the EEG is but one component of a brain state that is integrated with other biological features, past history, and features of the immediate context to create one of many possible psychological states (Coan & Allen, 2004).

This last statement may be generalizable. Information gathered on these children at age 15 revealed that a group of six boys who had been high-reactive infants and were extremely inhibited during a long interview in their home showed a unique profile. These six extremely inhibited boys showed right frontal activation, high sympathetic tone, a high ratio of beta to alpha power, and a large event-related potential to discrepant scenes at age 11. But, surprisingly, 15-year-old girls who had been low-reactive infants and were garrulous and sociable during the home interview also showed high sympathetic tone and a high ratio of beta to alpha power. Thus, the theoretical significance of these biological variables depends on the type of individual on whom the data are gathered.

Furthermore, 11-year-old high-reactive children were a little more likely than low-reactive children to possess light blue eyes and a small body size (24% of high-reactive but 7% of low-reactive children had both features). This result would not surprise scientists who study the physical characteristics that accompany domestication of fox, mink, and cattle. One team of scientists working at a field station in Russia selectively bred tame male silver fox with tame females for over 40 years (Trut, 1999). The wild form, which is not tame, has hairs that are black at the base and silver white at the outer edge, stiff erect ears, and a tail that turns down. However, the offspring of 20 generations of breeding tame with tame animals displayed distinct physical features that accompanied their increased tameness. The tame animals developed light spots on their coat that were free of melanin pigmentation, floppy, rather than stiff, ears, an upturned tail, and a broader face. These physical features are derivatives of neural crest cells. The offspring of the tame matings also had lower levels of cortisol and higher levels of serotonin metabolites. If minimal fear of unfamiliar adults is associated with distinct physical features in the fox, we should not be surprised to find that high- and low-reactive children differ in eye color and body size. Perhaps the genes that mediate the time of migration of the neural crest cells, along with molecular features of those cells, are pleiotropic and contribute to a cluster of physical and behavioral features.

Temperament Constraints

The main result of our longitudinal work is that very few high- or low-reactive children developed a profile of the complementary group. No more than one-third of the children in each group actualized the behavioral and biological profile in accord with theoretical expectation. The majority displayed patterns characteristic of randomly selected middle-class Caucasian children. Thus, the prediction that a high-reactive infant would not become a sociable, exuberant child with left frontal activation, a small Wave 5, and high vagal tone can be made with much greater confidence than the prediction that such a child will become a subdued, timid adolescent with high levels of arousal in cortical, brainstem, and autonomic targets. For the same reason, the prediction that a low-reactive infant will not become an extremely shy 11-year-old with signs of high biological arousal is more likely than the prediction that this child will be exuberant and show low levels of biological arousal.

The constraining power of initial conditions, whether biological or environmental, finds an analogy in a stone rolling down a steep mountain over a 5-minute interval. An observer would be able to eliminate a great many final locations after each 10 seconds of descent, but it is not until the final second that he or she will be able to predict exactly where the stone will come to rest. When the high promises of the genome project are met, and parents can request a complete genomic analysis of their newborn, an expert will be better able to tell parents what the child will *not* become than to inform them about the characteristics their infant will possess two decades later.

Persona and Anima

The concepts of high- and low-reactive, as well as inhibited and uninhibited, refer to behaviors and not to private feelings or brain states. As children grow, there is a dissociation between public behaviors and internal feeling states. Interviews with the 15-year-olds revealed that many high-reactive children who reported feeling uneasy with strangers and tense before examinations were not exceptionally shy when talking with an interviewer whom they did not know. Three of four clinically depressed adolescent girls in the group had been high-reactive infants, even though their behavior with the examiner did not reveal excessive inhibition. A few adolescents who had been high-reactive and appeared full of energy and vivacity told the interviewer that they disliked being touched, could not sleep before school examinations, worried about trips to unfamiliar places, and often experienced periods of deep sadness. The most salient feature in their self-descriptions was a profound uncertainty over future unfamiliar events for which they could not prepare in advance. One high-reactive adolescent girl confessed that she does not like spring because of its unpredictable changes in temperature and rainfall. The low-reactive children, by contrast, worried about the more realistic possibilities of failing an examination or performing poorly on the athletic field. The biology of these adolescents affected their feelings and concerns more than their social behaviors (Kagan et al., 2007).

IMPLICATIONS

Although some readers might regard a high-reactive temperament as less desirable than a low-reactive one, reflecting a bias for sociability in contemporary America, many 19th-century parents would have wanted their daughters to have the more cautious personality of a high-reactive. Furthermore, adolescents with a high-reactive temperament have some advantages in contemporary American society because they avoid excessive risk and conduct their lives with considerable caution, having learned that if they do not do so, they will feel tense and anxious. Hence, they are less likely to be injured in accidents, whether in automobiles or on skis, and, as adults, are likely to watch their diets, see their physician regularly, and probably will live a longer life. They are also more likely to be committed to a religious ideology; twice as many high- as low-reactive adolescents were deeply religious. The satisfaction derived from their faith may mute the more intense worry or depressed mood felt by high-reactive individuals who had no religious faith; none of the high-reactive girls who were religious was clinically depressed. Although high-reactive individuals are at a slightly greater risk for developing extreme anxiety when they anticipate meeting strangers, most will not become social phobics. We estimate that among the 10 of every 100 American adults diagnosed with social phobia, only five or six would have been a high-reactive, but probably no more than one would have been a low-reactive, infant.

By contrast, a relaxed, optimistic mood was a seminal feature of the adolescents who had been low-reactive infants. They talked freely, smiled often, and when asked to describe the last time they had felt happy answered more quickly than high-reactive children. A small number of adolescent boys who had been low-reactive infants comprised a unique category. They were supremely self-confident, almost immune to anxiety, pragmatic, realistic, had high goals for their lives, and showed left-hemispheric activation and a small Wave 5. When the interviewer asked the 15-year-olds what adult vocations they were considering, two from the entire sample of 146 adolescents replied, with a serious tone of voice, that they wanted to be president of the United States. Both had been low-reactive boys with the above profile. However, a particular level of amygdalar excitability does not, by itself, lead to any specific emotional state or personality. The brain state must be linked to a symbolic network constructed over many years, to produce a vulnerability to guilt, anxiety, loneliness, or anger. Thus, a brain state can be likened to verbs that can take different targets, such as the verbs *take*, *hit*, *give*, *kiss*, and *love*.

High-reactive adolescents with greater amygdalar reactivity are more likely than low-reactive adolescents to feel guilty over their thoughts than over actions that actually caused distress to another. When we asked the 15-year-olds to report the last time they had felt guilty, a majority cited a behavior that probably upset a friend or relative; for example, a rude comment or refusal to cooperate. A smaller group named an act of disloyalty that did not harm another; for example, gossiping about a person behind his or her back. More of the adolescents who displayed biological signs of amygdalar arousal were in this smaller group.

Psychopathology

Temperamental biases probably contribute to different forms of psychopathology. A group of fourth- and fifth-grade children living in south Florida had been assessed for the presence of an anxious mood over a year before Hurricane Andrew struck the area. The small proportion of children who were still anxious 7 months after the storm had passed had been anxious prior to the hurricane (La Greca, Silverman, & Wassastein, 1998). Although the absolute risk is low, children who are high-reactive have a greater risk than others for developing social phobia in adolescence or adulthood. The 3-month prevalence of any anxiety disorder in a large sample of North Carolina youth, ages 9–16 years, was between 2 and 3% (Costello, Mustillo, Erklani, Keeler, & Angold, 2003). However, Schwartz, Snidman, and Kagan (1999) found that 61% of a sample of 13-year-olds who had been inhibited in their second year had social phobia.

The risk categories for low-reactive individuals are failure to conform to community norms because of less uncertainty over criticism or the consequences of risky decisions. This trait is the best predictor of adult psychiatric problems in contemporary North American and European samples because it is correlated with academic failure in economically disadvantaged families. Six percent of a large sample of lower-class boys were persistently and seriously asocial from their second to their eighth year; the best predictor of membership in this small group was minimal fear when, in a laboratory, they heard the sounds of a gorilla while playing (Shaw, Gillion, Ingoldsby, & Nagio, 2003). Criminals show less, and social phobics more, amygdalar activity—as measured by fMRI—to neutral faces that were conditioned stimuli for a painful, unconditioned stimulus (Veit et al., 2002).

Implications for School and Family

We are less certain about the obvious implications of this research for teachers. Evidence indicates no fundamental difference in verbal or reasoning abilities between high- and low-reactive children, although high-reactive children are less impulsive, quieter, and less likely to raise their hands in class because they do not want to make a mistake. Teachers with extremely shy, quiet children should not assume that these children are resistant or unintelligent, but should entertain the possibility that they may have been high-reactive infants.

Parents should acknowledge their children's temperamental biases and not assume either that their rearing practices or the child's willfulness are the primary reasons for the behavior. They should also acknowledge the child's malleability and capacity for change; no temperamental profile determines a particular adult personality. Temperament is not destiny. Parents should accommodate their goals to the child's wishes. A regimen of rearing that takes into account both the parent's hopes and the child's desires can be found if parents are willing to search for it.

ACKNOWLEDGMENTS

The preparation of this chapter was supported by grants from the Bial Foundation, Metanexus Institute, and the COUQ Foundation.

REFERENCES

Abercrombie, H. C., Kalin, N. H., Thurow, M. E., Rosenkranz, M. A., & Davidson, R. J. (2003). Cortisol variation in humans affects memory for emotionally laden and neutral information. *Behavioral Neuroscience, 117,* 505–516.

Achenbach, T. M. (1985). *Assessment and taxonomy of child and adolescent psychopathology.* Newbury Park, CA: Sage.

Arbelle, S., Benjamin, J., Galin, M., Kremer, P., Belmaker, R. H., & Ebstein, R. P. (2003). Relation of shyness in grade school children to the genotype for the long form of the serotonin transporter promoter region polymorphism. *American Journal of Psychiatry, 160,* 671–676.

Auerbach, J., Geller, V., Lezer, S., Shinwell, E., Belmaker, R. H., Levin, J., et al. (1999). Dopamine D4 receptor (D4DR) and serotonin transporter promoter (5-HTTLPR) polymorphisms in the determination of temperament in two-month-old infants. *Molecular Psychiatry, 4,* 369–373.

Baas, J. M., Milstein, J., Donlevy, M., & Grillon, C. (2006). Brainstem correlates of a defensive states in humans. *Biological Psychiatry, 59,* 588–593.

Bates, J. E. (1989). Concepts and measures of temperament. In G. A. Kohnstamm,

J. E. Bates, & M. K. Rothbart (Eds.), *Temperament in childhood* (pp. 3–26). New York: Wiley.

Bates, J. E., & Wachs, T. D. (1994). *Temperament.* Washington, DC: American Psychological Association.

Birns, B., Barten, S., & Bridger, W. (1969). Individual differences in temperamental characteristics of infants. *Transactions of the New York Academy of Sciences, 31,* 1071–1082.

Buss, A. H., & Plomin, R. (1984). *Temperament: Early developing personality traits.* Hillsdale, NJ: Erlbaum.

Byrne, J., & Suomi, S. J. (2002). Cortisol reactivity and its relation to home cage behavior and personality ratings in tufted capuchin (*Cebux apella*) juveniles from birth to six years of age. *Psychoneuroendocrinology, 27,* 139–154.

Carey, W. B., & McDevitt, S. C. (1978). Revision of the infant temperament questionnaire. *Pediatrics, 61,* 735–739.

Caspi, A., & Silva, P. A. (1995). Temperamental qualities at age 3 predict personality traits in young adulthood. *Child Development, 66,* 486–498.

Cecchi, M., Khoshbouei, H., Javors, M., & Morilak, D. A. (2002). Modulatory effects of norepinephrine in the lateral bed nucleus of the stria terminalis on behavioral and neuroendocrine responses to acute stress. *Neuroscience, 112,* 13–21.

Chiappa, K. H. (1983). *Evoked potentials in clinical medicine.* New York: Raven Press.

Coan, J. A., & Allen, J. J. B. (2004). Frontal EEG asymmetry as a moderator and mediator of emotion. *Biological Psychology, 67,* 7–49.

Costello, E. J., Mustillo, S., Erkanli, A., Keeler, G., & Angold, A. (2003). Prevalence and development of psychiatric disorders in childhood and adolescence. *Archives of General Psychiatry, 60,* 837–844.

Davidson, R. J. (2003a). Affective neuroscience and psychophysiology. *Psychophysiology, 40,* 655–665.

Davidson, R. J. (2003b). Right frontal brain activity, cortisol, and withdrawal behavior in six-month-old infants. *Behavioral Neuroscience, 117,* 11–20.

Davidson, R. J., Ekman, P., & Saron, C. D. (1990). Approach, withdrawal, and cerebral asymmetry: Emotional expression and brain physiology. *Journal of Personality and Social Psychology, 58,* 330–341.

DiLalla, L. F., Kagan, J., & Reznick, J. S. (1994). Genetic etiology of behavioral inhibition among two-year-old children. *Infant Behavior and Development, 17,* 401–408.

Di Pietro, J. (1995, March). *Fetal origins of neurobehavioral function and individual differences.* Paper presented at the meeting of the Society for Research in Child Development, Indianapolis, IN.

Dyaglo, N. N., & Shishkina, G. Q. (2000). Genetic differences in the synthesis and reception of adrenaline in the mouse brain in behavior and novel environments. *Neuroscience and Behavioral Physiology, 30,* 327–330.

Eisenberg, N., Valiente, C., Morris, A. S., Fabes, R. A., Cumberland, A., Reiser, M., et al. (2003). Longitudinal relations among parental emotional expressivity, children's regulations, and quality of socioemotional functioning. *Developmental Psychology, 39,* 3–19.

Fanselow, M. S. (1994). Neural organization of the defensive behavior system responsible for fear. *Psychonomic Bulletin and Review, 1,* 429–438.

Feiring, C., & Lewis, M. (1980). Sex differences and stability in vigor, activity, and persistence in the first three years of life. *Journal of Genetic Psychology, 136,* 65–75.

Fish, S. E., & Fish, M. (1995, April). *Variability in neonatal heart rate during orientation tasks and its relation to later social and coping behavior.* Presented at the meeting of the Society for Research in Child Development, Indianapolis, IN.

Fox, N. A. (1989). Psychophysiological correlates of emotional reactivity during the first year of life. *Developmental Psychology, 25,* 364–372.

Fox, N. A. (1991). If it's not left, it's right: Electroencephalogram asymmetry and the development of emotion. *American Psychologist, 46,* 863–872.

Fox, N. A. (1994). Dynamic cerebral processes underlying emotion regulation. *Monographs of the Society for Research in Child Development, 59*(2–3), 152–166.

Fox, N. A., Henderson, H. A., Rubin, K. H., Calkins, S. D., & Schmidt, L. A. (2001). Continuity and discontinuity of behavioral inhibition and exuberance: Psychophysiological and behavioral influences across the first four years of life. *Child Development, 72,* 1–21.

Freedman, D. G., & Keller, B. (1963). Inheritance of behavior in infants. *Science, 140,* 196.

Fudge, J. L., Kunishio, K., Walsh, P., Richard, C., & Haber, S. N. (2002). Amygdaloid projections to ventromedial striatal subterritories in the primate. *Neuroscience, 110,* 257–275.

Goldsmith, H. H., & Campos, J. J. (1990). The structure of temperamental fear and pleasure in infants. *Child Development, 61,* 1944–1964.

Gortmaker, S. L., Kagan, J., Caspi, A., & Silva, P. A. (1997). Daylight during pregnancy and shyness in children. *Developmental Psychobiology, 31,* 107–114.

Gunnar, M. R. (1994). Psychoendocrine studies of temperament and stress in early childhood. In J. Bates & T. Wachs (Eds.), *Temperament: Individual differences at the interface of biology and behavior* (pp. 175–198). Washington, DC: American Psychological Association.

Hariri, A. R., Mattoy, V. S., Tessitore, A., Fera, F., Smith, W. G., & Weinberger, D. R. (2002). Dextroamphetamine modulates the response of the human amygdala. *Neurosystems Pharmacology, 27,* 1036–1040.

Henderson, H. A., Marshall, P. J., Fox, N. A., & Rubin, K. H. (2004). Psychophysiological and behavioral evidence for varying forms and functions of nonsocial behavior in preschoolers. *Child Development, 75,* 251–263.

Hyde, J. S. (2005). The gender similarities hypothesis. *American Psychologist, 60,* 581–592.

Insel, T. R., Wang, Z., & Ferris, C. (1994). Patterns of vasopressin receptor distribution associated with social organization in monogamous and non-monogamous microtine rodents. *Journal of Neuroscience, 14,* 5381–5392.

Kaasinen, V., Nagren, K., Hietala, J., Farde, L., & Rinne, J. O. (2001). Sex differences in extrastriatal dopamine D (2)-like receptors in the human brain. *American Journal of Psychiatry*, *158*, 308–311.

Kagan, J. (1971). *Change and continuity in infancy*. New York: Wiley.

Kagan, J. (1994). *Galen's prophecy*. New York: Basic Books.

Kagan, J., & Saudino, K. J. (2001). Behavioral inhibition and related temperaments. In R. N. Emde & J. K. Hewitt (Eds.), *Infancy to early childhood: Genetic and environmental influences on developmental change* (pp. 111–122). New York: Oxford University Press.

Kagan, J., & Snidman, N. (2004). *The long shadow of temperament*. Cambridge, MA: Harvard University Press.

Kagan, J., Snidman, N., Kahn, V., & Towsley, S. K. (in press). The preservation of two infant temperaments into adolescence. *Monographs of the Society for Research in Child Development*.

Kalin, N. H., Larson, C., Shelton, S. E., & Davidson, R. J. (1998). Asymmetric frontal brain activity, cortisol, and behavior associated with fearful temperament in Rhesus monkeys. *Behavioral Neuroscience*, *112*, 286–292.

Kalin, N. H., Shelton, S. E., & Davidson, R. J. (2000). Cerebrospinal fluid corticotropin-releasing hormone levels are elevated in monkeys with patterns of brain activity associated with fearful temperament. *Biological Psychiatry*, *47*, 579–585.

Kapp, B. S., Supple, W. F., & Whalen, R. (1994). Effects of electrical stimulation of the amygdaloid central nucleus on neocortical arousal in the rabbit. *Behavioral Neuroscience*, *108*, 81–93.

Klein, R. G. (1991). Parent–child agreement in clinical assessment of anxiety and other psychopathology. *Journal of Anxiety Disorders*, *5*, 182–198.

Kohnstamm, G. A., Bates, J. E., & Rothbart, M. K. (1989). *Temperament in childhood*. New York: Wiley.

Kumakiri, C., Kodama, K., Shimizu, E., Yamanouchi, N., Okada, S., Noda, S., et al. (1999). Study of the association between the serotonin transporter gene regulating polymorphism and personality traits in a Japanese population. *Neuroscience Letters*, *263*, 205–207.

La Bar, K. S., Gatenby, C., Gore, J. C., LeDoux, J. E., & Phelps, E. A. (1998). Human amygdala activation during conditioned fear acquisition and extinction. *Neuron*, *29*, 937–945.

La Greca, A. M., Silverman, W. K., & Wassastein, S. B. (1998). Children's predisaster functioning as a predictor of post-traumatic stress following Hurricane Andrew. *Journal of Consulting and Clinical Psychology*, *66*, 883–892.

Lee, Y., Schulkin, J., & Davis, M. (1994). Effect of corticosterone on enhancement of the acoustic startle reflex by corticotropin releasing factor (CRF). *Brain Research*, *666*, 93–98.

Lloyd, R. L., & Kling, A. S. (1991). Delta activity from amygdala in squirrel monkeys (*Saimiri sciureus*): Influence of social and environmental contexts. *Behavioral Neuroscience*, *105*, 223–229.

Maren, S., Yap, S. A., & Goosens, K. A. (2001). The amygdala is essential for the development of neuronal plasticity in the medial geniculate nucleus during auditory fear conditioning in rats. *Journal of Neuroscience*, *21*, RC135.

Marks, I. M. (1987). *Fears, phobias, and rituals.* New York: Oxford University Press.

Matheny, A. (1983). A longitudinal twin study of stability of components from Bayley's infant behavior record. *Child Development, 54,* 356–360.

McDougall, W. (1929). The chemical theory of temperament applied to introversion and extraversion. *Journal of Abnormal and Social Psychology, 24,* 293–309.

McGaugh, J. L., & Cahill, L. (2003). Emotion and memory. In R. J. Davidson, K. R. Scherer, & H. H. Goldsmith (Eds.), *Handbook of affective science* (pp. 93–116). New York: Oxford University Press.

McNally, G. P., & Westbrook, R. F. (2003). Opioid receptors regulate the extinction of Pavlovian fear conditioning. *Behavioral Neuroscience, 117,* 1292–1301.

Miyawaki, T., Goodchild, A. K., & Pilowsky, P. M. (2002). Activation of mu-opioid receptors in rat ventrolateral medulla selectively blocks baroreceptor reflexes while activation of delta opioid receptors blocks somato-sympathetic reflexes. *Neuroscience, 109,* 133–144.

Morley-Fletcher, S., Palanza, P., Parolaro, D., Vigano, D., & Laviola, G. (2003). Intra-uterine position has long term influences on brain mu-opioid receptor densities and behavior in mice. *Psychoneuroendocrinology, 28,* 386–400.

Nelson, E. E., Shelton, S. E., & Kalin, N. H. (2003). Individual differences in the responses of naïve rhesus monkeys to snakes. *Emotion, 3,* 3–11.

Pjerk, E., Winkler, D., Heiden, A., Praschak-Rieder, N., Willeit, M., Konstantinidis, A., et al. (2004). Seasonality of birth in seasonal affective disorder. *Journal of Clinical Psychiatry, 65,* 1389–1393.

Plomin, R., & McClearn, G. E. (Eds.). (1993). *Nature, nurture, and psychology.* Washington, DC: American Psychological Association.

Polak, C., Fox, N. A., Henderson, H. A., & Rubin, K. H. (2005). *Behavioral and physiological correlates of socially wary behavior in middle childhood: Does social wary behavior mediate the relation between infant temperament and later child maladjustment?* Unpublished manuscript.

Posner, M. I., & Petersen, S. E. (1990). The attention system of the human brain. *Annual Review of Neuroscience, 13,* 25–42.

Rattoni, F. B., Forthman, D. L., Sanchez, M. A., Perez, J. L., & Garcia, J. (1988). Odor and taste aversions conditioned in anesthetized rats. *Behavioral Neuroscience, 102,* 726–732.

Rebec, G. V., Christianson, J. R., Guevra, C., & Bardo, M. T. (1997). Regional and temporal differences in real time dopamine efflux in the nucleus accumbens during food choice novelty. *Brain Research, 776,* 61–67.

Reppucci, C. (1968). *Hereditary influences upon distribution of attention in infancy.* Unpublished doctoral dissertation, Harvard University, Cambridge, MA.

Rich, G. J. (1928). A biochemical approach to the study of personality. *Journal of Abnormal and Social Psychology, 23,* 158–175.

Roozendaal, B., & Cools, A. R. (1994). Influence of the noradrenergic state of the nucleus accumbens in basolateral amygdala mediated changes in neophobia of rats. *Behavioral Neuroscience, 108,* 1107–1118.

Rothbart, M. K. (1981). Measurement of temperament in infancy. *Child Development*, *52*, 569–578.

Rothbart, M. K., Ahadi, S. A., & Hershey, K. L. (1994). Temperament and social behavior in childhood. *Merrill–Palmer Quarterly*, *40*, 21–39.

Rothbart, M. K., Derryberry, D., & Posner, M. I. (1994). A psychobiological approach to the development of temperament. In J. E. Bates & T. D. Wachs (Eds.), *Temperament* (pp. 83–116). Washington, DC: American Psychological Association.

Rubin, K. H., Burgess, K. B., & Hastings, D. D. (2002). Stability and social behavioral consequences of toddlers' inhibited temperament and parenting behaviors. *Child Development*, *73*, 483–495.

Rubin, K. H., Cheah, C., & Fox, N. A. (2001). Emotion regulation, parenting, and display of social reticence in preschoolers. *Early Education and Development*, *12*, 97–115.

Sanders, S. K. (2001). Cardiovascular and behavioral effects of GABA manipulation in the region of the anterior basolateral amygdala of rats. *Dissertation Abstracts International, Section B, Sciences and Engineering*, *62*, 1060.

Saudino, K. J., & Cherny, S. S. (2001). Sources of continuity and change in observed temperament. In R. N. Emde & J. K. Hewitt (Eds.), *Infancy to early childhood: Genetic and environmental influences on developmental change* (pp. 85–100). New York: Oxford University Press.

Schmidt, L., & Fox, N. A. (1994). Patterns of cortical electrophysiology and autonomic activity in adults' shyness and sociability. *Biological Psychology*, *38*, 183–198.

Schwartz, C. E., Snidman, N., & Kagan, J. (1999). Adolescent social anxiety and outcome of inhibited temperament in childhood. *Journal of the American Academy of Child and Adolescent Psychiatry*, *38*, 1008–1015.

Schwartz, C. E., Wright, C. T., Shin, L. M., Kagan, J., & Rauch, S. L. (2003a). Inhibited and uninhibited infants "grown up": Adult amygdalar response to novelty. *Science*, *300*, 1952–1953.

Schwartz, C. E., Wright, C. E., Shin, L. M., Kagan, J., Whalen, P. J., McMullin, K. G., et al. (2003b). Differential amygdalar response to novel versus newly familiar neutral faces. *Biological Psychiatry*, *53*, 854–862.

Scott, J. P., & Fuller, S. (1965). *Genetics and the social behavior of the dog*. Chicago: University of Chicago Press.

Shaw, D. S., Gillion, M., Ingoldsby, E. M., & Nagio, P. S. (2003). Trajectories leading to school-age conduct problems. *Developmental Psychology*, *39*, 189–200.

Shumyatsky, G. P., Tsvetkov, E., Malleret, G., Vronskaya, S., Hatton, M., Hampton, L., et al. (2002). Identification of a signaling network in lateral nucleus of amygdala important for inhibiting memory specifically related to learned far. *Cell*, *11*, 905–918.

Smoller, J. W., Rosenbaum, J. F., Biederman, J., Kennedy, J., Dai, D., Racitte, S. R., et al. (2004). Association of the genetic marker at the corticotropin releasing hormone locus with behavioral inhibition. *Biological Psychiatry*, *54*, 1376–1381.

Spiker, D., Klebanov, P. K., & Brooks-Gunn, J. (1992, May). *Environmental and biological correlates of infant temperament.* Presented at the meeting of the International Society for Infant Studies, Miami, FL.

Stefanacci, L., & Amaral, D. G. (2002). Some observations on cortical inputs to the macaque amygdala. *Journal of Comparative Neurology, 451,* 301–323.

Stifter, C. A., Fox, N. A., & Porges, S. W. (1989). Facial expressivity and vagal tone in 5- and 10-month-old infants. *Infant Behavior and Development, 12,* 127–137.

Strelau, J., & Angleitner, A. (1991). *Explorations in temperament.* New York: Plenum Press.

Takahashi, L. K., & Rubin, W. W. (1994). Corticosteriod induction of threat-induced behavioral inhibition in preweanling rats. *Behavioral Neuroscience, 107,* 860–868.

Thomas, A., & Chess, S. (1977). *Temperament and development.* New York: Brunner/Mazel.

Tomarken, A. J., Davidson, R. J., & Henriques, J. B. (1990). Resting frontal brain asymmetry predicts affective responses to films. *Journal of Personality and Social Psychology, 59,* 791–801.

Treit, D., Pesold, C., & Rotzinger, S. (1993a). Dissociating the antifear effects of septal and amygdaloid lesions using two pharmacologically validated models of rat anxiety. *Behavioral Neuroscience, 107,* 770–785.

Treit, D., Pesold, C., & Rotzinger, S. (1993b). Noninteractive effects of diazepam and amygdaloid lesions in two animal models of anxiety. *Behavioral Neuroscience, 107,* 1099–1105.

Trut, L. N. (1999). Early canid domestication. *American Scientist, 87,* 160–169.

van Bockstaele, E. J., Bajic, D., Proudfit, H., & Valentino, R. J. (2001). Topographic architecture of stress-related pathways targeting the noradrenergic locus ceruleus. *Physiology and Behavior, 73,* 273–283.

Veit, R., Flor, H., Erb, M., Hermann, C., Lotze, M., Grudd, W., et al. (2002). Brain circuits involved in emotional learning in antisocial behavior and social phobia in humans. *Neuroscience Letters, 328,* 231–233.

Walker, D. L., Toufexis, D. J., & Davis, M. (2003). Role of the bed nucleus of the stria terminalis vs. the amygdala in fear, stress, and anxiety. *European Journal of Pharmacology, 463,* 199–216.

Wang, H., & Wessendorf, M. W. (2002). Mu- and delta-opioid receptor mRNAs are expressed in periaqueductal gray neurons projecting to the rostral ventromedial medulla. *Neuroscience, 109,* 619–634.

Williamson, D. E., Coleman, K., Bacanu, S., Devlin, B. J., Rogers, J., Ryan, N. D., et al. (2003). Heritability of fearful-anxious endophenotypes in infant rhesus macaques. *Biological Psychiatry, 53,* 284–291.

Wilson, F. A., & Rolls, E. T. (1993). The effect of stimulus novelty and familiarity on neuronal activity in the amygdala of monkeys performing recognition memory tasks. *Experimental Brain Research, 93,* 367–382.

CHAPTER 9

Frontal Lobe Development during Infancy and Childhood

CONTRIBUTIONS OF BRAIN ELECTRICAL ACTIVITY,
TEMPERAMENT, AND LANGUAGE
TO INDIVIDUAL DIFFERENCES
IN WORKING MEMORY AND INHIBITORY CONTROL

Martha Ann Bell
Christy D. Wolfe
Denise R. Adkins

It is a premise of developmental cognitive neuroscience that the foundations of many executive function skills are found in infancy and early childhood (Roberts & Pennington, 1996). Infants and young children readily perform tasks requiring working memory and inhibitory control (Diamond, Prevor, Callender, & Druin, 1997; Pelphrey et al., 2004) and exhibit the effortful control of attention (Posner & Rothbart, 2000; Ruff & Rothbart, 1996). Similarly, there is evidence that some aspects of cognition in infancy predict cognitive outcomes in childhood (Rose, Feldman, Wallace, & Cohen, 1991). Furthermore, it is well accepted that changes in cognition and the brain occur concurrently, although caution must be taken in interpreting these simultaneous developments as being causally linked (Casey, Tottenham, Liston, & Durston, 2005). Other factors such as infant/child temperament or parenting may affect developmental trajectories (Bell & Wolfe, 2004; Ruff & Rothbart, 1996).

The purpose of this chapter is to report findings from our program of research, in which we examine associations between developmental changes in brain electrical activity and cognitive changes in behavior from infancy to early childhood and, most recently, middle childhood. Thus, this chapter highlights our own changing research program, as our contribution to an earlier edition of this volume focused exclusively on infant work (Bell & Fox, 1994). We begin by defining the specific cognitive skills that are the focus of our research program and then offer brief comments regarding the use of developmentally appropriate cognitive tasks in longitudinal research studies that cross major developmental time periods. Because our research utilizes recordings of brain electrical activity that are tied to cognitive behaviors, we also offer brief comments on the use of the electroencephalogram (EEG) in brain–behavior research.

Most of the work we report here results from our longitudinal research study of the development of working memory and inhibitory control during infancy and childhood. We examine the findings separately for infancy (8 months of age), early childhood (4½ years of age), and middle childhood (8 years of age). At each age we highlight age-appropriate working memory/inhibitory control tasks as well as the brain processes and correlated EEG activity associated with these tasks. A major emphasis in our research program is on individual differences in cognitive development; thus, we focus on the contributions of EEG, temperament, and language to working memory performance during each age period. We also briefly discuss associations between the infancy and early childhood data and between the early childhood and middle childhood data. We begin by defining and linking the constructs of working memory and inhibitory control.

WORKING MEMORY AND INHIBITORY CONTROL

We focus on the construct of working memory as defined by Engle and colleagues in our program of research (Engle, Kane, & Tuholski, 1999; Kane & Engle, 2002). Engle defines working memory as a system consisting of those highly activated long-term memory traces that are active above threshold as short-term memory representational components. Included in this characterization of working memory are the procedures and skills necessary to achieve and maintain that activation, as well as a limited-capacity, domain-free controlled attention component. The attentional capacity allows maintenance of short-term memory representations in the presence of interference or response competition. Without this interference, information, goals, and response plans are easily retrieved from long-term memory.

In the face of interference, however, it is more likely that incorrect information and inaccurate responses will be retrieved (Kane & Engle, 2002). Thus, this executive attention component is not needed for all cognitive processing but is called into action in circumstances that require inhibition of prepotent responses, error monitoring and correction, and decision making and planning (Engle et al., 1999).

Individual differences in executive attention, called "working memory capacity" by Engle and colleagues (Engle et al., 1999; Kane & Engle, 2002, 2004), are associated with a wide variety of cognitive abilities and are revealed only in situations that encourage or require controlled attention. Individuals high in this controlled attention ability are more effective at blocking distracting, task-irrelevant information and maintaining a focus on pertinent information than individuals low in attention. Indeed, individuals ranked low on this attentional ability are more likely to break focus and orient to an irrelevant, attention-capturing external cue. Based on human and nonhuman primate literatures, Engle has hypothesized that individual differences in attentional control (i.e., working memory capacity) are associated with individual differences in the functioning of the dorsolateral prefrontal cortex (Engle et al., 1999; Kane & Engle, 2002).

DEVELOPMENTALLY APPROPRIATE TASKS

Working memory tasks offer the possibility of simultaneous brain–behavior assessments in both infants and young children. The comparability of working memory tasks for infants and preschool children is, of course, a concern for any longitudinal study that assesses participants across major periods of early development. We utilized developmentally appropriate tasks during infancy, early childhood, and middle childhood and later in this chapter we detail the task requirements at each time period. These requirements are comparable, with only the task response requiring different modalities (oculomotor for infants, verbal for early childhood, computer clicks for middle childhood).

USING EEG IN DEVELOPMENTAL RESEARCH ON BRAIN–BEHAVIOR RELATIONS

The recording of EEG is a brain imaging methodology that provides functional information about the developing brain. The EEG represents electrical activity recorded from the scalp, with the assumption that the origin of these electrical signals is in the brain itself. The EEG signal is spontaneous but context related; the signal generated during quiet rest is different from that generated during mental activity. The EEG signal has temporal resolution on the order of just hundreds of milliseconds. Thus, neuronal changes are reflected immediately in the EEG, making this methodology outstanding for tracking rapid shifts in brain functioning. Furthermore, these brain electrical signals are robust, and the techniques by which they are obtained are relatively simple, noninvasive, and comparatively inexpensive. These characteristics make the EEG one of the more favored methodologies for studying brain development in infants and children and for relating brain development to changes in behavior (Bell, in press; Casey & deHaan, 2002; Taylor & Baldeweg, 2002).

INFANCY

Our program of research has its foundation in investigations of working memory and inhibitory control (WMIC) during infancy. Largely influenced by Diamond's work (e.g., Diamond, 1985), we have examined these cognitive constructs in infants by employing age-appropriate tasks that require the utilization and integration of these two cognitive skills. We have reliably used the A-not-B reaching and A-not-B looking tasks. Successful performance on both of these tasks requires WMIC; the infant must *remember* where an object is hidden across multiple locations and *inhibit* a dominant response tendency.

WMIC Tasks for Infancy

Infant working memory tasks include the traditional delayed response task, which is perhaps the strongest and most consistently used measure of prefrontal functioning (Diamond, 2002; Luciana & Nelson, 1998), and its corollary, the Piagetian A-not-B task. Diamond (1990) has reported that human infants and nonhuman primate infants demonstrate identical developmental progression on delayed response and A-not-B tasks. The two tasks are very similar, with the only difference being the rule for deciding at which of two locations an attractive toy is to be hidden. The pattern of hidings for the A-not-B task is infant driven, whereas the pattern of hidings for the delayed response task is experimenter driven. During the infant working memory task, the research participants are required to remember information across a delay period and update memory representations of that information from trial to trial. As distraction, participants are not allowed to maintain attentional focus on the information during the delay and, furthermore, must attend in the presence of interference from information from the previous trial. These are requirements for classic working memory tasks and both the delayed response and the A-not-B tasks fulfill these requirements (Engle et al., 1999; Kane & Engle, 2002).

Diamond provided the basic behavioral neuroscience evidence that maturation of the dorsolateral prefrontal cortex (DLPFC) and corresponding skills of working memory and inhibitory control are major contributors to classic reaching performance on the A-not-B task as well as the delayed response task (Diamond, 2001; Diamond et al., 1997). We reasoned that the very same skills of working memory and inhibitory control would be needed on a *looking* version of the A-not-B task. Because cognitive skills are the same, with only response modality being different, performance on a reaching version of the A-not-B task should be comparable to a looking version of the task; and, indeed, it is (Bell & Adams, 1999; Matthews, Ellis, & Nelson, 1996; Pelphrey et al., 2004).

A-not-B Task

In our looking version of the classic A-not-B task, the infant searches for a hidden toy by making an eye movement to one of two possible hiding locations. The task requires the infant to constantly *update memory* of where the toy was hidden through a series of displacements and to *inhibit* looking back toward a previously rewarded hiding place. The testing apparatus that we use is a table, and the hiding sites are bright orange and blue plastic tubs. The infant sits on the parent's lap as the experimenter manipulates a toy and hides it under one of the two plastic tubs. Briefly, after the toy is hidden, the infant's gaze to the hiding site is broken and brought to midline by the experimenter calling the infant's name and asking, "Where's the toy?" The direction of the infant's first eye movement after being brought to midline is scored as either correct or incorrect. A video camera placed behind and above the experimenter's head is focused to maintain a closeup view of the infant's face. Because the infants are not allowed to manipulate the toys, the visual experience they receive from the toys and the smiles and praise ("Good job! You found it!") they receive from the experimenter after an eye movement to the correct tub have to provide the impetus to continue to search for the toy. For an eye movement to the incorrect tub, the infants receive a sigh and sad vocalizations from the experimenter ("Oh, no, it's not there").

The pattern of toy placement is determined by the infant's performance, with initial side of hiding randomized among infants. Two consecutive successful eye movements toward the same side (e.g., toward the infant's right) result in a reversal hiding, with the toy being hidden under the tub on the opposite side (toward the infant's left; i.e., right–right–left).

All infants receive reversal trials. Assessment ceases when the infant makes an eye movement toward the incorrect side in two reversal trials.

Brain Processes Associated with WMIC in Infancy

Significant changes in working memory processes are clearly identifiable during infancy and early childhood. These changes are inarguably associated with transformations in cortical function and organization. It has been suggested that the most salient modifications in brain anatomy (i.e., growth in brain weight, increased myelination, glucose utilization, and synaptic growth) take place in the first few years of life (see also, Lenroot & Giedd, Chapter 3, this volume).

The association between performance on the delayed response task and the DLPFC has been termed "one of the strongest brain–behavior relations in all of cognitive neuroscience" (Diamond, 2002, p. 468). The behavioral neuroscience work accomplished by Diamond and colleagues provided the initial evidence that the maturation and integrity of the DLPFC are also involved at some level in successful performance on Piaget's A-not-B reaching task (Diamond & Goldman-Rakic, 1989; Diamond, Zola-Morgan, & Squire, 1989). In her work with human infants, Diamond has emphasized maturation of this brain area (Diamond, 1990; Diamond et al., 1997) as well as the wide range of individual differences among infants in A-not-B performance (Diamond, 1985).

Electrophysiological Correlates of WMIC in Infancy

Infant EEG recorded during the A-not-B infant working memory task exhibits an increase in 6–9 hertz (Hz) power values, relative to baseline, at both anterior and posterior scalp locations at 8 months of age (Bell, 2001, 2002). Other researchers have employed a hiding task similar to the A-not-B task in that it requires attentional focus during delay. That task likewise results in increases in 6–9 Hz EEG power, relative to baseline, at multiple anterior and posterior scalp locations at 8–10 months of age (Orekhova, Stroganova, & Posikera, 2001). Thus, during infant performance of working memory tasks, brain electrical activity appears to be relatively widespread because changes in EEG power values across the entire scalp, rather than at specific scalp locations, are associated with cognitive processing.

More intriguing from a neuropsychological point of view is that the EEG recorded during task performance is highly informative (Bell, 2002). We are able to event-mark the EEG record to capture and delineate various aspects of our looking working memory task. For example, when we are displaying the toy to the infant prior to hiding it, we mark that particular portion of the EEG record and label it as the "attention" component of the task. We mark as the "memory" component of the task from the time the toy is hidden, we break the infant's gaze to the hiding site, and we count a delay to add further distraction until we allow the infant to make an eye movement to indicate the toy's location ("Where's the toy?"). Finally, we mark the portion of the record as "reward" that includes when we indicate to the infant that his or her choice was either correct or incorrect, varying our own facial expression and tone of voice to convey that the toy is indeed where he or she looked, or it isn't. We have already shown that the EEG changes from baseline to task. We have been able to further distinguish among the three stages of cognitive activity: attention, memory, and reward. The EEG was most active during the "memory" portion of the task, the most cognitively challenging phase. Most importantly, and most exciting for us, was that the EEG distinguished between correct and incorrect eye movement responses (Bell, 2002).

Individual Differences in WMIC in Infancy

Diamond has noted the dramatic improvements in WMIC abilities across infancy and hypothesized about the associated development of certain brain systems (Diamond, 1985, 1990, 2002). Yet all infants do not improve in their WMIC abilities at the same rate (Bell & Fox, 1992; Diamond, 1985). Our research program with infants includes an investigation of two variables that have been theoretically and empirically linked with WMIC: the EEG and infant temperament.

Electroencephalogram

We have recorded EEG during the infant A-not-B WMIC task from two different groups of 8-month-old infants during baseline and task (Bell, 2001, 2002, 2005). Of particular interest was a change in EEG values from baseline to task because this would be indicative of cortical involvement. In our initial study, only infants with high performance on the looking version of the infant WMIC task exhibited changes in EEG power from baseline to task; the low performers showed no change in EEG from baseline to task. These task-related changes were evident at frontal and posterior scalp locations (Bell, 2001, 2002). These data confirmed our previous cognitive neuroscience work associating frontal and posterior function with cognitive performance levels during infancy and strengthened our position that better performance was associated with greater brain maturation.

We have since replicated these findings with a second sample of 8-month-old infants (Bell, 2005). Again, changes in both frontal and posterior EEG from baseline to task were associated with task performance. More importantly, this particular sample of infants was followed longitudinally; thus, these children and their parents visited our research lab again at ages 4½ years and 8 years. We discuss those data later in this chapter.

Temperament

Rothbart and Bates (1998) defined temperament as biologically based individual differences in emotional reactivity and the emergence of self-regulation of that reactivity beginning late in the first year of life (see also Kagan & Snidman, Chapter 8, this volume). The emergence of these early regulatory processes is facilitated by the development of attention, which may have implications for cognitive development as well (Bush, Luu, & Posner, 2000; Ruff & Rothbart, 1996). We propose that the most pertinent example of this attentional regulation is the cognitive control infants begin to exhibit on WMIC tasks (Diamond, 1990; Diamond et al., 1997).

As noted when we defined the construct of working memory at the beginning of this chapter, individual differences associated with executive attention are the focus of Engle's model of working memory (Engle et al., 1999; Kane & Engle, 2002). These individual differences are considered to be a characteristic of the individual person and do not result from experience (Engle et al., 1999). Temperament, especially during early infancy, is considered to be a characteristic of the individual infant (Rothbart & Bates, 1998). Thus, Engle's attentional control and Rothbart's attentional regulation appear to be conceptually similar.

Our own infant studies have yielded correlations between temperamental characteristics associated with attentional self-regulation and working memory performance (Bell, 2005). In our 8-month-old infants, we have demonstrated associations between the temperamental characteristics of Activity Level and Distress to Limitations (measured using Rothbart's Infant Behavior Questionnaire) and performance on the A-not-B WMIC task. Infants rated by their parents as high on Activity or high on Distress performed better on the WMIC task. We hypothesized that infants with high Distress and Activity Levels may require more parental interaction than infants with lower Distress and Activity Levels. Accordingly, this counterintuitive finding may mean that these infants require more parental support in the development of their attentional skills, a result that may lead to enhanced cognitive skills as infants grow older if that support from the parent is appropriate and sensitive. Thus, parental behavior may be essential for cognition (Colombo & Saxon, 2002). This speculation deserves further attention, and we are currently investigating this notion with a longitudinal sample of infants.

Summary and Conclusion

As Diamond has demonstrated (1985, 1990; Diamond et al., 1997) and others have concurred (Bell & Fox, 1992; Matthews et al., 1996; Pelphrey et al., 2004), infancy is a time of extraordinary development in cognition, especially with respect to WMIC skills. Diamond's research program especially has contributed to our knowledge of the development of this cognitive skill in infancy, as well as to our knowledge about the development of the DLPFC. Research in our lab has added EEG data to this knowledge base and lent support to the involvement of the prefrontal cortex in these WMIC tasks in infancy (Bell, 2001, 2002). Our research has also demonstrated that individual differences in WMIC functioning are related to individual differences in brain electrical activity and temperament in infancy (Bell, 2001, 2005).

EARLY CHILDHOOD

Our program of research has also included an investigation of working memory and inhibitory control during the early childhood years. Again largely influenced by Diamond's work, we have examined these cognitive constructs in the preschool population by employing age-appropriate tasks that require the utilization and, importantly, the integration of these two cognitive skills. Two tasks that we have used reliably are the Stroop-like day–night task and the yes–no task. Successful performance on both of these tasks requires WMIC; that is, the child participant must *remember* two rules and *inhibit* a dominant response tendency.

WMIC Tasks for Early Childhood

Day–Night Task

The Stroop-like day–night task (Diamond et al., 1997; Diamond & Taylor, 1996; Gerstadt, Hong, & Diamond, 1994) was formulated in the manner of the traditional Stroop task (Stroop, 1935). In the classic color–word Stroop task, a participant is instructed to say the color of ink in which a color word is printed rather than read the color word aloud. Thus, this task requires the skills of working memory and inhibitory control: the participants must *remember* the rule or the goal for the task and also *inhibit* reading the word—a very dominant response tendency. Taking advantage of both accuracy scores and measures of reaction time as well as many different versions of the task, the classic Stroop paradigm has been used extensively in the adult cognitive and clinical literatures. However, this task has not been applicable to younger age groups, such as preschool populations, due to the reading requirement intrinsic to the task.

The day–night task lacks the reading component of the Stroop yet maintains the cognitive requirements of the classic task. This task challenges the child to *remember* two rules and *inhibit* a dominant response tendency. Specifically, a child is instructed to say *night* when shown a card with a bright yellow sun and to say *day* when shown a card with the moon and stars. The child is then given two learning trials, one with the sun card and one with the moon card. If the child is successful on both of these trials, then the task is continued for a total of 16 test trials, eight with the sun card and eight with the moon card arranged in a pseudo-random order. If the child is unsuccessful on either or both of the teaching trials, then the instructions are repeated and the child is asked to respond again. It is important that the child be successful on the first two trials to ensure that he or she has paid attention to the instructions and understands the rules as given. No feedback is generally given during testing unless the experimenter feels that the child needs prompting, such as, "What do you say for this card?", or nondirective encouragement, such as "Okay," after a response, to facilitate the completion of the task. For the day–night task, the child should be left to his or her own memory and inhibitory control abilities.

Research employing the day–night task indicates a great improvement in performance between 3½ and 7 years of age (Diamond et al., 1997; Diamond & Taylor, 1996; Gerstadt et al., 1994). With regard to accuracy—measured as percentage correct across the 16 trials—there is an almost linear increase in performance across the age groups of 3½, 4, 4½, 5, 5½, 6, 6½, and 7 years, with the most dramatic improvement between 3½ and 6 years of age. Decreases in reaction time are also seen, but the most radical improvement occurs early on, between the ages of 3½ and 4½. For the youngest children, a slower reaction time has been associated with increased performance, suggesting that cognitively the young children find the task more difficult than the older children and must take time to arrive at a correct response (Gerstadt et al., 1994). Indeed, Diamond, Kirkham, and Amso (2002) showed that if young children are encouraged to take their time in responding with an experimenter-imposed delay, their performance improves.

It is important to note that when control cards are used with abstract designs and the children are asked to say *day* to one design and *night* to the other, the youngest children perform as well as the oldest children, with high accuracy scores and low reaction times (Gerstadt et al., 1994). Thus, the crucial component of this task that taxes the desired cognitive ability is the presentation of stimuli that are meaningfully related to the instructed response. It is this particular scenario that creates a cognitive conflict requiring the integration of working memory and inhibitory control for resolution.

Researchers have also noted the high variability in performance on this task between the ages of 3½ and 5 years. That is, some children within this age range perform very well, whereas others have great difficulty. This phenomenon of individual differences is of great interest to us, and our research program includes an investigation of several variables that may be related to this particular type of cognitive ability. Just as Gerstadt and colleagues (1994) found that those children who had attended preschool performed better on their day–night task than children who had been cared for exclusively at home, we have found other variables associated with WMIC in early childhood, such as brain electrical activity (i.e., EEG), temperament, and language comprehension. These associations are discussed briefly at the end of this section.

Yes-No Task

The yes–no task is comparable to the Stroop-like day–night task and has also been used in the developmental literature with preschool children to assess WMIC (Wolfe & Bell, 2004). The yes–no task challenges children to *remember* two rules and to *inhibit* a dominant response tendency by instructing the children to say *no* when the experimenter nods her head yes and to say *yes* when the experimenter shakes her head no. Again, the children are given two learning trials, during which they are praised or corrected, and then 16 test trials with eight head nods and eight head shakes arranged in a pseudo-random order comparable to the day–night card sequence. Also, as with the day–night task, no feedback is generally given during testing, except under the conditions previously specified. It is important that the children rely on their own memories of the task rules and inhibitory capacities.

A recent study in our lab of 3½-, 4-, and 4½-year-old children indicated that performance on the yes–no task (i.e., accuracy) does improve across these three age groups (Wolfe & Bell, 2006). This pattern of change is comparable to that described by Diamond and colleagues for the day–night task (Diamond et al., 1997; Diamond & Taylor, 1996; Gerstadt et al., 1994). We have also directly compared children's performance on the day–night and yes–no tasks and found that performance on the two tasks is moderately to highly correlated (r = .598) and increases in parallel over developmental time (see Figure 9.1). We take this finding as evidence that the two tasks are tapping the same cognitive constructs (i.e., WMIC), even

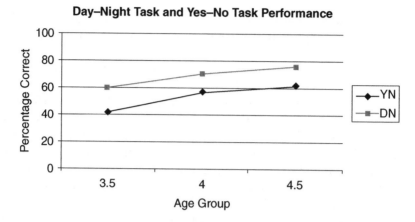

FIGURE 9.1. Performance on two early childhood WMIC tasks at different ages.

though the day–night task is reliably an easier task for the children (Wolfe & Bell, 2004, 2006).

One hypothesis to explain the greater difficulty of the yes–no task is that it involves highly familiar stimuli and responses. It is true that the day–night paradigm is indeed a familiar topic for young children, but the stimulus–response conflict is still less challenging to their cognitive resources than the yes–no conflict. Even the youngest children have been frequent participants in vocal and nonvocal dialogue that includes the particular behaviors involved in the yes–no task, and they are capable of comprehending gestures and language and associating the two. Thus, these behaviors are deeply entrenched in the child's behavioral and verbal repertoires. When the stimulus gesture is presented (e.g., a head shake) and the child is asked to respond (e.g., "yes"), great cognitive effort is required on the part of the child to override the wealth of experience with this particular stimulus and meaningfully associated response.

Brain Processes Associated with WMIC in Early Childhood

To date, there is no direct empirical evidence linking performance on the day–night and yes–no tasks with any particular brain system, as currently exists linking performance on the A-not-B and delayed response tasks with the functioning of the DLPFC (e.g., Diamond & Goldman-Rakic, 1989). It *is* known, however, that many advances are being made in higher-order cognitive processes between the ages of 3 and 7 years (e.g., Diamond & Taylor, 1996; Diamond et al., 1997; Gerstadt et al., 1994; Luciana & Nelson, 1998; Welsh, Pennington, & Groisser, 1991; Zelazo, Müller, Frye, & Marcovitch, 2003). These advances may reflect significant changes within the prefrontal cortex during this period of life (Diamond & Taylor, 1996). For example, the DLPFC is undergoing profound changes, such as increases in neuronal density, between the ages of 2 and 7 years (e.g., see Diamond, 2002, for a review of DLPFC development, including anatomical and biochemical evidence from infancy to young adulthood).

Although there is great theoretical support for the association between the day–night and yes–no tasks and DLPFC functioning (e.g., Diamond, 2001, 2002; Engle et al., 1999; Kane & Engle, 2002), there is only indirect empirical evidence (Diamond, 2001, 2002; Diamond et al., 1997; Luria, 1966; Wolfe & Bell, 2004, 2006). Providing some evidence of the association between WMIC and the DLPFC in early childhood, Diamond and colleagues have examined these cognitive constructs in a special population of children believed to have reduced levels of dopamine in the prefrontal cortex. Specifically, the day–night task has been examined in children treated early and continuously for phenylketonuria (PKU—Diamond, 2001; Diamond et al., 1997). The results of this longitudinal study suggest that the DLPFC is indeed involved in performance on this task during early childhood. Specifically, those children with higher phenylalanine levels (and consequently decreased amounts of dopamine available to the prefrontal cortex) performed more poorly than children with lower levels of phenylalanine and other control groups of children on this and other WMIC tasks. Importantly, these impairments were selective to those tasks that are theoretically associated with the DLPFC (i.e., those tasks requiring WMIC). Children with higher phenylalanine levels did not perform differently than the other children with PKU or any of the control groups on tasks that required areas of the cortex other than DLPFC or on other general cognitive measures.

Electrophysiological Correlates of WMIC in Early Childhood

Our research with young children also contributes evidence supporting a brain–behavior association between WMIC and prefrontal functioning. Specifically, we have investigated the electroencephalographic correlates of WMIC in the early childhood population by comparing baseline and WMIC task measures of EEG. The day–night and yes–no tasks have been particularly valuable for the electrophysiological avenue of our research program because they do not require any gross motor movement from the child and therefore do not introduce any intentional artifact into the physiological recording.

When the children in our infant sample were 4½ years of age, we examined WMIC task performance and EEG power using age-appropriate WMIC tasks (Wolfe & Bell, 2004). One of the research questions that guided this particular study was whether task-related power change at 6–9 Hz would be evident for preschool children as it had been for infants; that is, whether a similar increase in EEG power from the baseline measures to the task measures for multiple scalp locations would be evident in this population. (Previous longitudinal work had demonstrated that 6–9 Hz continues to be the dominant frequency band for preschool children during a baseline context and further purported that 6–10 Hz would be appropriate for older preschoolers; Marshall, Bar-Haim, & Fox, 2002.) In our study, EEG was recorded from the left and right hemispheres at eight scalp regions (frontal pole, medial frontal, lateral frontal, anterior temporal, posterior temporal, central, parietal, and occipital) during baseline and task periods. The baseline EEG data were collected as the children watched a 1-minute video clip, and the WMIC task EEG data were collected during the administration of the day–night and yes–no tasks.

The results of this study provided more indirect evidence for the involvement of the prefrontal cortex in WMIC in early childhood, thereby lending further support to both the early childhood brain–behavior associations purported by Diamond and the applicability of the Kane and Engle organizational framework of working memory to young children. Specifically, an increase in EEG power from baseline to task was evident for only one of the eight regions included in the investigation: the medial frontal region. The two scalp electrodes that comprise the medial frontal region (F3 and F4, the left and right medial frontal regions, respectively) are located above the prefrontal area. Although we are unable to unequivocally implicate the involvement of the prefrontal cortex, and specifically the DLPFC, these EEG data are consistent with the hypothesis of DLPFC involvement in these WMIC tasks in early childhood.

Individual Differences in WMIC in Early Childhood

Diamond has noted the dramatic improvements in WMIC abilities in the early childhood years and hypothesized about the associated development of certain brain systems. Yet all children do not improve in their WMIC abilities at the same rate. Furthermore, age does not seem to be a direct indicator of WMIC ability, in that some young children can outperform some older children on a given day (Wolfe & Bell, 2006). Our research program with preschoolers includes an investigation of three variables that have been linked both theoretically and empirically with WMIC: EEG, temperament, and language.

Electroencephalogram

Research in our lab has found differences in EEG power to be associated with performance on the day–night and yes–no WMIC tasks (Wolfe & Bell, 2004). Specifically, when children were divided into high and low performance groups based on their day–night and yes–no task performance, those children in the high WMIC performance group had higher EEG power values at both baseline and task than those children in the low WMIC performance group for the medial frontal, lateral frontal, and anterior temporal regions. These higher power values for the children in the high WMIC performance group are in accordance with the infant work showing higher power values for higher performing infants on a comparable WMIC task (Bell, 2001, 2002).

Additionally, we have consistently found recordings from the left medial frontal scalp location (i.e., F3) to be positively associated with performance on the WMIC tasks in the preschool population (Wolfe & Bell, 2004, 2006, in press). This association holds in bivariate analyses as well as in multivariate analyses in which power from the left medial frontal region contributes uniquely to the explanation of variance in WMIC performance (Wolfe & Bell, 2004, 2006, in press). Furthermore, power from the left medial frontal scalp location has been shown to explain variability in WMIC performance above and beyond the age variable (Wolfe & Bell, 2006). The brain electrical activity represented by the left medial frontal power measure may be associated with the functioning of the prefrontal cortex. The power values of the left medial frontal scalp electrode may also be indicative of neural activity associated with Broca's area. Broca's area is most often associated with speech production (a necessary component of the WMIC tasks employed in this study) and has many connections with the prefrontal cortex. Also, the left frontal lobe plays a substantial role in language-related planning and movement, such as speech, relative to the right frontal lobe (Kolb & Whishaw, 2003).

Temperament

In addition to the development in WMIC during the preschool years, an aspect of regulation that improves dramatically is the control of emotions and related behaviors (e.g., Kochanska, Murray, & Harlan, 2000; Kopp, 1982; Mischel & Mischel, 1983). Because of the conceptual similarity shared by the constructs of attentional control and emotional control, there has been increasing interest in comparing the development of these constructs and identifying common neural circuitry (Bell & Wolfe, 2004; Blair, 2002; Bush et al., 2000; Cacioppo & Berntson, 1999; Posner & Rothbart, 2000; Rothbart & Derryberry, 1981; Rothbart, Derryberry, & Posner, 1994; Rothbart & Posner, 2001; Ruff & Rothbart, 1996).

In fact, research is beginning to show that individual differences in behavioral style (i.e., temperament; Rothbart & Bates, 1998) are related to cognitive processing involving attentional control (Davis, Bruce, & Gunnar, 2002; Gerardi-Caulton, 2000). In general, positive associations have been found between measures of attentional control and the regulatory dimensions of temperament, such as the Effortful Control factor from the Children's Behavior Questionnaire (CBQ; Rothbart, Ahadi, Hershey, & Fisher, 2001) and its component scales (i.e., Inhibitory Control, Attentional Focusing, Perceptual Sensitivity, and Low Sensitivity Pleasure). Likewise, negative associations have been found between attentional control measures and the nonregulatory or surgent dimensions of temperament of the CBQ, such as Anger/Frustration, Impulsivity, and Approach/Anticipation.

Recent research and theorizing within our own lab (Bell & Wolfe, 2004; Wolfe & Bell, 2004) have corroborated these cognition–temperament findings. Specifically, we have demonstrated positive associations between collective performance on the day–night and yes–no tasks and the two scales of the Effortful Control factor that seem to draw on the more cognitive component of the factor; that is, the Attention Focusing and Inhibitory Control scales. Like Gerardi-Caulton (2000), we have demonstrated a negative relation between WMIC performance and the Anger/Frustration scale of the CBQ, suggesting that children who perform better on the WMIC tasks also have a greater ability to regulate their emotions of anger and frustration.

Finally, we have found an unexpected but rather robust relation between WMIC performance and parental ratings of Approach/Anticipation, a scale that is included in the Surgency factor of the CBQ. A consideration of the CBQ items that comprise the Approach/Anticipation scale provides some insight into this negative association; items include "gets very enthusiastic about the things s/he does," "shows great excitement about opening a present," and "gets so excited about things s/he has trouble sitting still." Although these findings are contrary to some work on temperament and cognition that reports that outgoing, sociable, and active children score higher on mental tasks, they are consistent with the findings of Davis and colleagues (2002), who reported a strong, but also unexpected, negative correlation between the Surgency factor of the CBQ and performance on inhibitory control tasks used by Casey and colleagues (e.g., Casey et al., 1997).

Language

The associations between language and memory are well established (e.g., Adams & Gathercole, 1995; Rose et al., 1991). We have found individual differences in WMIC to be related to individual differences in language comprehension (Wolfe & Bell, 2004, in press). Specifically, the children with the highest working memory scores also tend to have the highest receptive language abilities, as measured by the Peabody Picture Vocabulary Test–III (PPVT-III; Dunn & Dunn, 1997). A high score on the PPVT-III suggests strong comprehension and understanding of the spoken word— a skill that is advantageous for performance on our WMIC tasks in which following oral instructions is crucial.

Preliminary data from a very recent project in our lab indicate that language comprehension is *the* most valuable measure in the prediction and explanation of variance in WMIC performance when compared to EEG, temperament, or age (Wolfe & Bell, 2006). In fact, children's scores on the PPVT-III accounted for over 39% of the variance in WMIC performance for all three age groups (i.e., 3½-, 4-, and 4½-year-olds). Furthermore, when the association between WMIC performance and language comprehension was considered separately for each age group, the strength of the association tended to increase with age (i.e., age 3½, $r = .506$; age 4, $r = .621$; age 4½, $r = .758$).

What is it about knowing a lot of words that is associated with being able to perform these WMIC tasks well? Is language ability influencing WMIC skills? Or are WMIC skills allowing for the development of language? Or is there a third variable influencing both constructs? All of these explanations are conceivable. First, it is logical that the more words one knows, the better one can think through problems using private speech or self-talk. Second, it is also logical that the more WMIC one has, the better able to and more quickly one will learn words and associate them with their correct meanings. Finally, the third explanation is feasible and can be argued with the inclusion of many different factors. For example, parents could be influencing both WMIC and language comprehension. It is certain that parents are influencing word learning through their behaviors, such as reading and talking to their children and through other experiences that they provide. It is also certain that parents are facilitating the development of WMIC and the functioning of the prefrontal cortex through biological (genetic and cellular material) and environmental contributions, including the experiences they provide for their children, the way they talk to their children (e.g., Hoff-Ginsberg, 1991), and the way they perceive and interact with their children as independent thinkers (e.g., Landry, Smith, Swank, & Miller-Loncar, 2000).

Furthermore, theorists have suggested an association between self-regulatory aspects of temperament qualities and the development of language. It has been suggested that the development of language along with the continued development of the frontal cortex may underlie further advances in voluntary control of behavior and action (Ruff & Rothbart, 1996). In fact, an association between language and the self-regulatory aspects of development, especially those that involve higher-level attentional control, has been reported (Kaler & Kopp, 1990; Kopp, 1989).

Summary and Conclusion

Early childhood is a period of extraordinary change and advancement in many aspects of cognitive and social functioning. Our ability to track the developmental changes in WMIC has been made possible by the creation of age-appropriate cognitive tasks requiring the integration of working memory and inhibitory control, such as the day–night and yes–no tasks. Diamond's research program has contributed greatly to our knowledge of the development of WMIC skills in early childhood as well as to our understanding of the continued development of the DLPFC during this time period. Research in our lab has added EEG data to this knowledge base and lent support to the involvement of the prefrontal cortex in these WMIC tasks in early childhood. Our research has also demonstrated that individual differences in WMIC functioning are related to individual differences in brain electrical activity, temperament, and language comprehension in early childhood, and that knowing the age of the child is not necessarily sufficient to predict how the child will perform in terms of WMIC ability.

WMIC FROM INFANCY TO EARLY CHILDHOOD

With our longitudinal data set, we also wanted to explore the possibility that *infant* temperament would influence *childhood* cognition. There is some evidence that infant temperament may be related to general cognitive development in early childhood. For example, Lewis (1993) found that distress at 3 months in a maternal separation–reunion paradigm predicted lower scores on a general cognitive index of memory, motor, and verbal abilities at age 4 years. With our specific interests in WMIC, we hypothesized that the attentional and regulatory aspects of infant temperament would predict working memory performance during early childhood (Wolfe & Bell, in press).

In our longitudinal sample, both infant and child EEG and infant and child temperament were correlated; however, infant and child WMIC performance were not correlated. More importantly, as shown in Figure 9.2, infant temperament was a predictor of child language and child WMIC (Wolfe & Bell, in press). Specifically, Approach/Anticipation at age 4½ years mediated the relation between 8-month Soothability and 4½-year WMIC, with a positive correlation between Soothability and Approach/Anticipation. In essence, an infant difficult to soothe at 8 months may be low on Approach/Anticipation behaviors at 4½ years and thus more likely to perform well on WMIC tasks involving controlled, inhibitory processing. In supporting infants during distress or fussiness, many parents attempt to soothe infants by distracting them with visual and other stimuli. This distraction experience may aid in the development of attentional skills that are later key in relieving distress (Ruff & Rothbart, 1996). Attentional skills may also contribute to attentional and regulatory abilities, such as self-control during Approach/Anticipation, which is associated with the neural anterior attention system and later complex cognition, such as that required by WMIC tasks.

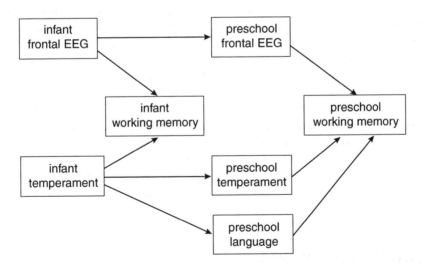

FIGURE 9.2. A diagram illustrating the effects of infant and early childhood frontal EEG, temperament, and language on early childhood WMIC performance. Adapted from Wolfe and Bell (in press).

The age of an infant when distress and soothability are assessed may be important. Lewis (1993) reported that distress of 3-month-olds in a maternal separation–reunion paradigm predicted lower scores on a general cognitive index. However, later measures of distress (i.e., 4–5½ months) did *not* predict cognitive competency at 4 years. It may be that at this slightly older age, infant soothability becomes a better predictor. Perhaps by 4 or 5 months of age the initial distress of earlier infancy is abated or perhaps parental intervention has aided in an initial development of attentional skills, which are hypothesized to be important to later cognition. Lewis suggested that temperamental influences on cognitive outcomes might be age specific. It may be that as temperament "develops" (Rothbart & Bates, 1998), its influence on other developmental processes develops as well.

The correlation between infant temperament and early childhood language was negative. Low levels of Approach and Duration of Orienting during infancy were associated with higher levels of language in childhood. Bloom (1993, 1998) proposed that neutral affect is more advantageous for language development. Both positive and negative affect may interfere with the cognitive capacity required for processing information. Although surgent children are more likely to approach a situation and initially engage in language interactions, their outgoing behaviors may interfere with their capacity to take advantage of these linguistic experiences. The more affectively neutral child may have the time and energy to focus attention on the language component of the interaction and thus benefit more from such encounters. In addition, we found that concurrent language and WMIC scores were positively correlated. Adams and Gathercole (1995) have also reported links between language and WMIC abilities.

With this longitudinal investigation from 8 months to 4½ years of age, we have made an initial attempt to link infant and early childhood brain–behavior data. By focusing on attentional and regulatory behaviors, we have shown that it may be possible to predict early childhood cognitive abilities not from infant cognitive performance, but from infant temperament characteristics. These findings suggest the value of early-learned regulatory and attentional behaviors and the impact of these early skills on later development.

MIDDLE CHILDHOOD

Very recently, we have begun to include investigations of WMIC during the middle childhood years in our program of research, as the children in our longitudinal study have reached 8 years of age (Adkins & Bell, 2006). Our work during this developmental time period has been largely influenced by the writings of Roberts and Pennington (1996), who have noted that much of the research on cognitive development past the early childhood period has focused on working memory and inhibitory control as *separate* cognitive constructs. Advocating the integration of these constructs in research on later development, Roberts and Pennington have indicated that many studies with older children employ tasks that are known to simultaneously tap both working memory and inhibitory control (e.g., the Wisconsin Card Sort Task, the traditional Stroop task, the antisaccade task, the Tower of Hanoi, and the counting go/no-go task), even though these cognitive skills are discussed separately in the research reports. In an examination of executive processes with children ages 8 and older, Luna and colleagues (Luna, Garver, Urban, Lazar, & Sweeney, 2004) have shown that whereas many executive function processes are independent, working memory and inhibitory control specifically appear to be interdependent. This finding lends credence to Roberts and Pennington's assertion that working memory and inhibitory control should be treated as an integrated process in developmental research. Likewise, Diamond (2002) has implicated the role of prefrontal areas in tasks that require older children (7 years onward) to maintain and manipulate information, use strategies, and exercise inhibition (i.e., WMIC tasks).

WMIC Tasks for Middle Childhood

In the 8-year-old children in our longitudinal sample, we used both the Wisconsin Card Sort Task (WCST) and the Stroop task as WMIC measures. All the children for whom we have data at 4½ years returned to our research laboratory at 8 years of age. We have begun initial analyses of these data; here we focus on the card sort task.

Wisconsin Card Sort Task

The WCST requires the individual to use feedback to determine the correct sorting principle (working memory) and to avoid sorting by the same principle when the sorting category changes (inhibition). The WCST has become commonly accepted as a measure of prefrontal functioning (Roberts & Pennington, 1996) and has multiple indices of performance. *Categories completed* has been used as a reflection of both working memory and inhibitory control (Sanz, Molina, Calcedo, Martin-Loeches, & Rubia, 2001) and *total correct* serves an index of overall task success on the WCST.

We used the second edition of the 64-card computerized version of the WCST with our 8-year-olds (WCST-64; Heaton & PAR staff, 2003). The

WCST-64 has the advantage of shortened administration time with retention of the original task demands. The children saw four key cards across the top of the computer screen and were instructed to match a stimulus card, which appeared at the bottom of the screen, to one of the four key cards at the top of the screen. As per WCST procedures, no details concerning the sorting principles were shared with the children, and the sorting could be accomplished by matching color, shape, or number. To move the card to the correct sorting location, the child used the computer mouse, and the computer provided feedback through a written "right" or "wrong" display. After every 10 consecutive correct responses, the matching criteria automatically changed. This process continued until all 64 cards had been sorted. Thus, the task was child driven with respect to the amount of time required for completion.

Individual Differences in WMIC in Middle Childhood

Electroencephalogram

For consistency with our previous EEG data, the same 6–9 Hz frequency band was used to predict WMIC functioning when the children were in middle childhood. We hypothesized that task performance would be associated with EEG only at frontal scalp locations. Indeed, successful performance on the WCST, as indexed by either categories completed or total correct, was associated with EEG power values at both F2 and F8, which are right frontal scalp locations (Adkins & Bell, 2006). Interestingly, this longitudinal sample is the first indication that right frontal power values are associated with task performance, as left frontal EEG was associated with task performance during the preschool assessment.

Temperament

Our previous work with this sample specifically showed that the regulatory and surgent dimensions of temperament were related to WMIC functioning at age 4½ years (Wolfe & Bell, 2004, in press). The self-regulatory temperament trait is referred to as Effortful Control on the Early Adolescent Temperament Questionnaire—Revised (EATQ-R; Ellis & Rothbart, 2001), normed on 9- to 16-year-olds but used successfully with children as young as 7 years of age. We focused on the scales of Inhibitory Control (i.e., the capacity to plan and suppress inappropriate responses), Attention (i.e., the capacity to focus attention as well as to shift attention when desired), and Activation Control (i.e., the capacity to perform an action when there is a strong tendency to avoid it) because they are included as subdimensions of the Effortful Control factor (Ellis & Rothbart, 2001).

With the 8-year-old children in our longitudinal sample, we had a unique opportunity to assess both child and parent reports of temperament. Only the children's self-report of Activation Control emerged as predictive of WMIC functioning. Interestingly, not only was parental report of Activation Control not predictive of WMIC functioning, it was not correlated with child report of Activation Control—contrary to the work of Ellis and Rothbart (2001), which showed that parent and child EATQ-R measures are highly correlated. Our finding is particularly intriguing because it was the parent report of temperament that predicted WMIC performance for our longitudinal sample in infancy and early childhood.

The other dimension of temperament that has been related to WMIC performance is surgency. High Intensity Pleasure (i.e., the pleasure derived from activities involving high intensity or novelty), low levels of Shyness (i.e., behavioral inhibition to novelty and challenge, especially social), and low levels of Fear (i.e., unpleasant affect related to anticipation of distress) make up the Surgent factor of the EATQ-R. With our 8-year-olds, only the child report of High Intensity Pleasure emerged from the Surgent dimension of temperament as predictive of WMIC functioning. Children rating themselves as higher on High Intensity Pleasure scored lower on the WMIC tasks. The parent report of High Intensity Pleasure failed to predict WMIC performance, despite the fact that it was positively correlated with the child report of High Intensity Pleasure.

The child report finding fits nicely with the 4½-year-old data from this sample showing the Surgent dimension of temperament to be negatively related to WMIC performance (Wolfe & Bell, 2004). Additionally, the Surgent dimension of temperament has been negatively related to academic performance in school-age children, such that low levels of fear and shyness paired with high levels of intensity pleasure are indicative of lower grades and more social problems (Rothbart & Jones, 1999). Perhaps the surgent child misses relevant information, both academically and socially, because he or she is easily excited, distracted, and often impulsive.

Language

Language comprehension was the strongest predictor of WMIC functioning in the current sample at age 4½ years (Wolfe & Bell, 2004). However, language comprehension, as tested by the PPVT-III, was not predictive of WMIC functioning at 8 years. It is possible that better language comprehension allowed for greater understanding of the task instructions in early childhood, but that this was not an issue by middle childhood.

Summary and Conclusion

Taken together, temperament (child report of Activation Control and High Intensity Pleasure) and EEG power values (at F2 and F8) explained 45% of the variance in WMIC functioning at 8 years of age. Right frontal EEG power at the F8 scalp location emerged as the strongest predictor of WMIC functioning at 8 years of age. Future planned analyses will serve to distinguish the relations between the predictors at 4½ years of age and performance at 8 years. Initial indications are that this study may provide important information about how individual differences in WMIC functioning may change from early childhood to middle childhood.

WMIC AND IMPLICATIONS FOR EDUCATION

The construct of working memory has been the focus of a great deal of attention in the adult cognitive literature, and with good reason: Working memory is an essential component of everyday adult cognition because it underlies higher-order cognitive processes such as reasoning, planning, cognitive control, problem solving, and decision making (Logie, 1993). Furthermore, individual difference measures of working memory in adulthood are predictive of language comprehension, learning, and fluid intelligence (Engle et al., 1999; Kane & Engle, 2002).

Much less attention has been given to the development of working memory. This is surprising because knowledge about the development of working memory is crucial to education, as school performance is closely tied to this cognitive skill. In preschool children between the ages of 2 and 5 years, both working memory and inhibitory control contribute to emerging mathematics skills (Espy et al., 2004). In young school-age children, working memory is associated with both English and mathematics achievement (Gathercole, Pickering, Ambridge, & Wearing, 2004). Predictably, children with poor working memory performance at age 5 score poorly on reading assessments at age 8 (Gathercole, Tiffany, Briscoe, & Thorn, 2005). Clearly, there appears to be a link between working memory, inhibitory control, and learning.

Because of the association between working memory and educational attainment, Gathercole and Alloway (2006) advocate screening children for working memory impairments and suggest a battery of working memory tasks suitable for that purpose. After identification, the effective management of working memory limitations can be accomplished by reducing working memory load; for example, by having children repeat back instructions and use nonverbal cues such as pictures or visual schematics. Gathercole and Alloway note that school-age children can be explicitly taught these self-help strategies that are likely to improve their learning success. It may be that these types of educational interventions to assist working memory performance actually influence the neural networks underlying learning (Posner & Rothbart, 2005).

Inhibitory control skills have also received some attention with respect to implications for educational achievement. School success is defined not only in terms of learning but also in terms of self-regulation. Thus, success in school depends on the ability to control one's own behavior and get along with others (Posner & Rothbart, 2005), as well as the ability to control action and thought (Riggs, Blair, & Greenberg, 2003). Because of its close conceptual association with inhibitory control skills, self-regulation recently has become the focus of much conceptual and empirical work on school readiness (e.g., Blair, 2002) and early school skills (e.g., Riggs et al., 2003). It is clear that children with stronger self-regulation abilities, including inhibitory control skills, tend to be at an advantage in the classroom and in the social environment of school.

According to Blair (2002), difficulties with inhibitory control and regulation may occur in a child who is otherwise developing in a typical manner. If that child is immersed in an environment that enhances reactive forms of regulation, then he or she is at risk for future difficulties in the development of executive function skills such as working memory, as well as at risk for inadequate school readiness. However, if that child is in a supportive environment that enhances self-regulatory capabilities, then he or she will likely demonstrate a tendency for better inhibitory control and self-regulation skills that contribute to school success (Blair, 2002). Thus, supportive home and preschool environments are potentially significant contributors to a child's educational readiness and achievement.

Clearly, self-regulated learning, along with the associated cognitive skills of working memory and inhibitory control, are crucial to school success. We propose that there is a need to examine the development of working memory and inhibitory control from their earliest origins, including possible contributors to individual differences. Our longitudinal program of research reported here, along with our most current longitudinal study with more frequent data collection points, represent our initial attempts to track these important developmental functions.

ACKNOWLEDGMENTS

Preparation of this chapter was supported in part by a grant from the National Institutes of Health (No. HD 43057) to Martha Ann Bell. Some of the research reported in this chapter was supported by grants from the College of Arts and Sciences at Virginia Tech.

REFERENCES

Adams, A. M., & Gathercole, S. E. (1995). Phonological working memory and speech production in preschool children. *Journal of Speech and Hearing Research, 38,* 403–414.

Adkins, D. R., & Bell, M. A. (2006). *Individual differences in working memory and inhibitory control during middle childhood.* Manuscript in preparation.

Bell, M. A. (2001). Brain electrical activity associated with cognitive processing during a looking version of the A-not-B task. *Infancy, 2,* 311–330.

Bell, M. A. (2002). Power changes in infant EEG frequency bands during a spatial working memory task. *Psychophysiology, 39,* 450–458.

Bell, M. A. (2005). *Individual differences in spatial working memory performance at 8 months: Contributions of electrophysiology and temperament.* Manuscript submitted for publication.

Bell, M. A. (in press). Tutorial on electroencephalogram methodology: EEG research with infants and young children. In D. L. Molfese & V. J. Molfese (Eds.), *Handbook of developmental neuropsychology.* Mahwah, NJ: Erlbaum.

Bell, M. A., & Adams, S. E. (1999). Comparable performance on looking and reaching versions of the A-not-B task at 8 months of age. *Infant Behavior and Development, 22,* 221–235.

Bell, M. A., & Fox, N. A. (1992). The relations between frontal brain electrical activity and cognitive development during infancy. *Child Development, 63,* 1142–1163.

Bell, M. A., & Fox, N. A. (1994). Brain development over the first year of life: Relations between electroencephalographic frequency and coherence and cognitive and affective behaviors. In G. Dawson & K.W. Fischer (Eds.), *Human behavior and the developing brain* (pp. 314–345). New York: Guilford Press.

Bell, M. A., & Wolfe, C. D. (2004). Emotion and cognition: An intricately bound developmental process. *Child Development, 75,* 366–370.

Blair, C. (2002). School readiness: Integrating cognition and emotion in a neurobiological conceptualization of children's functioning at school entry. *American Psychologist, 57,* 111–127.

Bloom, L. (1993). *The transition from infancy to language: Acquiring the power of expression.* New York: Cambridge University Press.

Bloom, L. (1998). Language acquisition in its developmental context. In W. Damon (Series Ed.), D. Kuhn & R. S. Siegler (Vol. Eds.), *Handbook of child psychology: Vol. 2. Cognition, perception, and language* (5th ed., pp. 309–420). New York: Wiley.

Bush, G., Luu, P., & Posner, M. I. (2000). Cognitive and emotional influences in anterior cingulate cortex. *Trends in Cognitive Sciences, 4,* 215–222.

Cacioppo, J. T., & Berntson, G. G. (1999). The affect system: Architecture and operating characteristics. *Current Directions in Psychological Science, 8,* 133–137.

Casey, B. J., & deHaan, M. (2002). Introduction: New methods in developmental science. *Developmental Science, 5,* 265–267.

Casey, B. J., Tottenham, N., Liston, C., & Durston, S. (2005). Imaging the developing brain: What have we learned about cognitive development? *Cognitive Sciences, 9,* 104–110.

Casey, B. J., Trainor, R. J., Orendi, J. L., Schubert, A. B., Nystrom, L. E., Giedd, J. N., et al. (1997). A developmental functional MRI study of prefrontal activation during performance of a go no-go task. *Journal of Cognitive Neuroscience, 9,* 835–847.

Colombo, J., & Saxon, T. F. (2002). Infant attention and the development of cognition: Does the environment moderate continuity? In H. E. Fitzgerald, K. H. Karraker, & T. Luster (Eds.), *Infant development: Ecological perspectives* (pp. 35–60). Washington, DC: Garland Press.

Davis, E. P., Bruce, J., & Gunnar, M. R. (2002). The anterior attention network: Associations with temperament and neuroendocrine activity in 6-year-old children. *Developmental Psychobiology, 40,* 43–56.

Diamond, A. (1985). Development of the ability to use recall to guide action, as indicated by infants' performance on AB. *Child Development, 56,* 868–883.

Diamond, A. (2001). A model system for studying the role of dopamine in the prefrontal cortex during early development in humans: Early and continuously treated phenylketonuria. In C. A. Nelson & M. Luciana (Eds.), *Handbook of developmental cognitive neuroscience* (pp. 433–472). Cambridge, MA: MIT Press.

Diamond, A. (2002). Normal development of prefrontal cortex from birth to young adulthood: Cognitive functions, anatomy, and biochemistry. In D. T. Stuss & R. T. Knight (Eds.), *Principles of frontal lobe function* (pp. 466–503). London: Oxford University Press.

Diamond, A., & Goldman-Rakic, P. S. (1989). Comparison of human infants and rhesus monkeys on Piaget's AB task: Evidence for dependence on dorsolateral prefrontal cortex. *Experimental Brain Research, 74,* 24–40.

Diamond, A., Kirkham, N., & Amso, D. (2002). Conditions under which young children can hold two rules in mind and inhibit a prepotent response. *Developmental Psychology, 38,* 352–362.

Diamond, A., Prevor, M. B., Callender, G., & Druin, D. P. (1997). Prefrontal cortex deficits in children treated early and continuously for PKU. *Monographs of the Society for Research in Child Development, 62*(4, Serial No. 252).

Diamond, A., & Taylor, C. (1996). Development of an aspect of executive control: Development of the abilities to remember what I said and to "Do as I say, not as I do." *Developmental Psychobiology, 29,* 315–334.

Diamond, A., Zola-Morgan, S., & Squire, L. R. (1989). Successful performance by monkeys with lesions of the hippocampal formation on AB and object retrieval, two tasks that mark developmental changes in human infants. *Behavioral Neuroscience, 103,* 526–537.

Dunn, L. M., & Dunn, L. (1997). *Peabody Picture Vocabulary Test* (3rd ed.). Circle Pines, MN: AGS.

Ellis, L. K., & Rothbart, M. K. (2001, April). *Revision of the Early Adolescent Temperament Questionnaire.* Poster presented at the biennial meeting of the Society for Research in Child Development, Minneapolis, MN.

Ellis, L. K., & Rothbart, M. K. (2001, April). *Revision of the Early Adolescent*

Temperament Questionnaire. Poster presented at the annual meeting of the Society for Research in Child Development, Minneapolis, MN.

Engle, R. W., Kane, M. J., & Tuholski, S. W. (1999). Individual differences in working memory capacity and what they tell us about controlled attention, general fluid intelligence and functions of the prefrontal cortex. In A. Miyake & P. Shah (Eds.), *Models of working memory: Mechanisms of active maintenance and executive control* (pp. 102–134). New York: Cambridge University Press.

Espy, K. A., McDiarmid, M. M., Cwik, M. F., Stalets, M. M., Hamby, A., & Senn, T. E. (2004). The contribution of executive functions to emergent mathematic skills in preschool children. *Developmental Neuropsychology, 26,* 465–486.

Gathercole, S. E., & Alloway, T. P. (2006). Practitioner review: Short-term and working memory impairments in neurodevelopmental disorders: Diagnosis and remedial support. *Journal of Child Psychology and Psychiatry, 47,* 4–15.

Gathercole, S. E., Pickering, S. J., Ambridge, B., & Wearing, H. (2004). The structure of working memory from 4 to 15 years of age. *Developmental Psychology, 40,* 177–190.

Gathercole, S. E., Tiffany, C., Briscoe, J., & Thorn, A. (2005). Developmental consequences of poor phonological short-term memory function in childhood: A longitudinal study. *Journal of Child Psychology and Psychiatry, 46,* 598–611.

Gerardi-Caulton, G. (2000). Sensitivity to spatial conflict and the development of self-regulation in children 24–36 months of age. *Developmental Science, 3,* 397–404.

Gerstadt, C. L., Hong, Y. J., & Diamond, A. (1994). The relationship between cognition and action: Performance of children 3½–7 years old on a Stroop-like day–night test. *Cognition, 53,* 129–153.

Heaton, R. K., & PAR staff. (2003). *WCST-64: Computer Version Scoring Program—Version 2 Research Edition (WCST-64: SP2)*. Lutz, FL: PAR.

Hoff-Ginsberg, E. (1991). Mother–child conversation in different social classes and communicative settings. *Child Development, 62,* 782–796.

Kaler, S. R., & Kopp, C. B. (1990). Compliance and comprehension in very young toddlers. *Child Development, 61,* 1997–2003.

Kane, M. J., & Engle, R. W. (2002). The role of prefrontal cortex in working-memory capacity, executive attention, and general fluid intelligence: An individual-differences perspective. *Psychonomic Bulletin and Review, 9,* 637–671.

Kochanska, G., Murray, K. T., & Harlan, E. T. (2000). Effortful control in early childhood: Continuity and change, antecedents, and implications for social development. *Developmental Psychology, 36,* 220–232.

Kolb, B., & Whishaw, I. Q. (2003). *Fundamentals of human neuropsychology* (5th ed.). New York: Worth.

Kopp, C. B. (1982). Antecedents of self-regulation: A developmental perspective. *Developmental Psychology, 18,* 199–214.

Kopp, C. B. (1989). Regulation of distress and negative emotions: A developmental view. *Developmental Psychology, 25,* 343–354.

Landry, S. H., Smith, K. E., Swank, P. R., & Miller-Loncar, C. L. (2000). Early maternal and child influences on children's later independent cognitive and social functioning. *Child Development, 71,* 358–375.

Lewis, M. D. (1993). Early socioemotional predictors of cognitive competency at 4 years. *Developmental Psychology, 29,* 1036–1045.

Logie, R. H. (1993). Working memory in everyday cognition. In G. M. Davies & R. H. Logie (Eds.), *Memory in everyday life* (pp. 173–218). Amsterdam: North-Holland.

Luciana, M., & Nelson, C. A. (1998). The functional emergence of prefrontally-guided working memory systems in four- to eight-year-old children. *Neuropsychologia, 36,* 273–293.

Luna, B., Garver, K. E., Urban, T. A., Lazar, N. A., & Sweeney, J. A. (2004). Maturation of cognitive processes from late childhood to adulthood. *Child Development, 75*(5), 1357–1372.

Luria, A. R. (1966). *The higher cortical functions in man.* New York: Basic Books.

Marshall, P. J., Bar-Haim, Y., & Fox, N. A. (2002). Development of the EEG from 5 months to 4 years of age. *Clinical Neurophysiology, 113,* 1199–1208.

Matthews, A., Ellis, A. E., & Nelson, C. A. (1996). Development of preterm and full-term infant ability on AB, recall memory, transparent barrier detour, and means–end tasks. *Child Development, 67,* 2658–2676.

Mischel, H. N., & Mischel, W. (1983). The development of children's knowledge of self-control strategies. *Child Development, 54,* 603–619.

Orekhova, E. V., Stroganova, T. A., & Posikera, I. N. (2001). Alpha activity as an index of cortical inhibition during sustained internally controlled attention in infants. *Clinical Neurophysiology, 112,* 740–749.

Pelphrey, K. A., Reznick, J. S., Davis Goldman, B., Sasson, N., Morrow, J., Donahoe, A., et al. (2004). Development of visuospatial short-term memory in the second half of the 1st year. *Developmental Psychology, 40,* 836–851.

Posner, M. I., & Rothbart, M. K. (2000). Developing mechanisms of self-regulation. *Development and Psychopathology, 12,* 427–441.

Posner, M. I., & Rothbart, M. K. (2005). Influencing brain networks: Implications for education. *Trends in Cognitive Sciences, 9,* 99–103.

Riggs, N. R., Blair, C. B., & Greenberg, M. T. (2003). Concurrent and 2-year longitudinal relations between executive function and the behavior of 1st and 2nd grade children. *Child Neuropsychology, 19,* 267–276.

Roberts, R. J., & Pennington, B. F. (1996). An interactive framework for examining prefrontal cognitive processes. *Developmental Neuropsychology, 12*(1), 105–126.

Rose, S. A., Feldman, J. F., Wallace, I. F., & Cohen, P. (1991). Language: A partial link between infant attention and later intelligence. *Developmental Psychology, 27,* 798–805.

Rothbart, M. K., Ahadi, S. A., Hershey, K. L., & Fisher, P. (2001). Investigations of temperament at three to seven years: The Children's Behavior Questionnaire. *Child Development, 72,* 1394–1408.

Rothbart, M. K., & Bates, J. C. (1998). Temperament. In N. Eisenburg (Ed.) & W. Damon (Series Ed.), *Handbook of child psychology: Vol. 3. Social, emotional, and personality development* (pp. 105–176). New York: Wiley.

Rothbart, M. K., & Derryberry, D. (1981). Development of individual differences in temperament. In M. E. Lamb & L. Brown (Eds.), *Advances in developmental psychology* (pp. 37–86). Hillsdale, NJ: Erlbaum.

Rothbart, M. K., Derryberry, D., & Posner, M. I. (1994). A psychobiological approach to the development of temperament. In J. E. Bates & T. D. Wachs (Eds.), *Temperament: individual differences at the interface of biology and behavior* (pp. 83–116). Washington, DC: American Psychological Association.

Rothbart, M. K., & Jones, L. B. (1999). Temperament, self-regulation and education. *School Psychology Review, 27,* 479–491.

Rothbart, M. K., & Posner, M. I. (2001). Mechanism and variation in the development of attentional networks. In C. A. Nelson & M. Luciana (Eds.), *Handbook of developmental cognitive neuroscience* (pp. 353–364). Cambridge, MA: MIT Press.

Ruff, H. A., & Rothbart, M. K. (1996). *Attention in early development: Themes and variations.* New York: Oxford University Press.

Sanz, M., Molina, V., Calcedo, A., Martin-Loeches, M., & Rubia, F. J. (2001). The Wisconsin Card Sorting Test and the assessment of frontal function in obsessive–compulsive patients: An event-related potential study. *Cognitive Neuropsychiatry, 6*(2), 109–129.

Stroop, J. R. (1935). Studies of interference in serial verbal reactions. *Journal of Experimental Psychology, 18,* 643–661.

Taylor, M. J., & Baldeweg, T. (2002). Application of EEG, ERP, and intracranial recordings to the investigation of cognitive functions in children. *Developmental Science, 5,* 318–334.

Welsh, M. C., Pennington, B. F., & Groisser, D. B. (1991). A normative-developmental study of executive function: A window on prefrontal function in children. *Developmental Neuropsychology, 7,* 131–149.

Wolfe, C. D., & Bell, M. A. (2004). Working memory and inhibitory control in early childhood: Contributions from physiology, temperament, and language. *Developmental Psychobiology, 44,* 68–83.

Wolfe, C. D., & Bell, M. A. (in press). The integration of cognition and emotion during infancy and early childhood: Regulatory processes associated with the development of working memory. *Brain and Cognition.*

Wolfe, C. D., & Bell, M. A. (2006). *Sources of variability in working memory performance in early childhood: A consideration of age, temperament, language, and EEG.* Manuscript submitted for publication.

Zelazo, P. D., Müller, U., Frye, D., & Marcovitch, S. (2003). The development of executive function in early childhood. *Monographs of the Society for Research in Child Development, 68*(3, Serial No. 274).

PART III

THE DEVELOPING BRAIN
AND BEHAVIOR IN SCHOOL-AGE
CHILDREN AND ADOLESCENTS

CHAPTER 10

Brain Bases of Learning and Development of Language and Reading

James R. Booth

The purpose of this chapter is to review what is known about the development of neurocognitive networks for language and reading. The chapter focuses on age-related changes in orthographic, phonological, semantic, and syntactical processing. Particular attention is paid to how these different representational systems are integrated by the posterior heteromodal cortex and how anterior systems in the inferior frontal gyrus may modulate these processes. Throughout this chapter, we examine whether learning mechanisms in adults are similar to developmental changes. Similarities between learning and development would support the skill-learning hypothesis that the neural basis of behavioral and cognitive development in children is the same as skill acquisition in adults (Johnson, 2001).

GENERAL MODEL OF FUNCTIONAL BRAIN DEVELOPMENT

Some have argued that a single cognitive process may involve the functional integration of many specialized areas (Friston & Price, 2001). Consistent with this premise, Johnson and colleagues have put forth the interactive specialization approach to functional brain development in humans (Johnson, 2003, 2005; Johnson & Munakata, 2005; see also Johnson, Chapter 5, this volume). According to this approach, over development, there is increasing specialization of brain regions and pathways into systems that have different computational principles. Once these specialized systems have started to develop, there is increasing integration among the systems. Studies have shown that abnormal interactions among systems affect their development (Maurer, Lewis, Brent, & Levin, 1999), so this integration is likely to involve a cascaded process. Increasing specialization with development is consistent with the finding that there is pruning of synapses over childhood into adolescence (Huttenlocher & Dabholkar, 1997). There is also behavioral evidence for lack of specialization in infants and young children, for example, in the processing of color and motion (Dobkins, 2006). Increasing integration with development is also consistent with the finding of gradual increases in white matter tracts over childhood into adolescence (Paus et al., 1999) and with electroencephalogram evidence showing increasing coherence among brain regions with age (Thatcher, Walker, & Guidice, 1987). There is also behavioral evidence for increasing integration between specialized systems, for example, in numerical development (Carey, 2001). This chapter presents data from neuroimaging research in language and reading that suggest that these processes of specialization and integration characterize functional brain development in humans.

MODEL OF LEXICAL PROCESSING

Over the past few years, my colleagues and I have developed a working model of how auditory and visual word representations may be processed in the brains of adults. This model suggests a left-lateralized network with orthographic processing involving visual association areas that include the fusiform gyrus, phonological processing involving auditory association areas that include the superior temporal gyrus, and semantic processing involving amodal association areas that include the middle temporal gyrus. Mappings between these representational systems seem to be mediated in part by heteromodal areas in the inferior parietal cortex (Booth et al., 2002a, 2002b). These posterior language processing systems are strongly interconnected with anterior systems in the frontal lobe. Figure 10.1 shows where these regions are located on the surface of the brain. Various studies have suggested that the anterior ventral portion of the inferior frontal gyrus is involved in semantic processing, whereas the dorsal posterior region of the inferior frontal gyrus is involved in phonological and grammatical pro-

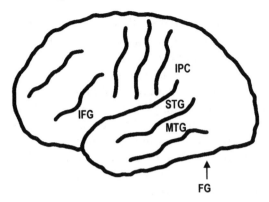

FIGURE 10.1. Brain regions involved in auditory and visual lexical processing: superior temporal gyrus (STG), fusiform gyrus (FG; not shown on this lateral view—it is located on the ventral portion of the temporal lobes), middle temporal gyrus (MTG), inferior parietal cortex (IPC), and inferior frontal gyrus (IFG).

cessing (Caplan, Alpert, & Waters, 1998; Poldrack, Desmond, Glover, & Gabrieli, 1998). This model of lexical processing was developed primarily through adult neuroimaging and patient studies, so research is needed to determine how well this model applies to development or learning.

Orthographic Processing in the Fusiform Gyrus

Reading acquisition is marked by greater elaboration of orthographic representations that involves increases in the number of lexical representations, in the precision of these representations, and in the interconnectivity among these representations (Perfetti, 1992). Adults show greater activation than children in the fusiform gyrus when presented with words in the visual modality (Booth, Burman, Meyer, Lei, et al., 2003), suggesting a greater functional elaboration of this system in response to task demands. Adults also show greater selective activation than children in the left fusiform gyrus when processing visual word forms as compared to auditory word forms, suggesting that adults have a more specialized system for orthographic processing. Plate 10.1a shows that adults have more activation during spelling, rhyming, and meaning tasks in the visual modality when compared to those same tasks in the auditory modality (Booth, Burman, Meyer, Lei, et al., 2003). When the same comparison is done for children, there is no selective activation. In contrast to adults, children show substantial overlap in brain activation when processing visual or auditory word forms. Plate 10.1b shows that adults have activation in the fusiform gyrus for words presented in the visual modality, but not when presented in the auditory modality (Booth et al., 2001). In contrast, Plate 10.1c shows that children have activation in the fusiform gyrus for both the visual and auditory modality (Booth et al., 2001).

Although orthographic representations seem to be more specialized in adults, there is also evidence that greater skill is associated with increasing interactivity between orthographic and phonological systems. Children who demonstrate higher accuracy show greater activation than children who demonstrate lower accuracy in the fusiform gyrus during an auditory rhyming task that does not require access to orthography for correct performance. The activation of representational systems that are unnecessary for performance may result from the higher accuracy children's greater experience with making mappings among representational systems. Plate 10.1d shows this correlation between accuracy and skill (Cone, Burman, Bitan, & Booth, submitted). Altogether, these results suggest that representations become more elaborated, specialized, and interconnected with development/skill.

Greater elaboration of the fusiform gyrus has also been shown in learning studies in adults, and greater specialization of the fusiform gyrus with development has been demonstrated in other cognitive domains. Training in face recognition results in increased activation in the fusiform gyrus (Gauthier, Tarr, Anderson, Skudlarski, & Gore, 1999), suggesting that elaboration of representations with learning occurs in other cognitive domains. In development, increasing specialization in the fusiform gyrus has also been shown during face processing (Passarotti et al., 2003). Although children and adults showed a similar amount of activation in the fusiform gyrus, it was distributed differently. Adults showed greater activation in the right medial as compared to the lateral fusiform gyrus, whereas children showed about an equal amount of activation in both lateral and medial regions. This difference resulted from a modest, nonsignificant developmental increase in activation in the medial fusiform gyrus, whereas the lateral fusiform gyrus showed a significant reduction of activation with development. These studies suggest that elaboration and specialization of representations may be general characteristics of learning and development in the brain.

A greater role of the left fusiform gyrus in orthographic processing seems to be associated with developmental and learning related reductions in activation in the right fusiform gyrus. Decreases in right fusiform gyrus activation with development have been shown for an implicit reading task that involved determining whether there was an ascending letter in visually presented words (Turkeltaub, Gareau, Flowers, Zeffiro, & Eden, 2003). Studies have also shown that adults' learning to read mirror-reversed text is associated with decreases in activation in the inferior temporal regions in the right hemisphere and increases of activation in the left fusiform gyrus (Poldrack et al., 1998). Some have suggested that reading acquisition is initially a right-hemispheric process that relies more on global visual forms, with greater engagement of the left hemisphere with increasing skill as analytic mappings are made between letters/symbols and phonemes/syllables (Orton, 1937).

Phonological Processing in the Superior Temporal Gyrus

As with orthographic processing, phonological processing seems to be characterized by increasing specialization of representations. Six-month-olds show large event-related potentials (ERPs) over both the left occipital and left temporal regions. Over the first 3 years of life, there is a gradual reduction of the left occipital response so that at 36 months, children show a reliable response to auditory stimuli only over the left temporal region (Neville, 1995; see also Mills & Sheehan, Chapter 7, this volume). In an ERP study that presented known and unknown auditory words to infants, 13- to 17-month-olds showed a differential response to these word types over frontal, parietal, and temporal sites in both hemispheres, whereas 20-month-olds showed a differential response only over temporal and parietal sites in the left hemisphere (Mills, Coffey-Corina, & Neville, 1997). Similar ERP effects have recently been reported when contrasting known words with nonsense words (Mills et al., 2004). The consolidation of the ERPs over the left auditory cortex in all of these studies suggests that this region is becoming specialized for processing speech early in development. However, this increasing specialization seems to continue through childhood. Older children (9- to 11-year-olds) show substantial overlap in brain activation associated with processing visual and auditory word forms. In contrast, adults show greater selective activation of the left superior temporal gyrus when processing auditory word forms as compared to visual word forms. Plate 10.1e shows this selective activation for the auditory modality for adults, and Plate 10.1f shows the overlap in activation between the visual and auditory modality for children (Booth et al., 2001). All of these results suggest that the superior temporal region becomes more specialized for phonological processing over development.

Developmental changes in the superior temporal region seem to depend on the task. Plate 10.1g shows developmental increases in activation for a rhyming task in the auditory modality, and this developmental increase for the lexical task did not overlap with activation associated with auditory processing of tones, suggesting that this increase was associated with linguistic processing (Cone et al., submitted). However, another study has recently shown developmental decreases in activation in the left superior temporal region when comparing rhyming judgments to visually presented words with nonlinguistic visual processing. Plate 10.1h shows these developmental decreases in Heschl's gyrus, and they are independent of both accuracy and reaction time differences on the rhyming task (Bitan et al., submitted). The greater activation in younger children may reflect greater reliance on unimodal auditory/phonological representations for the rhyming judgement. Activation in Heschl's gyrus and surrounding auditory processing areas has been associated with various acoustic parameters such as consonant perception and voice onset time processing (Binder et al., 2000; Jäncke, Wüstenberg, Scheich, & Heinze, 2002; Joanisse & Gati, 2003).

Although there are developmental decreases in auditory cortex activation, there are developmental increases in activation of the left inferior frontal gyrus during the visual rhyming task (Bitan et al., submitted). Older children may be relying more on phonological segmentation and covert articulation processes. Research suggests that the inferior frontal gyrus is involved in segmental processing and subvocal rehearsal (Clark & Wagner, 2003; Fiez, Balota, Raichle, & Petersen, 1999; Hagoort, Indefrey, Brown, Herzog, Steinmetz, & Seitz, 1999). Alternatively, developmental decreases in activation of the superior temporal region, combined with developmental increases in activation in the inferior frontal gyrus, may reflect a shift from reliance on whole-word phonological patterns in the superior temporal region in young children to a reliance on phonological segmentation in the inferior frontal gyrus in older children. This interpretation is supported by behavioral research that suggests a developmental progression from sensitivity to larger phonological units to smaller phonological units in speech processing (Stanovich, 1992). Most children master word-level skills before syllable-level skills, and syllable-level skills before onset-rime level skills, and onset-rime level skills before phoneme-level skills (Anthony, Lonigan, Driscoll, Phillips, & Burgess, 2003; Treiman & Zukowski 1996). Phoneme awareness appears to develop only when children are taught to read and write, perhaps because individual phonemes are less salient in speech and because reading highlights grapheme–phoneme correspondences (Goswami & Bryant, 1990).

Several studies with adults have shown increased activation in the superior temporal region associated with learning new phonological and auditory information. Adults learning Chinese tones, for example, show increased activation in the left superior temporal gyrus (Wang, Sereno, Jongman, & Hirsch, 2003). Increased activation in the left superior temporal sulcus has been observed in French speakers learning to associate English auditory words with pictures (Raboyeau et al., 2004). Widespread increases in activation in the bilateral superior temporal gyrus have been shown when native Japanese speakers learn the non-native /r–l/ contrast of English (Callan et al., 2003). Finally, magnetoencephalography (MEG) and ERP studies show enhanced auditory cortical representations in skilled musicians (Pantev et al., 1998) and in adults learning new phonemic distinctions (Tremblay, Kraus, & McGee, 1998). All of these studies indicate that learning new auditory information is associated with increased activation in the superior temporal regions, which may be associated with increasing elaboration of these sound-based representations. This learning-related increase in activation in the superior temporal gyrus is in apparent contrast to developmental studies that show age-related decreases in activation in the superior temporal gyrus. As discussed above, perhaps the developmental decreases reflect a qualitative shift from a reliance on larger to smaller phonological units when the subject is asked to perform a rhyming judgment.

Semantic Processing in the Middle Temporal Gyrus

As with orthographic and phonological processing, semantic processing seems to be characterized by increasing elaboration with development and learning. Behavioral studies have shown both a larger number of lexical entries and greater connections among these entries in older compared to younger children (McGregor, Friedman, Reilly, & Newman, 2002). Developmental increases in activation in the middle temporal gyrus have been observed during a narrative comprehension task in the auditory modality (Schmithorst, Holland, & Plante, 2006) and have also been reported for semantic association judgment tasks in both the visual and auditory modalities. Plate 10.1i shows that there are developmental increases in activation in the posterior region of the middle temporal gyrus (Chou, Booth, Bitan, et al., 2006; Chou, Booth, Burman, et al., 2006). Studies have also reported greater activation in the middle temporal gyrus for weakly associated word pairs as compared to strongly associated word pairs, suggesting that the developmental increases in this region are associated with semantic processing per se and not some other nonlexical process (Chou, Booth, Burman, et al., 2006). Greater activation for weakly associated pairs may result from more extensive activation of the semantic system to identify distant relationships. Learning studies suggest that the elaboration of semantic representations is not only associated with development, because studies on adults have shown that semantic training results in more activation in the left middle temporal gyrus (Sandak et al., 2004). Studies have also reported that higher accuracy among children on tasks that require a judgment of semantic association is correlated with greater activation in the middle temporal gyrus (Blumenfeld, Booth, & Burman, 2006), suggesting that children with lower accuracy have less elaborated semantic representations. Because children with lower accuracy seem to have underdeveloped semantic representations, they may rely more on retrieval and search mechanisms. A large body of research in adults suggests that more activation in the inferior frontal cortex is associated with more effortful retrieval or greater selection demands (Buckner et al., 1995; Thompson-Schill, D'Esposito, Aguirre, & Farah, 1997). The finding that lower skill is correlated with greater activation in the inferior frontal gyrus during semantic tasks (Blumenfeld et al., 2006) suggests that these children engage controlled processing in the prefrontal cortex to a greater degree.

Behavioral research suggests that as children become more skilled readers, they rely less on semantic representations for rapid word recognition. As the mapping between orthography and phonology becomes more automatic, semantic representations may have less opportunity to influence this rapid process (Plaut & Booth, 2000). This behavioral effect is supported by brain imaging studies that show that only children, and not adults, activate the left middle temporal gyrus during rhyming and spelling tasks in the visual and auditory modality (Booth & Burman, 2005). Plate 10.1j illustrates that children show more activation than adults in the left middle temporal gyrus during an auditory spelling task, and Plate 10.1k demonstrates that activation in this same region is present in both children and adults when they have to access semantic representations in an auditory meaning task. The middle temporal gyrus activation suggests that children are activating semantics during tasks that do not require access to these representations for correct performance. The reduction in activation in the middle temporal gyrus with development suggests that semantics plays a reduced compensatory role as reading acquisition proceeds. This reduced role is not to imply that high-skill readers have a less elaborated semantic system (Blumenfeld et al., 2006), but rather that their more developed orthographic and phonological processing allows semantics to have less influence on rapid word recognition.

Syntactic Processing in the Inferior Frontal Gyrus

Studies examining grammatical processing also suggest increasing specialization with development. An ERP study of toddlers examined activation associated with processing closed-class words (e.g., prepositions and conjunctions) that are purported to index syntactic processing. Twenty-month-olds showed similar negative potentials over the left and right hemispheres, and 28- to 30-month-olds showed a more prominent negative potential over the right hemisphere, whereas the 36- to 42-month-olds showed only a negative potential over the left frontal region (Neville & Bavelier, 2000).

Other studies suggest that these left anterior negativities associated with syntactic processing show a prolonged developmental time course, because they appear to be qualitatively different between children and adults until about 6 years of age (Hahne, Eckstein, & Friederici, 2004). Both the more diffuse bilateral activation in younger children and the consolidation of the evoked responses in left prefrontal regions suggest increasing specialization with development.

Greater involvement of the left inferior frontal gyrus in syntactic processing is also associated with language learning in adults. There is more activation in the left inferior frontal gyrus for grammatical as compared to ungrammatical strings after learning an artificial grammar (Lieberman, Chang, Chiao, Bookheimer, & Knowlton, 2004), and there is more activation in the left inferior frontal gyrus over training sessions when learning an artificial grammar (Opitz & Friederici, 2003). Studies suggest that the increase of the left inferior frontal gyrus activation with learning is specific to grammatical and not ungrammatical forms in these artificial languages (Tettamanti et al., 2002). Furthermore, learning syntactic rules that follow universal grammar results in increased activation in the left inferior frontal gyrus, but learning rules that do not follow universal grammar does not activate this brain region (Musso et al., 2003). Altogether, these results suggest that the left inferior frontal gyrus plays an increasing role in syntactic processing with learning and development.

Integration in the Inferior Parietal Cortex

One of the central skills associated with reading acquisition is the development of automatic and accurate mappings of orthographic forms to phonological forms (Booth, Perfetti, & MacWhinney, 1999). This increase in automaticity is associated with increasing elaboration of the connections between these systems at different levels, including grapheme–phoneme, onset-rime, and whole-word connections (Ehri, 1992). Several studies suggest that the inferior parietal cortex is involved in extracting the statistical regularities between orthography and phonology (Booth, Burman, Meyer, et al., 2002, 2003). Studies also show developmental differences in the inferior parietal cortex during cross-modal tasks that require mapping between orthography and phonology. Adults show more activation than children in this region during visual rhyming tasks, suggesting a developmental increase in the elaboration of the system for mapping between orthography and phonology (Booth et al., 2004).

Further support for the role of the inferior parietal lobule in the mapping process comes from a study that examined rhyming judgments to pairs of words in which orthographic and phonological similarity between the words in the pair was independently manipulated. In the nonconflicting pairs, both orthography and phonology of the words were either similar (e.g., *lime–dime*) or different (e.g., *staff–gain*). In conflicting pairs, words had similar phonology and different orthography (e.g., *jazz–has*) or different phonology and similar orthography (e.g., *pint–mint*). Plate 10.2a shows that a developmental increase in activation in the inferior parietal lobule overlaps with a region in which higher accuracy is associated with greater activation for conflicting pairs compared to nonconflicting pairs (Bitan et al., submitted). The correlation with accuracy for conflicting pairs suggests that the inferior parietal lobule is directly involved in mapping orthography to phonology, because this process is more demanding for conflicting pairs. Plate 10.2b shows that developmental increases in activation in the inferior parietal cortex are also observed when children have to make spelling judgments about words presented in the auditory modality (Booth, Cho, Burman, & Bitan, in press). This auditory spelling task requires mapping from phonological to orthographic representations, so greater activation in this region with development further suggests that this region, which is involved in mapping between representations, becomes more elaborated with development.

The change of activation in the inferior parietal cortex in adults when learning new relationships between orthography and phonology seems to be similar to the developmental differences reported for this region. Studies have shown that learning to associate new orthographic information with phonological information modulates activation in this region (Lee et al., 2003). For example, Japanese speakers learning to make associations between Korean letters and speech sounds produced more activation in the angular gyrus early in training, and functional connectivity of this region with the posterior inferior temporal gyrus increased with learning (Hashimoto & Sakai, 2004). Another study compared the neural correlates of three training approaches to learning nonwords (Sandak et al., 2004). Both phonological (rhyming judgments) and orthographic (letter judgments) training produced greater activation in the left angular gyrus as compared to semantic training, consistent with the involvement of this region in mapping between letters and sounds.

The inferior parietal cortex is a heteromodal region that appears to be involved in the integration of many different representational systems, not just orthography and phonology. Plate 10.2c shows a developmental increase in activation in the inferior parietal lobule during semantic association judgments to both visually and auditorily presented word pairs (Chou, Booth, Bitan, et al., 2006; Chou, Booth, Burman, et al., 2006). Activation in the inferior parietal lobule is also modulated by association strength, with strongly associated pairs producing greater activation in this region as

compared to weakly associated pairs (Chou, Booth, Bitan, et al., 2006).
The modulation by association strength suggests that the developmental
increase in activation of the inferior parietal lobule is directly related to
semantic processing and not to some other nonlexical process. The locus of
activation in the inferior parietal cortex for semantic tasks is more inferior
than the locus for rhyming tasks (compare Plate 10.2a–c), suggesting that
this region has distinct areas involved in different kinds of integration,
which both show developmental increases in activation. This specialization
within the inferior parietal cortex may be similar to that shown for the
anterior ventral inferior frontal gyrus in semantic processing and for the
posterior dorsal inferior frontal gyrus in phonological processing (Poldrack
et al., 1998).

Modulation by the Prefrontal Cortex

One of the most robust neuroimaging findings is that increased activation
of the inferior frontal gyrus is associated with both development and learning. Developmental increases in activation have been shown in cross-
sectional fMRI studies for silent verb generation to auditorily presented
concrete nouns (Holland et al., 2001), for verbal semantic fluency to
auditorily presented categories (Gaillard et al., 2003), for category judgments to visually presented words (Shaywitz et al., 2002), and for ascending letter judgments to visually presented words (Turkeltaub et al., 2003).
Developmental increases have also been shown in longitudinal fMRI studies during verb generation to auditorily presented words (Szaflarski et al.,
2006). Most artificial grammar learning studies in adults also show
increases in inferior frontal gyrus activation (Lieberman et al., 2004; Musso
et al., 2003; Opitz & Friederici, 2003; Tettamanti et al., 2002). Although
there are many studies showing acquisition and maturational effects in the
inferior frontal gyrus, the specific role of this region in learning and development has not yet been clearly defined.

One way of clarifying the meaning of the developmental increase in
inferior frontal gyrus activation is to use parametric manipulations. The
assumption is that if activation in a given brain region is correlated with
age and also sensitive to a parametric manipulation that taps into a specific
cognitive process, then perhaps the developmental effect is directly associated with that cognitive process. Consistent with many other studies that
have used a variety of language tasks (Gaillard et al., 2003; Holland et al.,
2001; Shaywitz et al., 2002; Turkeltaub et al., 2003), Plates 10.2d and
10.2e show developmental increases in activation in the inferior frontal
gyrus during a rhyming judgment task in both the auditory and visual
modalities (Bitan et al., submitted; Cone et al., submitted). The age-

activation correlation for the auditory rhyming task only emerged for the comparison between conflicting (e.g., *has–jazz, pint–mint*) and nonconflicting (e.g., *lime–dime, staff–gain*) conditions, and this developmental increase in activation overlapped with a cluster that showed greater activation in children with higher accuracy for all lexical conditions compared to a baseline. The age-activation correlation for the visual rhyming task for the lexical conditions compared to baseline overlapped with a region that produced more activation for conflicting than for nonconflicting conditions. Conflicting pairs presumably require more phonological processing as well as mapping of orthography to phonology, so the overlap with the age-activation correlation suggests that the ability for phonological access and manipulation develops with age.

Dynamic causal modeling has also been used to clarify the meaning of the developmental increase in activation in the inferior frontal gyrus. This technique allows for the examination of patterns of effective connectivity between brain regions by looking at how the directionally specific influence of one brain region on another is affected by an experimental manipulation. In a study with adults, a spelling task was marked by converging influence from other brain regions on the intraparietal sulcus, whereas a rhyming task was marked by converging influence on the superior temporal sulcus, suggesting that these regions are sites of integration for processing task-selective information–orthographic processing for the spelling task and phonological processing for the rhyming task (Bitan et al., 2005). In both tasks, modulating influences also converged on the inferior frontal gyrus. Because each task also modulated the influence of the inferior frontal gyrus on the task-selective region, it was proposed that the inferior frontal gyrus is involved in top-down modulation of task-selective regions in a way that differentially enhances their sensitivity to task-relevant information. Figure 10.2 presents a direct comparison of effective connectivity between adults and children during these rhyming and spelling tasks (Bitan et al., 2006). This study showed that the preferential influence of the inferior frontal gyrus on the task-specific integration site was stronger in adults. In other words, the modulation of the inferior frontal gyrus on the intraparietal sulcus for the spelling task and on the superior temporal sulcus for the rhyming task was stronger for adults as compared to children. This result suggests that greater activation in the inferior frontal gyrus in adults reflects their relatively effective top-down modulation of posterior task-selective regions. This weaker top-down modulation also suggests that children may be more strongly driven by the perceptual input, although there was no direct evidence for this in Bitan and colleagues (2006). The weak modulation of the prefrontal cortex on posterior regions in children may explain their ineffective cognitive control and increased

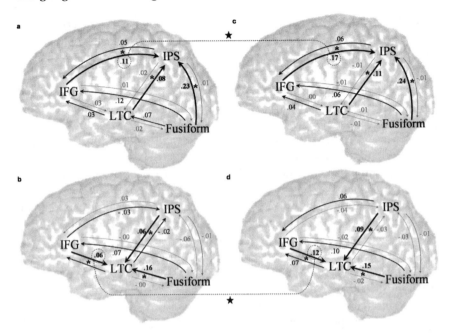

FIGURE 10.2. Adults show greater modulatory effects from the inferior frontal gyrus (IFG) to the task selective regions—intraparietal sulcus (IPS) for the visual spelling task and lateral temporal cortex (LTC) for the visual rhyming task. Effects of the spelling and rhyming tasks are shown in children (a, b respectively) and adults (c, d respectively). Average effects across individuals are presented. Black arrows, significant effects; gray arrows, nonsignificant effects; *, effects stronger in one direction; star, effects stronger in adults versus children. From Bitan et al., (2006). Copyright 2006. Reprinted with permission from Elsevier.

susceptibility to interference from irrelevant stimuli (Bunge, Dudukovic, Thomason, Vaidya, & Gabrieli, 2002; Casey, Galvan, & Hare, 2005). Weaker top-down modulation may also be the underlying mechanism for the diffuse and less fine-tuned brain activation patterns observed in children compared to adults (Booth et al., 2004; Casey et al., 2005). Similar to the developmental effects, learning in adults seems to be associated with increasing connectivity. Learning an artificial grammar is associated with increasing connectivity of the left inferior frontal gyrus with the left parietal lobe and the right inferior frontal gyrus (Fletcher, Büchel, Josephs, Friston, & Dolan, 1999). Increasing connectivity with learning has also been shown in other cognitive domains, such as spatial and object processing (Büchel, Coull, & Friston, 1999).

The developmental increase in connectivity, as revealed by dynamic causal modeling, is consistent with several other lines of research. Neuroimaging studies have shown developmental increases in white matter through adolescence in the left, but not right, arcuate fasiculus, which connects anterior and posterior language regions in the left hemisphere (Paus et al., 1999). Neuroimaging studies have also shown increases though adolescence in the white matter of the corpus callosum, which connects the right and left hemispheres (Thompson et al., 2000). Together, these studies suggest that development is characterized by prolonged increases in white matter, which may allow for more efficient and rapid communication among brain regions. Electroencephalogram studies have also shown increasing coherence among brain regions with age (Thatcher et al., 1987). Coherence essentially reflects the correlation of activation in one brain region with activation in another brain region; it therefore is a measure of functional connectivity. These developmental increases in coherence among brain regions seem to occur in growth spurts, and these spurts differ between brain regions (Hudspeth & Pribram, 1992; Somsen, van't Klooster, van der Molen, van Leeuwen, & Licht, 1997), so there seem to be nonlinearities in developmental processes that are not yet fully understood. The developmental differences in white matter are in contrast to synaptogenesis studies that show synaptic pruning throughout adolescence (Huttenlocher & Dabholkar, 1997), and neuroimaging studies that show complex patterns of increases and decreases of gray matter over development (Sowell, Thompson, Tessner, & Toga, 2001). These changes in synaptogenesis and gray matter may be more associated with specialization, rather than integration, processes.

EDUCATIONAL IMPLICATIONS

Understanding the processes of learning language and reading at multiple levels, including the neural and behavioral, will contribute to the knowledge base that lays the foundation for literacy education. Appreciating the complexity of the neurocognitive systems involved in language and reading development contributes to an understanding of the types of skills that might be addressed in language and reading education—orthographic, phonological, semantic, and syntactic skills, and their integration into fluent, literate behaviors.

A more thorough understanding of the development of the neural substrates for language and reading should have even more educational implications in the future. For example, neuroimaging may eventually be useful for diagnostic evaluation and remedial education. Neuroimaging can provide information beyond behavioral measurements because two children may be performing at similar levels on a behavioral test but be achieving that performance level in quite different ways. Neuroimaging could be useful in revealing alternate or compensatory mechanisms in the brain that underlie similar behavioral performances. In terms of remedial education, several studies have already demonstrated that targeted interventions result in the reorganization of brain networks in children with reading disorders (Aylward et al., 2003; Eden et al., 2004; Shaywitz et al., 2004; Temple et al., 2003). However, we are still far away from using neuroimaging in a systematic way for diagnosis or intervention.

Understanding how the learning process changes over development should also have educational implications. No neuroimaging studies in language and reading have examined whether the neural correlates of learning differ over development. However, some behavioral and neuroimaging studies suggest that nondeclarative learning (e.g., perceptual priming and procedural skill learning) shows small developmental differences, whereas declarative learning (e.g., conscious recollection) shows large developmental differences (Cycowicz, 2000; Meulemans, Van der Linden, & Perruchet, 1998; Naito, 1990; Thomas et al., 2004). Knowing how these learning processes differ over developmental time may suggest the most effective instructional methods for children of different ages.

CONCLUSIONS

This chapter has reviewed what is currently known about the neural correlates of reading and language development in children. Recurrent patterns across neuroimaging studies suggest that development involves increased connectivity, left-hemispheric prominence, and prefrontal control. Development also seems to be characterized by increasing elaboration and specialization of orthographic, phonological, semantic, and syntactic representations to specific regions in the left hemisphere. These principles of elaboration and specialization seem to be characteristic of other cognitive processing domains, and many of these age-related changes also seem to characterize learning of written and oral language in adults. However, studies are needed that directly compare learning in adults to developmental changes in order to more thoroughly evaluate the skill-learning hypothesis, which assumes that the neural basis of behavioral and cognitive development in children is the same as skill acquisition in adults (Johnson, 2001).

Measuring effective connectivity is an advance over conventional analyses because it can determine the directional influence of one brain region on another, and it allows the examination of the dynamics of neurocognitive networks. Work on effective connectivity suggests that the prefrontal cortex plays an increasing role in the top-down modulation of posterior representational systems in reading and language processing over development. The neuroimaging literature is consistent with the interactive specialization approach, which argues that human functional brain development is characterized by increasing specialization of brain regions as well as increasing integration among brain regions (Johnson, 2001; see also Johnson, Chapter 5, this volume). Further research should elucidate how the processes of specialization and integration influence one another, at different age points and in different brain regions, in reading and language development as well as in other domains.

ACKNOWLEDGMENTS

This research was supported by grants from the National Institute of Child Health and Human Development (No. HD042049) and the National Institute of Deafness and Other Communication Disorders (No. DC06149). I wish to thank Douglas D. Burman and Tali Bitan for very helpful comments on previous versions of this chapter.

REFERENCES

Anthony, J. L., Lonigan, C. J., Driscoll, K., Phillips, B. M., & Burgess, S. R. (2003). Phonological sensitivity: A quasi-parallel progression of word structure units and cognitive operations. *Reading Research Quarterly, 38*, 470–487.

Aylward, E. H., Richards, T. L., Berninger, V. W., Nagy, W. E., Field, K. M., Grimme, A. C., et al. (2003). Instructional treatment associated with changes in brain activation in children with dyslexia. *Neurology, 61*(2), 212–219.

Binder, J. R., Frost, J. A., Hammeke, T. A., Bellgowan, P. S., Springer, J. A., Kaufman, J. N., et al. (2000). Human temporal lobe activation by speech and nonspeech sounds. *Cerebral Cortex, 10*(5), 512–528.

Bitan, T., Booth, J. R., Choy, J., Burman, D. D., Gitelman, D. R., & Mesulam, M.-M. (2005). Shifts of effective connectivity within a language network during rhyming and spelling. *Journal of Neuroscience, 25*, 5397–5403.

Bitan, T., Burman, D. D., Lu, D., Cone, N., Gitelman, D. R., Mesulam, M.-M., et al. (2006). Weaker top-down modulation from left inferior frontal gyrus area in children. *NeuroImage, 33*, 991–998.

Bitan, T., Cheon, J., Lu, D., Burman, D. D., Gitelman, D. R., Marsel, M. M., et al. (submitted). *Developmental changes in the neural correlates of phonological processing.* Manuscript submitted for publication.

Blumenfeld, H. K., Booth, J. R., & Burman, D. D. (2006). Differential prefrontal–temporal neural correlates of semantic processing in children. *Brain and Language, 99*, 226–235.

Booth, J. R., & Burman, D. D. (2005). Using neuro-imaging to test developmental models of reading acquisition. In H. Catts & A. Kamhi (Eds.), *The connections between language and reading disabilities* (pp. 131–154). Mahwah, NJ: Erlbaum.

Booth, J. R., Burman, D. D., Meyer, J. R., Gitelman, D. R., Parrish, T. B., & Mesulam, M.-M. (2002). Functional anatomy of intra- and cross-modal lexical tasks. *NeuroImage, 16,* 7–22.

Booth, J. R., Burman, D. D., Meyer, J. R., Gitelman, D. R., Parrish, T. B., & Mesulam, M.-M. (2002). Modality independence of word comprehension. *Human Brain Mapping, 16,* 251–261.

Booth, J. R., Burman, D. D., Meyer, J. R., Gitelman, D. R., Parrish, T. B., & Mesulam, M.-M. (2003). The relation between brain activation and lexical performance. *Human Brain Mapping, 19,* 155–169.

Booth, J. R., Burman, D. D., Meyer, J. R., Gitelman, D. R., Parrish, T. B., & Mesulam, M.-M. (2004). Development of brain mechanisms for processing orthographic and phonological representations. *Journal of Cognitive Neuroscience, 16,* 1234–1249.

Booth, J. R., Burman, D. D., Meyer, J. R., Lei, Z., Choy, J., Gitelman, D. R., et al. (2003). Modality-specific and -independent developmental differences in the neural substrate for lexical processing. *Journal of Neurolinguistics, 16,* 383–405.

Booth, J. R., Burman, D. D., Van Santen, F. W., Harasaki, Y., Gitelman, D. R., Parrish, T. B., et al. (2001). The development of specialized brain systems in reading and oral-language. *Child Neuropsychology, 7*(3), 119–141.

Booth, J. R., Cho, S., Burman, D. D., & Bitan, T. (in press). Neural correlates of mapping from phonology to orthography in children performing an auditory spelling task. *Developmental Science.*

Booth, J. R., Perfetti, C. A., & MacWhinney, B. (1999). Quick, automatic, and general activation of orthographic and phonological representations in young readers. *Developmental Psychology, 35,* 3–19.

Büchel, C., Coull, J. T., & Friston, K. J. (1999). The predictive value of changes in effective connectivity for human learning. *Science, 283,* 1538–1541.

Buckner, R. L., Petersen, S. E., Ojemann, J. G., Miezin, F. M., Squire, L. R., & Raichle, M. E. (1995). Functional anatomical studies of explicit and implicit memory retrieval tasks. *Journal of Neuroscience, 15*(1, Pt. 1), 12–29.

Bunge, S. A., Dudukovic, N. M., Thomason, M. E., Vaidya, C. J., & Gabrieli, J. D. (2002). Immature frontal lobe contributions to cognitive control in children: Evidence from fMRI. *Neuron, 33,* 301–11.

Callan, D. E., Tajima, K., Callan, A. M., Kubo, R., Masaki, S., & Akahane-Yamada, R. (2003). Learning-induced neural plasticity associated with improved identification performance after training of a difficult second-language phonetic contrast. *NeuroImage, 19*(1), 113–124.

Caplan, D., Alpert, N., & Waters, G. (1998). Effects of syntactic structure and propositional number on patterns of regional cerebral blood flow. *Journal of Cognitive Neuroscience, 10*(4), 541–552.

Carey, S. (2001). Bridging the gap between cognition and developmental neuroscience: The example of number representation. In C. A. Nelson & M. Luciana

(Eds.), *Handbook of developmental cognitive neuroscience* (pp. 415–432). Cambridge, MA: MIT Press.

Casey, B. J., Galvan, A., & Hare, T. A. (2005). Changes in cerebral functional organization during cognitive development. *Current Opinion in Neurobiology, 15*(2), 239–244.

Chou, T. L., Booth, J. R., Bitan, T., Burman, D. D., Bigio, J. D., Cone, N. E., et al. (2006a). Developmental and skill effects on the neural correlates of semantic processing to visually presented words. *Human Brain Mapping, 27*, 915–924.

Chou, T. L., Booth, J. R., Burman, D. D., Bitan, T., Bigio, J. D., Lu, D., et al. (2006b). Developmental changes in the neural correlates of semantic processing. *NeuroImage, 29*, 1141–1149.

Clark, D., & Wagner, A. D. (2003). Assembling and encoding word representations: fMRI subsequent memory effects implicate a role for phonological control. *Neuropsychologia, 41*(3), 304–317.

Cone, N. E., Burman, D. D., Bitan, T., & Booth, J. R. (submitted). *Neural correlates of the interaction between phonological and orthographic processing in children during an auditory rhyme decision task*. Manuscript submitted for publication.

Cycowicz, Y. M. (2000). Memory development and event-related brain potentials in children. *Biological Psychology, 54*(1–3), 145–174.

Dobkins, K. R. (2006). Enhanced red/green color input to motion processing in infancy: Evidence for increasing dissociation of color and motion information during development. In Y. Munakata & M. H. Johnson (Eds.), *Processes of change in brain and cognitive development* (pp. 401–423). Oxford, UK: Oxford University Press.

Eden, G. F., Jones, K. M., Cappell, K., Gareau, L., Wood, F. B., Zeffiro, T. A., et al. (2004). Neural changes following remediation in adult developmental dyslexia. *Neuron, 44*(3), 411–422.

Ehri, L. C. (1992). Reconceptualizing the development of sight word reading and its relationship to recoding. In P. B. Gough & R. Treiman (Eds.), *Reading acquisition* (pp. 107–144). Hillsdale, NJ: Erlbaum.

Fiez, J. A., Balota, D. A., Raichle, M. D., & Petersen, S. E. (1999). Effects of lexicality, frequency, and spelling-to-sound consistency on the functional anatomy of reading. *Neuron, 24*, 205–218.

Fletcher, P., Büchel, C., Josephs, O., Friston, K., & Dolan, R. (1999). Learning-related neuronal responses in prefrontal cortex studied with functional neuroimaging. *Cerebral Cortex, 9*(2), 168–178.

Friston, K. J., & Price, C. J. (2001). Dynamic representations and generative models of brain function. *Brain Research Bulletin, 54*(3), 275–285.

Gaillard, W. D., Sachs, B. C., Whitnah, J. R., Ahmad, Z., Balsamo, L. M., Petrella, J. R., et al. (2003). Developmental aspects of language processing: fMRI of verbal fluency in children and adults. *Human Brain Mapping, 18*, 176–185.

Gauthier, I., Tarr, M. J., Anderson, A. W., Skudlarski, P., & Gore, J. C. (1999). Activation of the middle fusiform "face area" increases with expertise in recognizing novel objects. *Nature Neuroscience, 2*(6), 568–573.

Goswami, U., & Bryant, P. E. (1990). *Phonological skills and learning to read.* Hillsdale, NJ: Erlbaum.

Hagoort, P., Indefrey, P., Brown, C., Herzog, H., Steinmetz, H., & Seitz, R. J. (1999). The neural circuitry involved in the reading of German words and pseudowords: A PET study. *Journal of Cognitive Neuroscience, 11*(4), 383–398.

Hahne, A., Eckstein, K., & Friederici, A. D. (2004). Brain signatures of syntactic and semantic processes during children's language development. *Journal of Cognitive Neuroscience, 16*(7), 1302–1318.

Hashimoto, R., & Sakai, K. L. (2004). Learning letters in adulthood: Direct visualization of cortical plasticity for forming a new link between orthography and phonology. *Neuron, 42*(2), 311–322.

Holland, S. K., Plante, E., Weber Byars, A., Strawsburg, R. H., Schmithorst, V. J., & Ball, W. S., Jr. (2001). Normal fMRI brain activation patterns in children performing a verb generation task. *NeuroImage, 14*, 837–843.

Hudspeth, W. J., & Pribram, K. H. (1992). Psychophysiological indices of cerebral maturation. *International Journal of Psychophysiology, 12*(1), 19–29.

Huttenlocher, P. R., & Dabholkar, A. S. (1997). Regional differences in synaptogenesis in human cerebral cortex. *Journal of Comparative Neurology, 387*, 167–178.

Jäncke, L., Wüstenberg, T., Scheich, H., & Heinze, H. J. (2002). Phonetic perception and the temporal cortex. *NeuroImage, 15*(4), 733–746.

Joanisse, M. F., & Gati, J. S. (2003). Overlapping neural regions for processing rapid temporal cues in speech and nonspeech signals. *NeuroImage, 19*(1), 64–79.

Johnson, M. H. (2001). Functional brain development in humans. *Nature Reviews Neuroscience, 2*(7), 475–483.

Johnson, M. H. (2003). Development of human brain functions. *Biological Psychiatry, 54*(12), 1312–1316.

Johnson, M. H. (2005). Sensitive periods in functional brain development: Problems and prospects. *Developmental Psychobiology, 46*(3), 287–292.

Johnson, M. H., & Munakata, Y. (2005). Processes of change in brain and cognitive development. *Trends in Cognitive Sciences, 9*(3), 152–158.

Lee, H. S., Fujii, T., Okuda, J., Tsukiura, T., Umetsu, A., Suzuki, M., et al. (2003). Changes in brain activation patterns associated with learning of Korean words by Japanese: An fMRI study. *NeuroImage, 20*(1), 1–11.

Lieberman, M. D., Chang, G. Y., Chiao, J., Bookheimer, S. Y., & Knowlton, B. J. (2004). An event-related fMRI study of artificial grammar learning in a balanced chunk strength design. *Journal of Cognitive Neuroscience, 16*(3), 427–438.

Maurer, D., Lewis, T. L., Brent, H. P., & Levin, A. V. (1999). Rapid improvement in the acuity of infants after visual input. *Science, 286*, 108–110.

McGregor, K. K., Friedman, R. M., Reilly, R. M., & Newman, R. M. (2002). Semantic representation and naming in young children. *Journal of Speech, Language, and Hearing Research, 45*(2), 332–346.

Meulemans, T., Van der Linden, M., & Perruchet, P. (1998). Implicit sequence learning in children. *Journal of Experimental Child Psychology, 69*(3), 199–221.

Mills, D. L., Coffey-Corina, S., & Neville, H. J. (1997). Language comprehension and cerebral specialization from 13 to 20 months. *Developmental Neuropsychology, 13*(3), 397–445.

Mills, D. L., Prat, C., Zangl, R., Stager, C. L., Neville, H. J., & Werker, J. F. (2004). Language experience and the organization of brain activity to phonetically similar words: ERP evidence from 14- and 20-month-olds. *Journal of Cognitive Neuroscience, 16*(8), 1452–1464.

Musso, M., Moro, A., Glauche, V., Rijntjes, M., Reichenbach, J., Büchel, C., et al. (2003). Broca's area and the language instinct. *Nature Neuroscience, 6*(7), 774–781.

Naito, M. (1990). Repetition priming in children and adults: Age-related dissociation between implicit and explicit memory. *Journal of Experimental Child Psychology, 50*(3), 462–484.

Neville, H. J. (1995). Developmental specificity in neurocognitive development in humans. In M. Gazzaniga (Ed.), *The cognitive neurosciences* (pp. 219–231). Cambridge, MA: MIT Press.

Neville, H. J., & Bavelier, D. (2000). Specificity and plasticity in neurocognitive development in humans. In M. S. Gazzaniga (Ed.), *The new cognitive neurosciences* (pp. 93–98). Cambridge, MA: MIT Press.

Opitz, B., & Friederici, A. D. (2003). Interactions of the hippocampal system and the prefrontal cortex in learning language-like rules. *NeuroImage, 19*(4), 1730–1737.

Orton, S. T. (1937). *Reading, writing and speech problems in children and selected papers.* Baltimore: International Dyslexia Association.

Pantev, C., Oostenveld, R., Engelien, A., Ross, B., Roberts, L. E., & Hoke, M. (1998). Increased auditory cortical representation in musicians. *Nature, 392,* 811–814.

Passarotti, A. M., Paul, B. M., Bussiere, J. R., Buxton, R. B., Wong, E. C., & Stiles, J. (2003). The development of face and location processing: An fMRI study. *Developmental Science, 6*(1), 100–117.

Paus, T., Zijdenbos, A., Worsley, K., Collins, D. L., Blumenthal, J., Giedd, J. N., et al. (1999). Structural maturation of neural pathways in children and adolescents: In vivo study. *Science, 283,* 1908–1911.

Perfetti, C. A. (1992). The representation problem in reading acquisition. In P. B. Gough & R. Treiman (Eds.), *Reading acquisition* (pp. 145–174). Hillsdale, NJ: Erlbaum.

Plaut, D. C., & Booth, J. R. (2000). Individual and developmental differences in semantic priming: Empirical findings and computational support for a single-mechanism account of lexical processing. *Psychological Review, 107*(4), 786–823.

Poldrack, R. A., Desmond, J. E., Glover, G. H., & Gabrieli, J. D. E. (1998). The neural basis of visual skill learning: An fMRI study of mirror reading. *Cerebral Cortex, 8*(1), 1–10.

Raboyeau, G., Marie, N., Balduyck, S., Gros, H., Demonet, J. F., & Cardebat, D. (2004). Lexical learning of the English language: A PET study in healthy French subjects. *NeuroImage, 22*(4), 1808–1818.

Sandak, R., Mencl, W.E., Frost, S. J., Rueckl, J. G., Katz, L., Moore, D. L., et al. (2004). The neurobiology of adaptive learning in reading: A contrast of different training conditions. *Cognitive, Affective and Behavioral Neuroscience, 4*(1), 67–88.

Schmithorst, V. J., Holland, S. K., & Plante, E. (2006). Cognitive modules utilized for narrative comprehension in children: A functional magnetic resonance imaging study. *NeuroImage, 29*(1), 254–66.

Shaywitz, B. A., Shaywitz, S. E., Blachman, B. A., Pugh, K. R., Fulbright, R. K., Skudlarski, P., et al. (2004). Development of left occipitotemporal systems for skilled reading in children after a phonologically-based intervention. *Biological Psychiatry, 55*, 926–933.

Shaywitz, B., Shaywitz, S., Pugh, K. R., Mencl, W. E., Fulbright, R. K., Skudlarski, P., et al. (2002). Disruption of posterior brain systems for reading in children with developmental dyslexia. *Biological Psychiatry, 52*(2), 101–110.

Somsen, R. J., van't Klooster, B. J., van der Molen, M. W., van Leeuwen, H. M., & Licht, R. (1997). Growth spurts in brain maturation during middle childhood as indexed by EEG power spectra. *Biological Psychology, 44*(3), 187–209.

Sowell, E. R., Thompson, P. M., Tessner, K. D., & Toga, K. W. (2001). Mapping continued brain growth and gray matter density reduction in dorsal frontal cortex: Inverse relationships during postadolescent brain maturation. *Journal of Neuroscience, 21*(22), 8819–8829.

Stanovich, K. E. (1992). Speculations on the causes and consequences of individual differences in early reading acquisition. In P. B. Gough, L. C. Ehri, & R. Treiman (Eds.), *Reading acquisition* (pp. 307–342). Hillsdale, NJ: Erlbaum.

Szaflarski, J. P., Schmithorst, V. J., Altaye, M., Byars, A. W., Ret, J., Plante, E., et al. (2006). A longitudinal functional magnetic resonance imaging study of language development in children 5 to 11 years old. *Annals of Neurology, 59*(5), 796–807.

Temple, E., Deutsch, G. K., Poldrack, R. A., Miller, S. L., Tallal, P., Merzenich, M. M., et al. (2003). Neural deficits in children with dyslexia ameliorated by behavioral remediation: Evidence from functional MRI. *Proceedings of the National Academy of Sciences, 100*(5), 2860–2865.

Tettamanti, M., Alkadhi, H., Moro, A., Perani, D., Kollias, S., & Weniger, D. (2002). Neural correlates for the acquisition of natural language syntax. *NeuroImage, 17*(2), 700–709.

Thatcher, R. W., Walker, R. A., & Giudice, S. (1987). Human cerebral hemispheres develop at different rates and ages. *Science, 236*, 1110–1113.

Thomas, K. M., Hunt, R. H., Vizueta, N., Sommer, T., Durston, S., Yang, Y., et al. (2004). Evidence of developmental differences in implicit sequence learning: An fMRI study of children and adults. *Journal of Cognitive Neuroscience, 16*(8), 1339–1351.

Thompson, P. M., Giedd, J. N., Woods, R. P., MacDonald, D., Evans, A. C., &

Toga, A. W. (2000). Growth patterns in the developing brain detected by using continuum mechanical tensor maps. *Nature, 404,* 190–193.

Thompson-Schill, S. L., D'Esposito, M., Aguirre, J. K., & Farah, M. J. (1997). Role of left inferior prefrontal cortex in retrieval of semantic knowledge: A reevaluation. *Proceedings of the National Academy of Sciences, 94,* 14792–14797.

Treiman, R., & Zukowski, A. (1996). Children's sensitivity to syllables, onsets, rimes, and phonemes. *Journal of Experimental Child Psychology, 61,* 193–215.

Tremblay, K., Kraus, N., & McGee, T. (1998). The time course of auditory perceptual learning: Neurophysiological changes during speech–sound training. *NeuroReport, 9*(16), 3557–3560.

Turkeltaub, P. E., Gareau, L., Flowers, D. L., Zeffiro, T. A., & Eden, G. F. (2003). Development of the neural mechanisms for reading. *Nature Neuroscience, 6*(6), 767–773.

Wang, Y., Sereno, J. A., Jongman, A., & Hirsch, J. (2003). fMRI evidence for cortical modification during learning of Mandarin lexical tone. *Journal of Cognitive Neuroscience, 15*(7), 1019–1027.

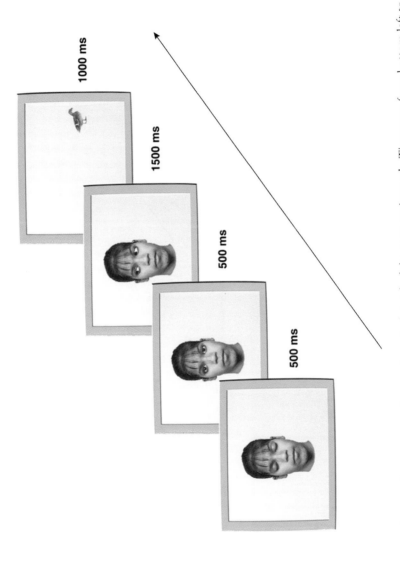

PLATE 5.1. A graphic showing the sequence of events in a single trial of the gaze-cueing task. Time runs from bottom left to top right. The trial illustrated is an incongruent trial in which eye gaze is directed to a location opposite that in which the target object appears. From Farroni, Johnson, Brockbank, and Simion (2000). Reprinted with permission from Psychology Press (http://www.psypress.co.uk/journals.asp).

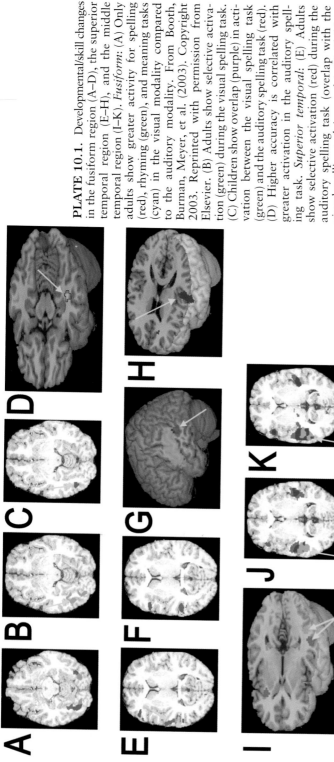

PLATE 10.1. Developmental/skill changes in the fusiform region (A–D), the superior temporal region (E–H), and the middle temporal region (I–K). *Fusiform:* (A) Only adults show greater activity for spelling (red), rhyming (green), and meaning tasks (cyan) in the visual modality compared to the auditory modality. From Booth, Burman, Meyer, et al. (2003). Copyright 2003. Reprinted with permission from Elsevier. (B) Adults show selective activation (green) during the visual spelling task. (C) Children show overlap (purple) in activation between the visual spelling task (green) and the auditory spelling task (red). (D) Higher accuracy is correlated with greater activation in the auditory spelling task. *Superior temporal:* (E) Adults show selective activation (red) during the auditory spelling task (overlap with the visual spelling task in purple). (F) Children show overlap (purple) between the auditory spelling task and the visual spelling task. (G) Developmental increases in activation (red) during the auditory rhyming task do not overlap much (purple) with activation due to auditory perceptual processing (green). (H) Developmental decreases in activation (blue) during the visual rhyming task. *Middle temporal:* (I) Developmental increases in activation for the visual (green) and auditory (red) meaning tasks. (J) Children (green) show more activation than adults (red) in the middle temporal region during the auditory spelling task (overlap in purple). (K) Both children (green) and adults (red) show activation in the middle temporal region during the auditory meaning task (overlap in purple). Plate 10.1B, C, E, and F from Booth et al. (2001). Reprinted with permission from Psychology Press (http://www.psypress.co.uk/journals.asp).

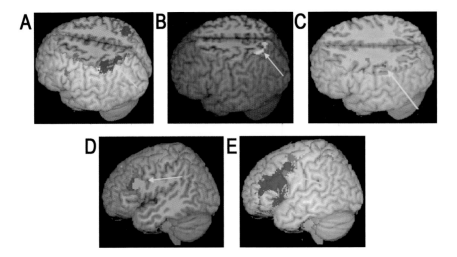

PLATE 10.2. Developmental changes in the inferior parietal region (A–C) and the inferior frontal region (D–E). *Inferior parietal*: (A) Developmental increase in activation (red) for the visual rhyming task overlaps (purple) with correlation (blue) of behavioral performance (higher accuracy) with the difference between the conflicting and nonconflicting conditions (e.g., *jazz–has* vs. *ball–wall*). (B) Developmental increase in activation for the auditory spelling task. (C) Developmental increase in activation for the visual (green) and auditory (red) meaning task (overlap in purple). *Inferior frontal*: (D) Developmental increase in activation (green) for the auditory rhyming task for the comparison of the conflicting to the nonconflicting conditions overlaps (purple) with the correlation of higher accuracy with greater activation in all lexical conditions compared to baseline (red). (E) Developmental increase in activation (red) for the visual rhyming task overlaps (purple) with greater activation for the conflicting compared to the nonconflicting conditions (blue).

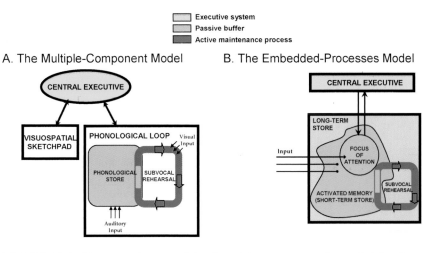

PLATE 11.1. Two prominent models of working memory, color-coded for three theoretical components: executive system (yellow), passive buffer (pink), and active maintenance process (blue). (A) The main structural and processing components of the multiple-component model (Baddeley, 1986; modified with permission from Chein et al., 2003). (B). The main features of the embedded-processes model (Cowan, 1995; modified with permission from Chein et al., 2003).

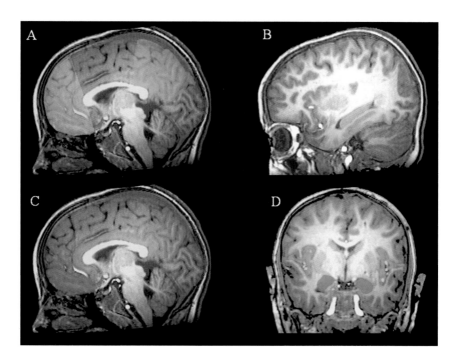

PLATE 12.1. The approximate locations of regions described in this chapter are shown here in the brain of a 10-year-old child. In A, the prefrontal cortex (yellow) and parietal cortex (orange) are involved in linking attention to behavioral regulation. In B, the temporal cortex (pink) contains the superior temporal sulcus and fusiform gyrus, which, together with the amygdala (red) and insular cortex (green) shown in D, are involved in linking emotion perception with behavioral responses. Memories, associations, and emotional experiences are also linked to the insular cortex as well as to the regions shown in C, including the orbitofrontal cortex (purple) and anterior cingulate cortices (blue). See Wismer Fries and Pollak (Chapter 12, this volume) for further discussion.

Development of Verbal Working Memory

Gal Ben-Yehudah
Julie A. Fiez

Working memory is broadly defined as the temporary storage and manipulation of information needed to perform complex everyday cognitive activities, such as reasoning (Baddeley, 1986) and language comprehension (Just & Carpenter, 1992). The aim of this chapter is to explore one domain of working memory, the maintenance of verbal information, and its development during the preschool and early school years. Behavioral effects of working memory have been explored for over three decades, with earlier research on short-term memory (the cognitive predecessor of working memory) dating back to the 19th century (James, 1890). The advent of neuroimaging techniques in the 1980s provided scientists with new non-invasive methodologies with which to explore the relationship between brain and behavior. Our aim is to bridge the gap between brain and behavior by examining both behavioral and neural evidence for the development of verbal working memory and the interrelationship between verbal working memory and language.

WORKING MEMORY

The distinction between short-term and long-term representation of information can be attributed to the renowned psychologist William James

(1890), who stated that a person's "secondary memory" could hold an unlimited amount of knowledge, whereas a person's "primary memory" could hold only a small amount of knowledge in consciousness at any one time. Cognitive theories in the 20th century divided memory into limited capacity short-term stores and virtually unlimited long-term stores (Baddeley, 1986; Ericsson & Kintsch, 1995). One of the best known accounts of short-term memory capacity is George Miller's (1956) "magical number 7, plus or minus 2," the number of items (i.e., chunks of information) that people can maintain for a short duration. The term *working memory* (Miller, Galanter, & Pribram, 1960) was coined to emphasize the *active* role of short-term memory in everyday cognition, in contrast to the prevailing view that it functioned as a *passive* mediator between perception and long-term memory (Broadbent, 1958).

In the 1970s Baddeley and Hitch (1974) adopted the term *working memory* to distinguish between their multicomponent model of short-term memory and the earlier unitary models. One such unitary model proposed that information was first processed by a series of sensory registers and then moved to a limited capacity short-term memory store, which fed information into and out of long-term memory (Atkinson & Shiffrin, 1968). Multicomponent models, in contrast, argued in favor of several limited capacity stores for different types of information, such as verbal and visuospatial information (Baddeley, 1986; Monsell, 1984; Shah & Miyake, 1996) and more recently for episodic information (Baddeley, 2000).

To date, Baddeley's multiple-component model of working memory remains a highly influential theoretical framework (for a review, see Baddeley, 2003) that has prompted numerous studies on the behavioral, neural, and developmental manifestations of working memory (e.g., Gathercole & Pickering, 2000; Gathercole, Pickering, Ambridge, & Wearing, 2004; Henson, 2001; Jones, Macken, & Nicholls, 2004; Larsen & Baddeley, 2003; Logie, 1995; Paulesu, Frith, & Frackowiak, 1993). Although some findings can be explained within the framework of this model, other results are not easily accounted for by Baddeley's theory (e.g., Chein & Fiez, 2001; Jones et al., 2004). The complex behavioral manifestations of working memory have spurred a broad range of theoretical models with a variety of structural constructs (Miyake & Shah, 1999). Moreover, even theories that share a basic assumption can differ dramatically in their view of these basic structural components. For example, the assumption that working memory and attention are closely related is shared by several prominent theories (Baddeley & Logie, 1999; Cowan, 1995; Engle, Kane, & Tuholski, 1999; Lovett, Reder, & Lebiere, 1999), yet differences in the interpretation of this relationship have resulted in different structural layouts for working memory.

Despite fundamental differences across models of working memory, most theories agree on a basic division of verbal working memory into three components (Plate 11.1). One component is the *passive buffer*, which holds representations of task-relevant information either in a functionally separate verbal short-term store (Baddeley, 1986) or as an activated subset of verbal information stored in long-term memory (Cowan, 1995; Ericsson & Kintsch, 1995). The second component is the *active maintenance process*, a mechanism that prevents the decay of task-relevant information. Examples of two proposed maintenance processes are a verbally specific subvocal rehearsal process (Baddeley, 1986) and a domain-general attentional process (Cowan, 1995). These active maintenance processes may not be mutually exclusive (Cowan, 1999b). A third component found in most models is a domain-general control system, often termed the *executive system* (Baddeley, 1996, 1998). In our consideration of working memory development we use a loose terminology that fits the broad assumptions of most models. However, we concentrate on the models developed by Baddeley (1986) and Cowan (1995) because most developmental studies of verbal working memory have been interpreted within these two frameworks (respectively, Plate 11.1a and 11.1b). We first discuss developmental effects that may arise from changes in executive control and then evaluate changes in verbally specific passive buffer and active maintenance processes.

Throughout this chapter, we also consider the relationship between verbal working memory and language. We discuss traditional perspectives on this relationship, including theories that individual differences in attentional resources affect both verbal working memory and high-level language processing (such as comprehension), and that verbal working memory may serve as a language-learning device. We also evaluate the possibility that there is a tight link between verbal working memory and the phonological representations that support reading. This perspective is motivated, in part, by findings from neuroimaging and provides a novel view of patterns of developmental change in verbal working memory and speech production.

DEVELOPMENTAL CHANGES
IN DOMAIN-GENERAL PROCESSES

Developmental change in working memory is commonly seen as an increase in the size of memory span. Span is typically measured with an immediate serial recall paradigm, in which participants are presented with a series of items (e.g., pictures of objects, digits, or visual patterns) and are then asked to recall them in order of presentation. The longest series of items recalled correctly is the span (or capacity) of working memory. Generally, memory span increases steeply from 4 to 8 years of age and then shows a more gradual improvement up to about 12 years, when performance asymptotes around adult levels (Gathercole, 1999). This developmental trajectory is common to the recall of both verbal and visuospatial information (Chuah & Maybery, 1999; Isaacs & Vargha-Khadem, 1989; Nichelli, Bulgheroni, & Riva, 2001). Indeed, developmental studies have shown that there is a significant amount of shared variance between tasks that are thought to tap into spatial versus verbal working memory (Chuah & Maybery, 1999; Nichelli et al., 2001).

The similar growth of verbal and nonverbal working memory may reflect a common mediation of working memory by verbal mechanisms. Although the perceptual input differs, both types of information may be recoded to a phonological form for maintenance and retrieval. Indeed, there is some evidence that older children and adults verbally recode spatial and object information in order to boost working memory performance (Hitch, Halliday, Dodd, & Littler, 1989; Hitch, Halliday, Schaafstal, & Schraagen, 1988). Unique processing of verbal and visuospatial information in separate memory systems may occur, but only in young children, as indicated by separate factor analysis loadings of visual and verbal subtests from the Wide Range Assessment of Memory and Learning battery (Adams & Sheslow, 1990). For children 9 years of age and older, visual memory subtests load equally strongly onto a visuospatial and a verbal factor, suggesting the emergence of verbal recoding to improve memory span.

An alternative explanation for the similar developmental profile of verbal and nonverbal working memory is that both share at least some processing resources that continue to mature through adolescence. For instance, many models of working memory posit an executive control system that allocates attentional resources, manipulates and integrates information, and inhibits irrelevant information across both verbal and nonverbal domains (Baddeley, 1986; Engle et al., 1999; Just & Carpenter, 1992). To probe the development of an executive control system, Luciana, Conklin, Hooper, and Yarger (2005) examined performance on a series of nonverbal working memory tasks thought to make increasing demands on executive control (e.g., recall of a spatial sequence in forward vs. backward order). Based on differences in accuracy across different age groups, they argued that performance on tasks with low executive demands stabilizes early (11–12 years), whereas performance on more demanding tasks continues to improve throughout adolescence. Similar findings were reported in a study that examined executive functions in older children (8 years) through adulthood (30 years) across a wide range of tasks (Luna, Graver, Urban, Lazar, & Sweeney, 2004).

The prefrontal cortex is a potential neural substrate for domain-general changes in working memory. Numerous neuroimaging studies of adults have found increased activation in the dorsolateral prefrontal cortex during working memory tasks that manipulated load (e.g., set size, concurrent task) but not the type of information (e.g., D'Esposito et al., 1995; Smith & Jonides, 1999). The dorsolateral prefrontal cortex also shows age-related increases in activation, as do other regions associated with working memory, such as the left inferior frontal, left premotor, and posterior parietal cortices (Kwon, Reiss, & Menon, 2002). Kwon and colleagues (2002) used multiple linear regression to examine whether age (7–22 years) and two task performance measures (reaction time and accuracy) predicted the extent and reliability of brain activation during a two-back visuospatial working memory task. Age was the significant predictor of brain activity in the above-mentioned regions.

Changes in the functional activation of the dorsolateral prefrontal cortex may reflect underlying neuroanatomical changes. It is well documented that the prefrontal cortex undergoes continued structural and neurochemical refinement throughout childhood and into adolescence (Chugani, 1998; Spear, 2000; see also Lenroot & Giedd, Chapter 3, and Spear, Chapter 13, this volume). Brain volume and gross structure are relatively stable by the age of 5 (Giedd et al., 1996; Paus et al., 2001; Reiss, Abrams, Singer, Ross, & Denckla, 1996), but gray matter loss occurs at a protracted rate in the prefrontal cortex due to synaptic pruning—a process thought to enhance the speed and precision of information processing (Sowell, Thompson, Tessner, & Toga, 2001; Sowell et al., 2003). In addition, white matter conductivity increases due to axon myelination (Klingberg, Vaidya, Gabrieli, Moseley, & Hedehus, 1999; Paus, Marrett, Worsley, & Evans, 1996). A recent study in children 8–18 years old examined both structural and functional data within the same group of subjects by combining an index of white matter growth with an analysis of neural activity for a visuospatial working memory task (Olesen, Nagy, Westerberg, & Klingberg, 2003). Consistent with previous findings from this group (Klingberg, Forssberg, & Westerberg, 2002), this study indicated that there is joint maturation of white and gray matter in a frontoparietal network. Taken together, gray matter loss and white matter myelination allow for more efficient processing associated with the development of cognitive functions.

The development of executive control processes should have important implications for higher-level aspects of language processing. For instance, Carpenter and Just (1992) proposed a theoretical framework, the "capacity theory of comprehension," in which working memory is a pool of operational resources that plays a critical role in language comprehension. They showed that individual differences in performance across a range of higher-level comprehension tasks (e.g., syntactic ambiguity) were accounted for by a measure of complex verbal working memory, the reading span test. This test requires simultaneous storage and processing of verbal material, which heavily taxes executive functions. Although the "capacity theory" has been challenged (MacDonald & Christiansen, 2002; Waters & Caplan, 1996), it continues to provide one framework for the relationship between working memory and language (Just, Carpenter, & Keller, 1996). Findings from a recent neuroimaging study of adults suggest that individual differences in complex working memory (as measured by the listening span test) are manifested in levels of activation in the anterior cingulate cortex, a region implicated in cognitive control (Osaka et al., 2003). Although few studies have examined the development of complex working memory, one recent study found an age-related increase in complex memory span that was similar across tasks that assessed the storage and processing of either words (i.e., sentence span) or digits (i.e., operation span; Conlin, Gathercole, & Adams, 2005).

Studies in patients with traumatic brain injury provide an additional perspective on the interrelationship between executive control, memory, and language. Traumatic brain injury is most often caused by motor vehicle accidents; the overall injury is often diffuse, but due to the acceleration–deceleration forces typically associated with such accidents, there is a characteristic profile of injury (for a review, see McAllister, 1992). Specifically, focal damage is often found in prefrontal and anterior temporal cortices, along with injury to axonal fiber pathways such as the corpus callosum (McAllister, 2002; Povlishock & Katz, 2005). Behaviorally, long-lasting impairments in executive control are observed, with the magnitude of deficit a significant predictor of long-term employment success (Ownsworth & McKenna, 2004). Impairments of delayed memory functions, such as consolidation, retention, and retrieval, characterize different subgroups of traumatic brain injury patients; impairments in verbal working memory span, on the other hand, do not characterize a specific subgroup of patients (Curtiss, Vanderploeg, Spencer, & Salazar, 2001). Basic language skills are usually preserved (Capruso & Levin, 1992), but higher-level skills, such as those involved in discourse processing, are affected (Body & Perkins, 2004; Snow & Douglas, 2000). Children with a history of traumatic brain injury tend to have a similar neuropsychological profile (for a review, see Levin & Hanten, 2005). For instance, Chapman and colleagues (2004) found that such children were less able to extract the high-level content of a short written paragraph, relative to normally developing children. In contrast, performance on basic memory and language tasks was comparable across the brain-injured and normally developing groups, and not significantly correlated with performance on the discourse task.

DEVELOPMENTAL CHANGES
IN VERBAL REPRESENTATION AND PROCESSES

Despite a similar developmental curve, memory span for verbal items is slightly larger (by about 1.5 items) than for visuospatial items (Gathercole, 1998; Nichelli et al., 2001). Other behavioral (Fastenau, Conant, & Lauer, 1998; Gould & Glencross, 1990) and neuropsychological (reviewed in Vallar & Papagano, 2002) evidence for a dissociation between verbal and visuospatial working memory suggests that each process is mediated by separate memory systems (or representations). Baddeley's theoretical fractionation of working memory into a "phonological loop" (i.e., verbal subsystem) and a "visuo-spatial sketchpad" (i.e., visuospatial subsystem) reflects this modular view of working memory (Baddeley, 2003). In this section we focus on developmental changes that are specific to the buffering and rehearsal of verbal information.

Several lines of evidence indicate that some developmental changes are specific to the verbal domain. For instance, one behavioral marker of verbal working memory in adults, the phonological similarity effect (i.e., a reduced span for items that share similar sounds), has a different behavioral profile in young children (Hulme, 1987). Four-year-old children do not show a reduction in span for similarly named pictures (Conrad, 1971) or acoustically presented words (Hulme, Thompson, Muir, & Lawrence, 1984), whereas older children show a classic phonological similarity effect in both modalities, with age-related increases in effect size for acoustically presented items (Hulme, 1987). Although the origin of this effect is still debated (Baddeley, 2003; Hulme & Mackenzie, 1992), its presence in adults but not in young children suggests specificity in developmental change to the representation and maintenance of verbal information. Based on our review of working memory models, there are two candidate structures for developmental change in verbal working memory: the passive buffer and the active maintenance process. In the following sections, we examine developmental evidence for a quantitative change in the number of items held within the passive buffer (e.g., Baddeley, 2003) and for a decrease in the rate of decay of information from the buffer, which is associated with developmental changes in the active maintenance process. Candidates for change in a maintenance process range from the amount of interference between items in the buffer (Neath & Nairne, 1995) to the speed of articulation (Baddeley, 1986) and attentional scanning (Cowan, 1999b), both of which may reactivate decaying representations. Finally, we discuss the novel idea that qualitative changes in the representations subserving the passive buffer contribute to the observed developmental growth in verbal working memory span.

Changes in the Capacity of a Passive Buffer

Late-20th-century theories of working memory can be classified according to their depiction of the passive buffer, its content, and capacity limits. One class of theories equates the passive buffer with an activated portion of long-term memory that contains verbal information in various formats, such as phonological, orthographic, or semantic (Cowan, 1988; Ericsson & Kintsch, 1995). A second class of theories views the passive buffer as a domain-specific short-term store that is functionally separable from long-term memory and specializes in the temporary maintenance of phonological information (e.g., Baddeley, 1986). Although the notion of buffer capacity differs across theoretical models of working memory, it is useful to examine possible avenues of developmental change in this construct.

As noted above, advocates of the first class of theories, such as Cowan's embedded-processes model (Cowan, 1995, 1999b), equate the passive buffer with an activated subset of long-term memory. The capacity of the buffer is limited by the scope of the mechanism that activates relevant representations. In Cowan's model, the amount of active long-term memory is unlimited; however, the activated subset of this memory (i.e., working memory buffer) is limited by the "focus of attention" (Cowan, 1995, 1999b). Capacity, therefore, can be conceptualized as the amount of information that can be sustained by this attentional spotlight. Furthermore, whereas the attentional spotlight is domain-general, the content of the buffer depends upon the type of material that is currently in the activated subset of long-term memory (e.g., the activated representations that encode the phonological forms for a set of presented words). Similar to Baddeley's model, these representations are subject to decay (Cowan, 1988) unless refreshed by limited-capacity maintenance mechanisms such as attentional scanning and subvocal rehearsal (Cowan, 1999b).

Cowan's model associates developmental change in the capacity of the buffer with the scope of the attentional mechanism (Cowan, Saults, & Elliott, 2002). In a series of developmental studies, Cowan and colleagues (Cowan, Nugent, Elliott, Ponomarev, & Saults, 1999; Cowan, Nugent, Elliott, & Saults, 2000) investigated the focus of attention using a unique paradigm, the ignored-speech procedure. In this procedure, participants performed an auditory serial recall task and a distracting visual rhyme-matching task, both separately and concurrently. The auditory memory task consisted of rapidly presented digits that the participant had to recall in order when a visual cue interrupted the distracting task. In the visual distracting task, four pictures of familiar items were simultaneously presented and the participant had to point to the picture that rhymed with a target picture presented at the center of the screen. The rationale behind this procedure was that rehearsal of the auditory digits would be prevented by their rapid sequential presentation and the demanding concurrent verbal task, but because the auditory digits would be in the focus of attention, their memory trace would persist. Memory span measured with this procedure is therefore argued to be an index of the number of items that can be maintained within the focus of attention (i.e., buffer capacity). Based on their findings and those of other classic studies (e.g., Sperling, 1960), Cowan (2001) proposed that the capacity of the passive buffer is fixed at 4 ± 1 chunks of information. Consistent with this hypothesis is the observation that memory span in preschool children (~4 items) is equivalent to the size of Cowan's proposed fixed capacity of the focus of attention; furthermore, a recent study with adults using a training procedure to induce associations between word pairs found that although training increased the number of two-word chunks recalled, the total chunk span remained constant at about three to four items (Cowan, Chen, & Rouder, 2004). Although the passive buffer remains a candidate for developmental change, converging evidence from the adult and developmental literatures suggests that this change may not be quantitative because the size of the buffer remains constant (e.g., Cowan et al., 2004). Rather, the increase in verbal memory span with age might result from a qualitative change in the ability to recode larger amounts of verbal items into fewer chunks of information or to more effectively implement active rehearsal and control strategies. Similar arguments have been made to explain developmental changes in the ability to perform complex cognitive tasks (Chi, 1978; Simon, 1974).

Baddeley's (1986) multiple-component model belongs to the second class of theories. In this model the passive buffer is termed the "phonological store," and its capacity is limited by the rate at which stored representations decay. Because an active maintenance mechanism prevents (or slows) this decay via "articulatory rehearsal," the *effective capacity* of the store is constrained by the individual's subvocal speech rate (i.e., span = the number of words one can repeat in 2 seconds; Baddeley, Thomson, & Buchanan, 1975). In Baddeley's model, the phonological store and the articulatory rehearsal process make up the "phonological loop," one of the domain-specific slave systems of working memory (Baddeley, 2003). Developmental changes in effective capacity therefore depend upon maturation of the speech production system (which we discuss in the next section).

Changes in the effective size of the passive buffer, via either faster rehearsal or more efficient chunking, may have important ramifications for language development. As noted above, during normal development children's verbal memory span increases by almost three-fold between 4 and 14 years of age (Gathercole, 1999). This dramatic increase in span has also been shown to correlate with the rapid growth of vocabulary in preschool children (e.g., Gathercole, Service, Hitch, Adams, & Martin, 1999; Gathercole, Willis, Emslie, & Baddeley, 1992), suggesting a link between language acquisition and verbal working memory. This link has been explored in studies of word learning, which have found that children's ability to learn phonologically unfamiliar names (Gathercole & Baddeley, 1990; Michas & Henry, 1994) and word–pseudoword pairs (Gathercole, Service, et al., 1999) is related to their memory span. To account for these observations, Baddeley and colleagues (Baddeley, Gathercole, & Papagno, 1998) proposed that the phonological loop (i.e., the verbal slave-system of working memory) plays a role in language acquisition. They postulated that the phonological loop boosts new word learning by temporarily storing unfamiliar sound traces until a long-term representation is formed. Further evidence for the role of verbal working memory in language learning comes from a longitudinal study of second-language acquisition in 9-year-old Finnish children. Service (1992) reported a significant correlation between nonword repetition scores (i.e., the ability to repeat an unfamiliar sequence of speech sounds) assessed at the beginning of foreign language instruction and second-language proficiency assessed 2.5 years after the initial testing period. He concluded that the ability to represent unfamiliar phonology in working memory underlies the ability to acquire new vocabulary in a foreign language.

Changes in Active Rehearsal

Both Baddeley (Baddeley & Logie, 1999) and Cowan (1999b) agree that items in the passive buffer are subject to decay but can be refreshed by an inner speech mechanism, which we refer to as *active rehearsal*. Historically, two arguments have been made about developmental changes in active rehearsal.

The first claim is that only older (> 4 years) children engage in active rehearsal. Support for this claim comes from evidence that young children do not always show classic behavioral effects that have been linked to speech-based rehearsal. For instance, young children's memory span is not correlated with speech rate, which some suggest is an index of active rehearsal (Gathercole, Willis, Baddeley, & Emslie, 1994; Henry, 1991). On the other hand, in older children (Cohen & Heath, 1990; Cowan et al., 1994, 1998; Henry, 1994; Kail & Park, 1994) and adults (Cowan et al., 1998; Gathercole et al., 1994) memory span is positively correlated with speech rate. Another marker of active rehearsal is the word-length effect, which is the reduction in span for words with longer articulatory durations (e.g., three-syllable as compared to one-syllable words). The traditional account of the word-length effect is that the increased length of individual items increases the time required to rehearse ("loop through") the items in the memory sequence, and thus greater decay in the passive buffer occurs. The word length effect should emerge once children begin to use rehearsal as a maintenance mechanism. Several studies have found that children around 4 years of age show a word-length effect (Henry, 1991; Hulme, Maughan, & Brown, 1991; Hulme et al., 1984; Hulme & Tordoff, 1989). To our knowledge word-length effects in younger children have not been examined; therefore, the age at which this effect emerges is unknown.

To complicate matters, the age at which children begin to use an active rehearsal strategy may also depend upon the modality in which the stimuli are presented. Speech is thought to have privileged access to a buffer that contains phonological representations, and this may in turn result in the more natural engagement of active rehearsal for auditory stimuli (Baddeley, 1986). Visual information, on the other hand, is thought to require recoding into a phonological form, potentially through the same processes that support active rehearsal. A finding that supports this hypothesis is that preschool children do not appear to recode visual pictures into phonological forms (Henry, Turner, Smith, & Leather, 2000; Hitch et al., 1989; Hulme, 1987). The failure to recode visual items is consistent with evidence that word-length effects for visually presented items emerge at a later age (> 6 years) than they do for acoustically presented items (Hitch & Halliday, 1983). However, a more recent study reported an opposite effect of modality on word length, with a word-length effect emerging earlier for visual drawings of objects than for spoken words in children 4 years of age (Henry et al., 2000). Thus, the effect of presentation modality on the use of active rehearsal in children is not resolved.

A second claim about the development of active rehearsal is that it becomes more effective with increasing age. It is well established that there are developmental changes in speech rate that may reflect continued maturation of the speech production system (e.g., Hasselhorn & Grube, 2003). As a consequence of this increased speech rate, the time required to rehearse a set of items using covert ("inner") speech is thought to decrease, thereby decreasing the decay of information in the passive buffer and increasing effective memory capacity. Thus, this account provides a mechanism to explain why speech rate and memory span are positively correlated in older (> 5 years) children and adults (Cowan et al., 1998).

According to this hypothesis, the size of the word-length effect for speech and working memory tasks should change as a function of age because the difference in the time to articulate long versus short words changes. A recent study examined the size of the word-length effect as a function of age in 5-, 8-, and 10-year-old children in the context of two speeded speech tasks and a serial recall task (Jarrold, Hewes, & Baddeley, 2000). As expected, the word-length effect in speech was age-dependent for the two measures of articulation rate: That is, the difference between the time to articulate short versus long words changed with age. Furthermore, consistent with prior results (Henry, 1991; Hulme et al., 1984, 1991; Hulme & Tordoff, 1989), a significant word-length effect for serial recall was present in all age groups. Surprisingly, however, the size of this effect for accurate recall was age invariant. This result challenges the simple assumption that maturation of the speech production system affects working memory solely by changing the speed of active rehearsal.

A more complex account of speech rate and its relationship to working memory offers additional insight. Cowan (1999a) argues that the total duration of a speeded articulation consists of two separate components of speech production. One component is the time it takes to say an individual word (i.e., word duration). The second component is the duration of the silent pauses between words (i.e., interword pauses). Interword pauses and word duration both predict variance in memory span; however, they are not correlated with each other (Cowan, 1992; Cowan et al., 1994; Jarrold et al., 2000). Cowan speculated that interword pauses measure the retrieval time of the correct word to be recalled from a passive memory buffer, whereas duration reflects spoken output time.

In a series of developmental studies, Cowan and colleagues found that interword pauses decreased with development (Cowan, 1992; Cowan et al., 1994). Reanalysis of data collected from children in grades 1, 3, and 5 (Cowan et al., 1998) further established that rapid speech rates (a "cleaner" measure of word duration) and interword pauses have different developmental profiles (Cowan, 1999a). Within-age-group correlations showed that memory span and rapid speech rates were significantly correlated only within first graders, whereas span and interword pauses were significantly correlated only within fifth graders. These speech processing measures therefore appear to be influenced by independent operations of rehearsal and retrieval that have different patterns of maturation. Thus, speech rate as a marker of active rehearsal may reflect both the accessibility of phonological forms and the time needed to articulate these forms.

Representational Changes in the Passive Buffer

The relationship between interword pauses and memory span suggests that there may be developmental changes in the phonological representations that are accessed during speech output, which may also be related to the age-dependent increases in memory span. Another source of the developmental increase in memory span is the quality of input representations in the passive buffer. Traditionally, these representations have been probed with a well-known behavioral marker, the phonological similarity effect (PSE), which is the reduction in span typically observed for items that share similar sounds (e.g., rhyming items). Classic studies in the 1970s and 1980s examined the age at which the phonological similarity effect first appears in young children and whether the emergence of a PSE is modulated by presentation modality. Because the PSE was initially associated with phonological confusions within the passive buffer, its presence in young children marked the age at which phonological recoding of visual items began (Baddeley, 1986). However, the source of the PSE in adults, as well as in children, has been the focus of an ongoing debate in the literature (e.g., Jones et al., 2004). For instance, studies in the 1990s have attributed the PSE to confusions between articulatory plans during active rehearsal (e.g., Hulme & Mackenzie, 1992), whereas more recent studies have related this effect to the reconstruction of decaying representations from long-term memory, known as the redintegration process (e.g., Hasselhorn & Grube, 2003).

The PSE thus appears to be another manifestation of a complex relationship between phonological representation, speech production, and memory span. Regardless of the source of the PSE, there are well-documented changes across development that merit consideration. As noted above, researchers in the 1970s were interested in the age at which the PSE first appears. The first study to examine this question found that from the age of 5 and upward, children's memory span was sensitive to phonological similarity. School-age children recalled a set of pictures with nonrhyming names better than a set of pictures with rhyming names, whereas younger children recalled both sets equally well (Conrad, 1971). Other studies argued that the PSE for visually presented items emerged earlier. For example, Hulme (1987) reported a PSE for children as young as 4 years of age when he used black and white drawings and a nonverbal response, instead of the colorful drawings and spoken recall that Conrad (1971) had employed. Because these behavioral studies are difficult to conduct with very young children, the presence of a PSE, to our knowledge, has not been examined in children younger than 4 years old. Later studies examined the effect of presentation modality on the size of the PSE. For visual presentation, Hulme reported a similar PSE in 4-, 7-, and 10-year-old children. When an auditory presentation was used, 4-year-olds either did not show a statistically significant effect (Hulme et al., 1984) or the effect size was small; however, in older children the PSE increased significantly in an age-dependent manner (Hulme et al., 1984; Hulme & Tordoff, 1989). Interestingly, the directionality of a modality effect on the PSE is opposite to the pattern observed for the word-length effect, in which length effects emerge first (age 4) for auditory items and later (ages 7–8) for visual items (Hitch & Halliday, 1983; though see Henry et al., 2000).

Despite a possible differential effect of modality on the phonological similarity and word-length behavioral markers of verbal working memory, several studies in the 1990s have attributed both effects to active rehearsal. Because the developmental trajectory of active rehearsal is similar to that of the PSE, Hulme and Mackenzie (1992) proposed that the age-dependent increase in the PSE reflects a developmental shift and improvement in the strategy used to maintain verbal information from a visuospatial (or echoic) trace to an active rehearsal strategy. Their proposal was based on a number of behavioral observations: (1) the PSE was age dependent (Hulme, 1987); (2) in older children the size of the PSE was correlated with speech rate (Hulme & Tordoff, 1989); and (3) in adults the PSE was reduced under concurrent articulation to a level similar to that of 5-year-olds (Cowan, Cartwright, Winterowd, & Sherk, 1987). Taken together, these findings suggested that the PSE might be due to confusability between similar articulatory plans during active rehearsal and not between representations within the store.

More recent working memory studies challenge this hypothesis, because they did not find age-dependent increases in the PSE. Hasselhorn and Grube (2003) carefully matched German words for syllable number and frequency while manipulating phonetic similarity. Auditory memory span and speech rate for these words were tested in large groups of children ranging in age from 7 to 13 years old (Hasselhorn & Grube, 2003). In this study a significant PSE was found; however, the PSE was age invariant, and it did not correlate with speech rate (which showed the expected gradual increase with age). Furthermore, the PSE was significantly smaller in the concurrent articulation condition, but it was not eliminated, suggesting that subvocal rehearsal is not the sole contributor to the phonological similarity effect (Hasselhorn & Grube, 2003; see Jones et al., 2004, for a review of concurrent articulation and PSE in adults). To account for these and other findings, Hasselhorn and Grube and others (Cowan, Saults, Winterowd, & Sherk, 1991; Gathercole, Frankish, Pickering, & Peaker, 1999; Li, Schweickert, & Gandour, 2000) have proposed an alternative explanation of the PSE that is based on the theoretical idea that the decaying memory trace is reconstructed by retrieving information from long-term memory. This reconstruction (or redintegration) process would be less accurate for items that share similar phonology (or articulatory plans) than for distinct items, because these items have more competition between long-term representations that are candidates for reconstruction.

A recent developmental study examined redintegration in 5-, 7-, and 10-year-old children (Turner, Henry, Smith, & Brown, 2004). In an auditory probed recall task, the use of a redintegration process, as shown by the presence of lexicality effects (i.e., better recall for familiar than less familiar words, and for less familiar words than nonwords), increased with age. Interestingly, this age-related increase in the use of redintegration coincides with an age-related increase in the size of the PSE for recall of auditory items (as described above). Based on additional evidence from an auditory item recognition task with rhyming and nonrhyming foils, Turner and colleagues (2004) suggest that older children rely on smaller (sublexical) chunks of information to reconstruct the decaying memory trace, whereas younger children do not have this fine-grain level of representation upon which to draw. Taken together, these findings support the hypothesis that representational changes in the passive buffer underlie the developmental increase in the capacity of verbal working memory. The following section explores one possible source for the change in the quality of phonological representations and its impact on verbal working memory.

Literacy Effects on Verbal Working Memory

The emerging role of the speech perception system in the reconstruction of decaying memory traces suggests, along with correlations between inter-word pauses and memory span, that some developmental changes in verbal working memory result from qualitative changes in long-term representations of phonological information (Ericsson & Kintsch, 1995). The most dramatic changes in verbal working memory span occur between the preschool and early school years, the time during which children typically learn to read. Is the acquisition of reading a catalyst for this observed growth in memory span?

Although the influence of reading on memory span has received some attention in the literature (e.g., Baddeley, 1986), most of the discussion has revolved around the question of whether the acquisition of reading promotes the use of an active rehearsal strategy, which thereby increases measured span. However, the acquisition of reading skill appears to be intimately related to profound changes in phonological processing and representation, as measured by tasks that involve both visual and auditory stimulus presentation. One key change appears to be the emergence of (or accessibility to) more precise phonological representations that capture information at a smaller grain size, such as individual phonemes and subphonemic units (e.g., articulatory features; Snowling & Hulme, 1994; Ziegler & Goswami, 2005). In one model of reading development, these changes in grain size are thought to emerge as a consequence of interactions between brain regions involved in speech perception (in left temporo-parietal cortex) and speech production (in left inferior frontal cortex). Fur-thermore, the integrated activation of areas involved in speech perception, speech production, and orthographic representation during reading acqui-sition may alter both the strength of connectivity between these regions and the degree to which the encoding of visual and auditory stimuli automati-cally give rise to robust phonological representations (Sandak, Mencl, Frost, & Pugh, 2004).

Several lines of evidence support the hypothesis that reading may have an impact on the quality of phonological representations, thereby improv-ing working memory span. First, neuroimaging and neuropsychological studies of adults provide strong evidence that phonological representations are shared across verbal working memory and reading. Reviews of func-tional imaging studies in both domains strongly implicate the inferior fron-tal gyrus (Broca's area) and the temporoparietal cortex in phonological processes that support skilled performance (e.g., Chein, Ravizza, & Fiez, 2003; Fiez & Petersen, 1998; Paulesu et al., 2000; Turkeltaub, Eden, Jones, & Zeffiro, 2002). For instance, a specific subregion of the inferior frontal gyrus responds more strongly when subjects attempt to maintain a set of pronounceable nonwords as compared to words, and this same region is also more active when subjects attempt to read aloud nonwords as com-pared to words (Chein, Fissell, Jacobs, & Fiez, 2002). Patients with focal damage to this brain region show impairments in both nonword reading and verbal working memory (Fiez, Tranel, Seger-Frerichs, & Damasio, 2006). Second, individuals with reading disabilities often have both lower memory spans relative to age-matched normal readers (Wilson & Lesaux, 2001) and abnormal patterns of functional activation within the inferior frontal gyrus and temporoparietal cortex (Shaywitz & Shaywitz, 2005). A third source of evidence is studies with illiterate adults, who supposedly have a fully matured verbal working memory system but have not been taught to read for cultural reasons (Castro-Caldas, Petersson, Reis, Stone-Elander, & Ingvar, 1998; Loureiro et al., 2004). Illiterate adults relative to literate adults from the same sociocultural background have both poorer phonological abilities and lower verbal spans (Castro-Caldas et al., 1998; Loureiro et al., 2004). This finding strongly suggests that literacy affects verbal working memory and not vice versa. Loureiro and colleagues (2004) have replicated these results in a different group of illiterate adults. In their study, measures of phonological memory tracked with the degree of literacy—specifically, the most illiterate group had the poorest memory spans. An imaging study of illiterate adults corroborates the conclusion that learning to read changes the functional organization of the brain (Castro-Caldas et al., 1998). Taken together, these findings suggest that brain regions supporting phonological processes subserve both reading and verbal working memory. Some changes to brain structures are developmental, but literacy may play an important role in reshaping phonology and consequently have an impact on verbal working memory abilities.

SUMMARY AND FUTURE DIRECTIONS

The developmental growth in the capacity of verbal working memory during early childhood is dramatic. Many studies have documented the steep increase in memory span that occurs from 4 to 8 years of age and the gradual increase in span up to about 12 years of age. In this chapter, we reviewed two main sources for this developmental increase in verbal working memory span: changes in domain-general processes and changes in verbal representations and processes. To ground these components in a theoretical framework, we associated each source of developmental change with theoretical constructs that are generally agreed upon in the literature and then examined the evidence for and against developmental changes in these constructs.

To summarize our review of the literature, changes in domain-general processes are associated with the maturation of an executive control system. Ample behavioral and neuronal evidence suggests that the continued development of the prefrontal cortex throughout puberty underlies some changes in working memory abilities. The second source of developmental change is the representation and processing of verbal information. Generalizing across models of working memory, two potential theoretical constructs for change during development are the passive buffer and the active maintenance process. Although numerous studies have examined the developmental trajectory of behavioral effects traditionally associated with these constructs (e.g., phonological similarity and word-length effects), the adult literature has begun to question the sources of these effects as postulated by earlier studies of working memory (Jones et al., 2004; Nairne, Neath, & Serra, 1997; Neath, 2000). In light of this ongoing debate, we feel that it is premature to draw firm conclusions about the underlying cause of developmental change in working memory. Having acknowledged this caveat, however, we point to several sources that may contribute to the developmental increase in verbal working memory span. Since the capacity of the passive buffer appears to be fixed (at 4 ± 1), the age-related increase in span reflects a change in the effective capacity of the buffer, which is influenced by maturation of the speech production system and changes in the ability to access representations subserving the buffer. At the theoretical construct level, these developmental changes translate into a more efficient active maintenance process and more robust phonological representations.

Several lines of evidence support developmental change in one particular process of active maintenance: subvocal rehearsal. Maturation of the speech production system and an increase in the speed of retrieval from the passive buffer both contribute to more efficient subvocal rehearsal in older children (Cowan, 1999a). Evidence for a qualitative change in the passive buffer includes age-related changes in the ability to access smaller units (grain size) of phonological representations (Ziegler & Goswami, 2005) and in the growing strength of associations between phonology and other lexical constituents (Perfetti, Liu, & Tan, 2005). Taken together, these changes may increase the speed of rehearsal and improve the accuracy of a redintegration process. As research in this area continues, advances in the use of neuroimaging techniques in children (Brown & Chiu, 2006; Toga, Thompson, & Sowell, 2006) should provide a new direction to examine open questions about the development of verbal working memory. For instance, developmental neuroimaging studies of visuospatial working memory have provided evidence for structural (white matter) maturation of a superior frontoparietal network that is positively correlated with cortical activation in these regions during spatial span tasks (Klingberg, 2006).

A second goal of this review was to examine the relationship between developmental changes in verbal working memory and related changes in language processing. We briefly discussed the "capacity theory of comprehension," which posits that individual differences in executive control influence higher-level aspects of language processing (Just & Carpenter, 1992). It is interesting to note that the developmental research community has only recently begun to study this relationship in children (Conlin et al., 2005). The main focus of our discussion, however, was on the link between verbal working memory development and changes in verbal representations during the early school years. We suggest a novel view in which learning to read is the catalyst for the observed increase in children's memory span between 4 and 8 years of age. Reading acquisition is thought to change the ability to explicitly access smaller units of phonological representations (Ziegler & Goswami, 2005), which, we argue, will consequently influence the quality of the representations used to reconstruct (and maintain) the decaying memory trace.

The hypothesis that learning to read changes the capacity of verbal working memory has several implications for educational practice and future research directions. Developmental studies in the 1980s examined the diagnostic value of verbal working memory tests as a tool to assess reading readiness. Some longitudinal studies found that reading skills were correlated with serial recall performance measured at a younger age (Mann & Liberman, 1984). However, other studies reported that span measures predicted later reading skill only after the child had at least 1 year of formal reading instruction. For instance, Ellis and Large (1988) found that pre-school verbal recall scores on a standardized test, the Digit Span subtest of the Wechsler Intelligence Scale for Children—Revised (WISC-R; Wechsler, 1974), were not a good predictor of single-word reading at age 6, but beyond this age the two measures shared a reciprocal relationship.

Another perspective on developmental predictors of reading skill comes from studies that have examined nonword repetition, which has also been portrayed as a measure of verbal working memory (though termed *phonological memory*). In nonword repetition tests (Dollaghan & Campbell, 1998; Gathercole et al., 1994), the child hears a single nonword, which increases in syllable length on subsequent sets, and is asked to repeat it immediately. Although serial recall and nonword repetition tests have been used interchangeably in the developmental literature (Gathercole & Baddeley, 1993), we speculate that performance on these tests may be sensitive to different sources of variance that may have different relationships to reading. Potentially, nonword repetition tests may provide a more focused probe of the passive buffer. To the extent that phonological representations within the buffer are also accessed to support skilled reading, correlations between nonword repetition and various aspects of reading skill should persist from childhood to adulthood. Results from children (Gathercole, Willis, & Baddeley, 1991) provide consistent support for this claim, as do preliminary results from adults (Ben-Yehudah, Moore, & Fiez, 2006). Thus, nonword repetition may be a better diagnostic tool of reading readiness, although more research is needed to fully understand the underlying processes measured by this test.

Serial recall tests, on the other hand, may invoke the use of additional processes to support recall, such as articulatory recoding, redintegration, and mnemonic strategies. Some of these additional processes may also play a role in the acquisition of skilled reading (e.g., effortful decoding may involve articulatory recoding), but become less important as phonology becomes automatically generated from print (Perfetti & Bell, 1991). This could explain why span measures correlate with reading performance in children (Ellis & Large, 1988) but not in skilled adult readers (Ben-

Yehudah et al., 2006). Understanding the complex relationship among various measures of verbal working memory, such as serial recall and nonword repetition, and reading skill is an important direction for future research.

ACKNOWLEDGMENTS

We would like to acknowledge the following sources of National Institutes of Health support: to Gal Ben-Yehudah, a postdoctoral National Research Service Award No. 1 F32 HD051390-01, and to Julie Fiez, National Institutes of Health Grant No. 2 R01 MH059256.

REFERENCES

Adams, W., & Sheslow, D. (1990). *WRAML: Wide Range Assessment of Memory and Language.* Wilmington, DE: Jastak.

Atkinson, R. C., & Shiffrin, R. M. (1968). Human memory: A proposed system and its control processes. In K. W. Spence & J. T. Spence (Eds.), *The psychology of learning and motivation: Advances in research and theory* (Vol. 2, pp. 89–195). New York: Academic Press.

Baddeley, A. D. (1986). *Working memory.* Oxford, UK: Clarendon Press.

Baddeley, A. D. (1996). Exploring the central executive. *Quarterly Journal of Experimental Psychology: Human Experimental Psychology A, 49*(1), 5–28.

Baddeley, A. D. (1998). The central executive: A concept and some misconceptions. *Journal of the International Neuropsychological Society, 4*(5), 523–526.

Baddeley, A. D. (2000). The episodic buffer: A new component of working memory? *Trends in Cognitive Sciences, 4*(11), 417–423.

Baddeley, A. D. (2003). Working memory: Looking back and looking forward. *Nature Reviews Neuroscience, 4*(10), 829–839.

Baddeley, A. D., Gathercole, S., & Papagno, C. (1998). The phonological loop as a language learning device. *Psychological Review, 105*(1), 158–173.

Baddeley, A. D., & Hitch, J. (1974). Working memory. In G. Bower (Ed.), *Recent advances in learning and motivation* (Vol. 8, pp. 47–90). New York: Academic Press.

Baddeley, A. D., & Logie, R. H. (1999). Working memory: The multiple-component model. In A. Miyake & P. Shah (Eds.), *Models of working memory: Mechanisms of active maintenance and executive control* (pp. 28–61). New York: Cambridge University Press.

Baddeley, A. D., Thomson, N., & Buchanan, M. (1975). Word length and the structure of short-term memory. *Journal of Verbal Learning and Verbal Behavior, 14*(6), 575–589.

Ben-Yehudah, G., Moore, M. W., & Fiez, J. A. (2006). *Individual differences in adult reading skill: A role for verbal working memory?* Paper presented at the 47th annual meeting of the Psychonomic Society, Houston, TX.

Body, R., & Perkins, M. R. (2004). Validation of linguistic analyses in narrative discourse after traumatic brain injury. *Brain Injury, 18*(7), 707–724.

Broadbent, D. E. (1958). *Perception and communication.* London: Pergamon Press.

Brown, R. D., & Chiu, C. Y. (2006). Neural correlates of memory development and learning: Combining neuroimaging and behavioral measures to understand cognitive and developmental processes. *Developmental Neuropsychology, 29*(2), 279–291.

Capruso, D. X., & Levin, H. S. (1992). Cognitive impairment following closed head injury. *Neurologic Clinics, 10*(4), 879–893.

Castro-Caldas, A., Petersson, K. M., Reis, A., Stone-Elander, S., & Ingvar, M. (1998). The illiterate brain: Learning to read and write during childhood influences the functional organization of the adult brain. *Brain, 121*(6), 1053–1063.

Chapman, S. B., Sparks, G., Levin, H. S., Dennis, M., Roncadin, C., Zhang, L., et al. (2004). Discourse macrolevel processing after severe pediatric traumatic brain injury. *Developmental Neuropsychology, 25,* 37–60.

Chein, J. M., & Fiez, J. A. (2001). Dissociating verbal working memory system components using a delayed serial recall task. *Cerebral Cortex, 11*(11), 1003–1014.

Chein, J. M., Fissell, K., Jacobs, S., & Fiez, J. A. (2002). Functional heterogeneity within Broca's area during verbal working memory. *Physiology and Behavior, 77*(4–5), 635–639.

Chein, J. M., Ravizza, S., & Fiez, J. A. (2003). Using neuroimaging to evaluate models of working memory and their implications for language processing. *Journal of Neurolinguistics, 16*(4–5), 315–339.

Chi, M. T. H. (1978). Knowledge structures and memory development. In R. S. Siegler (Ed.), *Children's thinking: What develops?* (pp. 73–96). Hillsdale, NJ: Erlbaum.

Chuah, L., & Maybery, M. T. (1999). Verbal and spatial short-term memory: Common sources of developmental change? *Journal of Experimental Child Psychology, 73,* 7–44.

Chugani, H. T. (1998). The critical period of brain development: Studies of cerebral glucose utilization with PET. *Preventive Medicine, 27,* 184–188.

Conlin, J. A., Gathercole, S. E., & Adams, J. W. (2005). Stimulus similarity decrements in children's working memory span. *Quarterly Journal of Experimental Psychology A, 58*(8), 1434–1446.

Conrad, R. (1971). The chronology of the development of covert speech in children. *Developmental Psychology, 5,* 398–405.

Cowan, N. (1988). Evolving conceptions of memory storage, selective attention, and their mutual constraints within the human information-processing system. *Psychological Bulletin, 104*(2), 163–191.

Cowan, N. (1992). Verbal memory span and the timing of spoken recall. *Journal of Memory and Language, 31*(5), 668–684.

Cowan, N. (1995). *Attention and memory: An integrated framework.* New York: Oxford University Press.

Cowan, N. (1999a). The differential maturation of two processing rates related to digit span. *Journal of Experimental Child Psychology, 72*(3), 193–209.

Cowan, N. (1999b). An embedded-processes model of working memory. In A. Miyake & P. Shah (Eds.), *Models of working memory: Mechanisms of active maintenance and executive control* (pp. 62–101). New York: Cambridge University Press.

Cowan, N. (2001). The magical number 4 in short-term memory: A reconsideration of mental storage capacity. *Behavioral and Brain Sciences, 24*(1), 87–185.

Cowan, N., Cartwright, C., Winterowd, C., & Sherk, M. (1987). An adult model of preschool children's speech memory. *Memory and Cognition, 15*, 511–517.

Cowan, N., Chen, Z., & Rouder, J. N. (2004). Constant capacity in an immediate serial-recall task. *Psychological Science, 15*(9), 634–640.

Cowan, N., Keller, T. A., Hulme, C., Roodenrys, S., McDougall, S., & Rack, J. (1994). Verbal memory span in children: Speech timing clues to the mechanisms underlying age and word length effects. *Journal of Memory and Language, 33*, 234–350.

Cowan, N., Nugent, L. D., Elliott, E. M., Ponomarev, I., & Saults, J. S. (1999). The role of attention in the development of short-term memory: Age differences in the verbal span of apprehension. *Child Development, 70*, 1082–1097.

Cowan, N., Nugent, L. D., Elliott, E. M., & Saults, J. S. (2000). Persistence of memory for ignored lists of digits: Areas of developmental constancy and change. *Journal of Experimental Child Psychology, 76*, 151–172.

Cowan, N., Saults, J. S., & Elliott, E. M. (2002). The search for what is fundamental in the development of working memory. *Advances in Child Development and Behavior, 29*, 1–49.

Cowan, N., Saults, J. S., Winterowd, C., & Sherk, M. (1991). Enhancement of 4-year-old children's memory span for phonologically similar and dissimilar word lists. *Journal of Experimental Child Psychology, 51*, 30–52.

Cowan, N., Wood, N. L., Wood, P. K., Keller, T. A., Nugent, L. D., & Keller, C. V. (1998). Two separate verbal processing rates contributing to short-term memory span. *Journal of Experimental Psychology: General, 127*(2), 141–160.

Curtiss, G., Vanderploeg, R. D., Spencer, J., & Salazar, A. M. (2001). Patterns of verbal learning and memory in traumatic brain injury. *Journal of the International Neuropsychological Society, 7*(5), 574–585.

D'Esposito, M., Detre, J. A., Alsop, D. C., Shin, R. K., Atlas, S., & Grossman, M. (1995). The neural basis of the central executive system of working memory. *Nature, 378*, 279–281.

Dollaghan, C., & Campbell, T. F. (1998). Nonword repetition and child language impairment. *Journal of Speech, Language, and Hearing Research, 41*, 1136–1146.

Ellis, N., & Large, B. (1988). The early stages of reading: A longitudinal study. *Applied Cognitive Psychology, 2*, 47–76.

Engle, R. W., Kane, M. J., & Tuholski, S. W. (1999). Individual differences in working memory capacity and what they tell us about controlled attention, general fluid intelligence, and functions of the prefrontal cortex. In A. Miyake & P. Shah (Eds.), *Models of working memory: Mechanisms of active mainte-*

nance and executive control (pp. 102–134). New York: Cambridge University Press.

Ericsson, K. A., & Kintsch, W. (1995). Long-term working memory. *Psychological Review, 102*(2), 211–245.

Fastenau, P. S., Conant, L. L., & Lauer, R. E. (1998). Working memory in young children: Evidence from modality-specificity and implications for cerebral reorganization in early childhood. *Neuropsychologia, 36*(7), 643–652.

Fiez, J. A., & Petersen, S. E. (1998). Neuroimaging studies of word reading. *Proceedings of the National Academy of Sciences, 95*(3), 914–921.

Fiez, J. A., Tranel, D., Seger-Frerichs, D., & Damasio, H. (2006). Specific reading and phonological processing deficits are associated with damage to the left frontal operculum. *Cortex, 42*(4), 624–643.

Gathercole, S. E. (1998). The development of memory. *Journal of Child Psychology and Psychiatry and Allied Disciplines, 39*(1), 3–27.

Gathercole, S. E. (1999). Cognitive approaches to the development of short-term memory. *Trends in Cognitive Sciences, 3*, 410–419.

Gathercole, S. E., & Baddeley, A. D. (1990). The role of phonological memory in vocabulary acquisition: A study of young children learning new names. *British Journal of Psychology, 81*(4), 439–454.

Gathercole, S. E., & Baddeley, A. D. (1993). *Working memory and language.* Hove, UK: Erlbaum.

Gathercole, S. E., Frankish, C. R., Pickering, S. J., & Peaker, S. (1999). Phonotactic influences on short-term memory. *Journal of Experimental Psychology: Learning, Memory, and Cognition, 25*(1), 84–95.

Gathercole, S. E., & Pickering, S. (2000). Assessment of working memory in six- and seven-year-old children. *Journal of Educational Psychology, 92*(2), 377–390.

Gathercole, S. E., Pickering, S., Ambridge, B., & Wearing, H. (2004). The structure of working memory from 4 to 15 years of age. *Developmental Psychology, 40*(2), 177–190.

Gathercole, S. E., Service, E., Hitch, G., Adams, A. M., & Martin, A. (1999). Phonological short-term memory and vocabulary development: Further evidence on the nature and the relationship. *Applied Cognitive Psychology, 13*, 65–77.

Gathercole, S. E., Willis, C. R., & Baddeley, A. (1991). Differentiating phonological memory and awareness of rhyme: Reading and vocabulary development in children. *British Journal of Psychology, 82*, 387–406.

Gathercole, S. E., Willis, C. S., Baddeley, A. D., & Emslie, H. (1994). The Children's Test of Nonword Repetition: A test of phonological working memory. *Memory, 2*(2), 103–127.

Gathercole, S. E., Willis, C. S., Emslie, H., & Baddeley, A. D. (1992). Phonological memory and vocabulary development during the early school years: A longitudinal study. *Developmental Psychology, 28*, 887–898.

Giedd, J. N., Snell, J. W., Lange, N., Rajapakse, J. C., Casey, B. J., Kozuch, P. I., et al. (1996). Quantitative magnetic resonance imaging of human brain development: Ages 4–18. *Cerebral Cortex, 6*, 551–560.

Gould, J. H., & Glencross, D. J. (1990). Do children with a specific reading disability have a general serial-ordering deficit? *Neuropsychologia, 28*, 271–278.

Hasselhorn, M., & Grube, D. (2003). The phonological similarity effect on memory span in children: Does it depend on age, speech rate, and articulatory suppression? *International Journal of Behavioral Development, 27*(2), 145–152.

Henry, L. (1994). The relationship between speech rate and memory span in children. *International Journal of Behavioral Development, 17*, 37–56.

Henry, L. A. (1991). The effects of word length and phonemic similarity in young children's short-term memory. *Quarterly Journal of Experimental Psychology: Human Experimental Psychology A, 43*(1), 35–52.

Henry, L. A., Turner, J. E., Smith, P. T., & Leather, C. (2000). Modality effects and the development of the word length effect in children. *Memory, 8*(1), 1–17.

Henson, R. (2001). Neural working memory. In J. Andrade (Ed.), *Working memory in perspective* (pp. 151–173). Philadelphia: Psychology Press.

Hitch, G. J., & Halliday, M. S. (1983). Working memory in children. *Philosophical Transactions of the Royal Society of London B, 302*, 325–340.

Hitch, G. J., Halliday, M. S., Dodd, A., & Littler, J. E. (1989). Development of rehearsal in short-term memory: Differences between pictorial and spoken stimuli. *British Journal of Developmental Psychology, 7*(4), 347–362.

Hitch, G. J., Halliday, M. S., Schaafstal, A. M., & Schraagen, J. M. C. (1988). Visual working memory in young children. *Memory and Cognition, 16*, 120–132.

Hulme, C. (1987). The effects of acoustic similarity on memory in children: A comparison between visual and auditory presentation. *Applied Cognitive Psychology, 1*(1), 45–51.

Hulme, C., & Mackenzie, S. (1992). *Working memory and severe learning difficulties.* Hove, UK: Erlbaum.

Hulme, C., Maughan, S., & Brown, G. D. (1991). Memory for familiar and unfamiliar words: Evidence for a long-term memory contribution to short-term memory span. *Journal of Memory and Language, 30*(6), 685–701.

Hulme, C., Thomson, N., Muir, C., & Lawrence, A. (1984). Speech rate and the development of short-term memory span. *Journal of Experimental Child Psychology, 38*(2), 241–253.

Hulme, C., & Tordoff, V. (1989). Working memory development: The effects of speech rate, word length, and acoustic similarity on serial recall. *Journal of Experimental Child Psychology, 47*(1), 72–87.

Isaacs, E. B., & Vargha-Khadem, F. (1989). Differential course of development of spatial and verbal memory span: A normative study. *British Journal of Developmental Psychology, 7*, 377–380.

James, W. (1890). *Principles of psychology.* New York: Holt.

Jarrold, C., Hewes, A. K., & Baddeley, A. D. (2000). Do two separate speech measures constrain verbal short-term memory in children? *Journal of Experimental Psychology: Learning, Memory, and Cognition, 26*(6), 1626–1637.

Jones, D. M., Macken, W. J., & Nicholls, A. P. (2004). The phonological store of working memory: Is it phonological and is it a store? *Journal of Experimental Psychology, 30*(3), 656–674.

Just, M. A., & Carpenter, P. A. (1992). A capacity theory of comprehension: Individual differences in working memory. *Psychological Review*, 99(1), 122–149.

Just, M. A., Carpenter, P. A., & Keller, T. A. (1996). The capacity theory of comprehension: New frontiers of evidence and arguments. *Psychological Review*, 103(4), 773–780.

Kail, R., & Park, Y. S. (1994). Processing time, articulation time and memory span. *Journal of Experimental Child Psychology*, 57, 281–291.

Klingberg, T. (2006). Development of superior frontal-intraparietal network for visuo-spatial working memory. *Neuropsychologia*, 44(11), 2171–2177.

Klingberg, T., Forssberg, H., & Westerberg, H. (2002). Increased brain activity in frontal and parietal cortex underlies the development of visuospatial working memory capacity during childhood. *Journal of Cognitive Neuroscience*, 14(1), 1–10.

Klingberg, T., Vaidya, C. J., Gabrieli, J. D., Moseley, M. E., & Hedehus, M. (1999). Myelination and organization of the frontal white matter in children: A diffusion tensor MRI study. *NeuroReport*, 10(13), 2817–2821.

Kwon, H., Reiss, A. L., & Menon, V. (2002). Neural basis of protracted developmental changes in visuo-spatial working memory. *Proceedings of the National Academy of Sciences*, 99(20), 13336–13341.

Larsen, J. D., & Baddeley, A. (2003). Disruption of verbal STM by irrelevant speech, articulatory suppression, and manual tapping: Do they have a common source? *Quarterly Journal of Experimental Psychology: Human Experimental Psychology A*, 56(8), 1249–1268.

Levin, H. S., & Hanten, G. (2005). Executive functions after traumatic brain injury in children. *Pediatric Neurology*, 33(2), 79–93.

Li, X., Schweickert, R., & Gandour, J. (2000). The phonological similarity effect in immediate serial recall: Positions of shared phonemes. *Memory and Cognition*, 28, 1116–1125.

Logie, R. H. (1995). *Visuo-spatial working memory*. Hillsdale, NJ: Erlbaum.

Loureiro, C. d. S., Braga, L. W., Souza, L. d. N., Filho, G. N., Queiroz, E., & Dellatolas, G. (2004). Degree of illiteracy and phonological and metaphonological skills in unschooled adults. *Brain and Language*, 89, 499–502.

Lovett, M. C., Reder, L. M., & Lebiere, C. (1999). Modeling working memory in a unified architecture: An ACT-R perspective. In A. Miyake & P. Shah (Eds.), *Models of working memory: Mechanisms of active maintenance and executive control* (pp. 135–182). New York: Cambridge University Press.

Luciana, M., Conklin, H. M., Hooper, C. J., & Yarger, R. S. (2005). The development of nonverbal working memory and executive control processes in adolescents. *Child Development*, 76(3), 697–712.

Luna, B., Graver, K. E., Urban, T. A., Lazar, N. A., & Sweeney, J. A. (2004). Maturation of cognitive processes from late childhood to adulthood. *Child Development*, 75(5), 1357–1372.

MacDonald, M. C., & Christiansen, M. H. (2002). Reassessing working memory: Comment on Just and Carpenter (1992) and Waters and Caplan (1996). *Psychological Review*, 109(1), 35–54.

Mann, V. A., & Liberman, I. Y. (1984). Phonological awareness and verbal short-term memory. *Journal of Learning Disabilities, 17*, 592–599.

McAllister, T. W. (1992). Neuropsychiatric sequelae of head injuries. *Psychiatric Clinics of North America, 15*(2), 395–413.

McAllister, T. W. (2002). Evaluation and treatment of neurobehavioral complications of traumatic brain injury: Have we made progress? *NeuroRehabilitation, 17*(4), 263–264.

Michas, I. C., & Henry, L. A. (1994). The link between phonological memory and vocabulary acquisition. *British Journal of Developmental Psychology, 12*, 147–163.

Miller, G. A. (1956). The magical number seven, plus or minus two: Some limits on our capacity for processing information. *Psychological Review, 63*, 81–97.

Miller, G. A., Galanter, E., & Pribram, K. H. (1960). *Plans and the structure of behavior.* New York: Holt, Rinehart & Winston.

Miyake, A., & Shah, P. (Eds.). (1999). *Models of working memory: Mechanisms of active maintenance and executive control.* New York: Cambridge University Press.

Monsell, S. (1984). Components of working memory underlying verbal skills: A "distributed capacities" view. In H. Boumo & D. G. Bouwhuis (Eds.), *Attention and performance X: Control of language processes* (pp. 327–350). Hillsdale, NJ: Erlbaum.

Nairne, J. S., Neath, I., & Serra, M. (1997). Proactive interference plays a role in the word-length effect. *Psychonomic Bulletin and Review, 4*(4), 541–545.

Neath, I. (2000). Modeling the effects of irrelevant speech on memory. *Psychonomic Bulletin and Review, 7*(3), 403–423.

Neath, I., & Nairne, J. S. (1995). Word-length effects in immediate memory: Overwriting trace decay theory. *Psychonomic Bulletin and Review, 2*(4), 429–441.

Nichelli, F., Bulgheroni, S., & Riva, D. (2001). Developmental patterns of verbal and visuospatial spans. *Neurological Science, 22*, 377–384.

Olesen, P. J., Nagy, Z., Westerberg, H., & Klingberg, T. (2003). Combined analysis of DTI and fMRI data reveals a joint maturation of white and grey matter in a fronto-parietal network. *Cognitive Brain Research, 18*, 48–57.

Osaka, M., Osaka, N., Kondo, H., Morishita, M., Fukuyama, H., Aso, F., et al. (2003). The neural basis of individual difference in working memory capacity: An fMRI study. *NeuroImage, 18*, 789–797.

Ownsworth, T., & McKenna, K. (2004). Investigation of factors related to employment outcome following traumatic brain injury: A critical review and conceptual model. *Disability and Rehabilitation, 26*(13), 765–783.

Paulesu, E., Frith, C. D., & Frackowiak, R. S. (1993). The neural correlates of the verbal component of working memory. *Nature, 362*, 342–345.

Paulesu, E., McCrory, E., Fazio, F., Menoncello, L., Brunswick, N., Cappa, S. F., et al. (2000). A cultural effect on brain function. *Nature Neuroscience, 3*, 91–96.

Paus, T., Marrett, S., Worsley, K., & Evans, A. (1996). Imaging motor-to-sensory discharges in the human brain: An experimental tool for the assessment of functional connectivity. *NeuroImage, 4*, 78–86.

Perfetti, C. A., & Bell, L. (1991). Phonemic activation during the first 40 ms of word identification: Evidence from backward masking and priming. *Journal of Memory and Language, 30*, 473–485.

Perfetti, C. A., Liu, Y., & Tan, L. H. (2005). The lexical constituency model: Some implications of research on Chinese for general theories of reading. *Psychological Review, 112*(1), 43–59.

Povlishock, J. T., & Katz, D. I. (2005). Update of neuropathology and neurological recovery after traumatic brain injury. *Journal of Head Trauma Rehabilitation, 20*(1), 76–94.

Reiss, A. L., Abrams, M. T., Singer, H. S., Ross, J. L., & Denckla, M. B. (1996). Brain development, gender and IQ in children: A volumetric imaging study. *Brain, 119*, 1763–1774.

Sandak, R., Mencl, W. E., Frost, S. J., & Pugh, K. (2004). The neurobiological basis of skilled and impaired reading: Recent findings and new directions. *Scientific Studies of Reading, 8*(3), 273–292.

Service, E. (1992). Phonology, working memory, and foreign-language learning. *Quarterly Journal of Experimental Psychology: Human Experimental Psychology A, 45*(1), 21–50.

Shah, P., & Miyake, A. (1996). The separability of working memory resources for spatial thinking and language processing: An individual differences approach. *Journal of Experimental Psychology: General, 125*(1), 4–27.

Shaywitz, S. E., & Shaywitz, B. A. (2005). Dyslexia (specific reading disability). *Biological Psychiatry, 57*, 1301–1309.

Simon, H. A. (1974). How big is a chunk? *Science, 183*, 482–488.

Smith, E. E., & Jonides, J. (1999). Storage and executive processes in the frontal lobes. *Science, 283*, 1657–1661.

Snow, P. C., & Douglas, J. M. (2000). Conceptual and methodological challenges in discourse assessment with TBI speakers: Towards an understanding. *Brain Injury, 14*(5), 397–415.

Snowling, M., & Hulme, C. (1994). The development of phonological skills. *Philosophical Transactions of the Royal Society of London B, 346*, 21–27.

Sowell, E. R., Peterson, B. S., Thompson, P. M., Welcome, S. E., Henkenius, A. L., & Toga, A. W. (2003). Mapping cortical change across the human lifespan. *Nature Neuroscience, 6, 309–315.*

Sowell, E. R., Thompson, P. M., Tessner, K. D., & Toga, A. W. (2001). Mapping continued brain growth and gray matter density reduction in dorsal frontal cortex: Inverse relationships during postadolescent brain maturation. *Journal of Neuroscience, 21*, 8819–8829.

Spear, L. P. (2000). The adolescent brain and age-related behavioral manifestations. *Neuroscience and Biobehavioral Reviews, 24*, 417–463.

Sperling, G. (1960). The information available in brief visual presentation. *Psychological Monographs, 74*(11, Whole No. 498), 29.

Toga, A. W., Thompson, P. M., & Sowell, E. R. (2006). Mapping brain maturation. *Trends in Neuroscience, 29*(3), 148–159.

Turkeltaub, P. E., Eden, G. F., Jones, K. M., & Zeffiro, T. A. (2002). Meta-analysis of the functional neuroanatomy of single-word reading: Method and validation. *NeuroImage, 16*(3, Pt. 1), 765–780.

Turner, J. E., Henry, L. A., Smith, P. T., & Brown, P. A. (2004). Redintegration and lexicality effects in children: Do they depend upon the demands of the memory task? *Memory and Cognition, 32*(3), 501–510.

Vallar, G., & Papagano, C. (2002). Neuropsychological impairments of verbal short-term memory. In A. D. Baddeley, M. D. Kopelman, & B. A. Wilson (Eds.), *The handbook of memory disorders* (pp. 249–270). Chichester, UK: Wiley.

Waters, G. S., & Caplan, D. (1996). The capacity theory of sentence comprehension: Critique of Just and Carpenter (1992). *Psychological Review, 103*(4), 761–772.

Wechsler, D. (1974). *Manual for the Wechsler Intelligence Scale for Children— Revised.* New York: Psychological Corporation.

Wilson, A. M., & Lesaux, N. K. (2001). Persistence of phonological processing deficits in college students with dyslexia who have age-appropriate reading skills. *Journal of Learning Disabilities, 34*(5), 394–400.

Ziegler, J. C., & Goswami, U. (2005). Reading acquisition, developmental dyslexia, and skilled reading across languages: A psycholinguistic grain size theory. *Psychological Bulletin, 131*(1), 3–29.

Emotion Processing
and the Developing Brain

Alison B. Wismer Fries
Seth D. Pollak

Emotions are complex sets of processes that individuals use to evaluate and respond to environmental demands. Successful emotional functioning requires that children learn to express their feelings to others and accurately attend to, recognize, and interpret the emotions expressed by others. The core feature of emotion processing is the child's developing ability to sense and assess the value, meaning, and significance of environmental cues and appropriately regulate behavior; in higher-order primates, this ability is heavily based on interpersonal exchanges of emotional cues within social contexts. These functions engage multiple neural circuits, which are distributed across many different cortical and subcortical brain regions. Over the course of (normative) development, these functions and processes interact seamlessly and rapidly. The goal of this chapter is to highlight brain–behavior relations relevant to the development of emotion processing. However, at present, the field of developmental affective neuroscience is still in infancy (or at least toddlerhood). Therefore, we draw upon studies of human adults and nonhuman animals for the many areas in which knowledge about the biology of emotional development of children is still sparse. However, it is important to note that the limitations of such a translational approach are significant because both biological substrates

329

and emotional experiences are not identical across species, and similarities between mature and immature organisms have not yet been thoroughly investigated.

The recent growth in the field of affective neuroscience has led to a tremendous increase in our understanding of brain systems associated with emotion processing abilities. But, as noted above, the state of the field is such that these data rarely involve studies of human children. As a result, we speculate about the implications of nonhuman animal, human adult lesion, and imaging studies of adult subjects for understanding the putative neural underpinnings of these processes in children. Although an exhaustive list of all of the brain systems potentially involved in emotion processing is beyond the scope of this chapter, we have selected key neurobiological findings that cast new light on how children learn to process emotional information. In our consideration of the brain–behavioral systems that subserve emotional development we find it helpful to consider two categories of biological systems: (1) mechanisms through which emotional information is processed via operations such as perception, attention, memory, and motor responses, and (2) mechanisms that moderate, or up- or down-regulate, how emotional information is processed. This chapter focuses on the first category of these systems. We discuss early sensory processing of emotional stimuli and how potentially emotional cues from the environment are selectively attended to or filtered out. We also review how the cues to which a child attends may be connected with relevant memories of past experiences, contextual knowledge, motivational significance, and subjective feelings. Next we present data about how the associations that become activated by stimuli in the environment may influence the interpretation and evaluation of subsequent incoming stimuli and lead to enactment of behavioral responses.

Attempts to present unified summaries of the brain systems underlying emotional behavior always run the risk of being oversimplified, overly speculative, or just plain incorrect because of the variability in what can count as "emotion." In large part, emotion processing is difficult to capture because the neural circuitry involved likely operates in both a serial and parallel fashion. It is easy to think about an emotional response being triggered by an environmental event and proceeding along a linear chain of reactions. For example, a child who is playing notices a babysitter arrive at the front door and associates this cue with a parent leaving, which triggers the onset of a stress response in anticipation of separation, the onset of crying, and a decision to increase proximity to the parent. But because emotional processes function as continual loops, multiple stages of emotion processing overlap. Each response potentially leads to a change in the social environment (e.g., as the child's stress increases, what he or she sees and hears will be constrained, or as crying starts, the behavior of the parent and babysitter may change) and all of these physiological and behavioral changes will then require further evaluation of the environment and different kinds of regulatory responses. And since an individual's emotional reactivity and ability to regulate emotion have important implications for which aspects of the environment will be attended to, the associations that will be made to those stimuli are always being updated and will be reflected in the nature of the child's subsequent behavioral responses. For example, some kind of reward produced as the babysitter arrives may redirect attention and emotion, and the child's experiences during the episode are likely to trigger new associations the next time he or she sees a babysitter arrive at the door (for better or worse . . .).

The general point here is that children (and adults) are likely to engage multiple neural circuits at the same time when processing emotional information. As one example, visual cortices, the amygdala, and prefrontal cortex are highly interconnected, dynamic regions that operate in a parallel fashion. As a result, individuals may be concurrently experiencing an emotion, perceiving a continually changing stream of potentially relevant emotional information, and regulating a behavioral response to previously attended cues. This means that we can be enacting a behavioral response while still perceiving changes in the environment. As we present facets of emotion processing, we assume that each process feeds both forward and backward to other stages of processing. For example, activation of particular associations and memories in response to available emotion cues not only influences the nature of the individual's behavioral response, but also influences perception and selective attention to subsequent emotional information. Although we have organized this chapter in a sequential manner for heuristic purposes, readers should be aware of the complex and parallel functioning of brain systems involved in emotion. The major brain regions discussed are depicted in Plate 12.1.

PERCEPTION OF EMOTIONAL SIGNALS

Emotional processing begins with a child's perception of some change in the environment. The process of perceiving emotional signals entails detecting something that is present in the environment that may require further evaluation and, potentially, a response, and depends on the development of separate sensory systems (Walker-Andrews, 1988). These early sensory and perceptual evaluations generally help the organism to assess the overall valence or desirability of the change. For example, what we remember most are not mundane aspects of stimuli we encountered in our environments, but things that made us especially happy or sad, or things that repelled us or elicited our interest and delight. In fact, individuals assess changes in their environments even when attentional resources are limited, reflecting coordination of circuitry in the amygdala and prefrontal cortex, a region with a protracted period of development in humans (Anderson & Phelps, 2001; Armony & Dolan, 2002; see also Kagan & Snidman, Chapter 8, this volume).

At birth, human perceptual systems are already sensitive to information from the environment, and this sensitivity appears to be especially true for social stimuli. For example, neonates look longer at images that are configured like faces, attend more to people and animated objects than to nonanimated objects (Johnson, Dziurawiec, Bartrip, & Morton, 1992), and are predisposed to mimic facial expressions (Field, Woodson, Greenberg, & Cohen, 1982). Early in postnatal life, human infants are also able to detect and prefer information relevant for the discrimination and later recognition of social and emotional information, such as changes in frequency, intensity, and temporal structure of auditory information, patterned visual stimuli, moving figures, and multimodal presentations of cues, such as faces that are also paired with voices (see Walker-Andrews, 1997, for review). We find it helpful to distinguish between the initial perceptions of emotion cues and the process of recognition, which is discussed below. According to this view, perception involves detection and discrimination of emotional stimuli (person A has wide eyes and an open mouth as compared to person B), whereas recognition involves imparting meaning to the perceived emotion cues, such that the perceiver will be able to predict how someone else will act, based on the emotional cues (in this example, recognizing that person A may be scared but person B is not; Walker-Andrews, 1988). Basic perceptual processing emerges early in life and marks the entry point of emotional stimuli into the brain's emotion processing network.

Visual Perception and Occipitotemporal Regions

Perceptual information arrives via visual, auditory, tactile, gestural, and olfactory sensory modalities, each of which carries cues relevant to emotion processing. Here we focus on visual and auditory perception because of the importance of facial expressions and tone of voice in human emotional and social communication. Circuitry involving the occipital and posterior temporal cortices plays a crucial role in the perceptual encoding of emotionally relevant visual information (Adolphs, 2002). For example, in humans, increased activation in the superior temporal sulcus (STS) is found in response to changeable aspects of the face, including eye gaze (Hoffman & Haxby, 2000), mouth movements (Puce, Allison, Bentin, Gore, & McCarthy, 1998; Puce & Perrott, 2003), and facial expressions (Phillips et al., 1998). Similarly, human patients with lesions in the occipitotemporal regions show selective deficits in perceiving faces (De Renzi, 1997).

Additionally, face perception in general (of both neutral and emotional expressions) has been found to differentially involve right-hemispheric activation, particularly in the STS and fusiform gyrus (Kesler et al., 2001). In healthy adults, the fusiform gyrus responds more to images of faces than to animate stimuli, including pictures of human hands (Kanwisher, McDermott, & Chun, 1997). The fusiform cortex also appears to be involved in the perception of detailed, high spatial frequency information in faces, as compared to the amygdala, which is more activated to low spatial frequency facial information (Vuilleumier, Armony, Driver, & Dolan, 2003). This pattern of results suggests that these circuits integrate information as the individual moves beyond noticing a face in order to process more specific information such as the identity of the face or the emotional expression conveyed by the face.

There are also different processes involved in actually viewing faces as compared to thinking about emotions more abstractly. For example, in comparing the neural correlates of visual perception versus visual imagery, the temporal cortex (which includes regions such as the fusiform gyrus, inferior temporal gyrus, right middle temporal gyrus, and the parahippocampal gyrus) and the occipital lobe respond with greater activation during perception than imagery (Ganis, Thompson, & Kosslyn, 2004). This finding suggests that sensory input drives activation of key perceptual areas more than input from information stored in memory. Interestingly, similar brain regions are activated in both static and dynamic perception of facial emotions (Sato, Kochiyama, Yoshikawa, Naito, & Matsumura, 2004).

Auditory Perception

Less frequently studied than visual information, but also a central aspect of emotion communication, is children's understanding of auditory affective cues. The human voice contains in its acoustic structure a wealth of information about the speaker's identity and emotional state, yet little is known about the neural basis of vocal emotion communication. Voice-selective regions along the upper bank of the STS show greater neuronal activity in response to human voices than to matched control stimuli (Belin, Zatorre, Lafaille, Ahad, & Pike, 2000). These voice-selective areas in the STS may represent the counterpart of the face-selective areas in the human visual cortex and appear critical for understanding children's perception of auditory emotional signals. Indeed, the distributed neural networks involved in

auditory emotion perception are very similar to those activated in response
to visual emotional cues, including the caudate, amygdala, insula, and ventral prefrontal cortices (Morris, Scott, & Dolan, 1999). If anything, these
regions show more activation when facial expressions of emotion and emotional voices are presented together than when either type of cue is presented alone (Pourtois, de Gelder, Bol, & Crommelinck, 2005).

Perception, Emotion, and Development

The results of many studies converge in suggesting that perceptual processing of emotional stimuli occurs early in the stream of information processing and that neural responses to emotional signals also occur especially rapidly in the brain, across widespread regions (Kawasaki et al., 2001). Less is
known about how this processing occurs, although preliminary magnetoencephalographic (MEG) and functional magnetic resonance imaging (fMRI)
data indicate that the amygdala modulates processing of environmental signals that the perceiver may find significant. This modulation appears to
occur through inputs from ventral visual and auditory pathways to the
amygdala and feedback sent from the amygdala via widely distributed projections to all relevant brain regions, essentially through a noncortical,
rapid response pathway in the brain (LeDoux, 1992; Morris et al., 1998;
Vuilleumier, Armony, Driver, & Dolan, 2001). The psychological manifestation of this pathway is illustrated by studies of adults who have sustained
brain damage: Following damage to the amygdala, the ability to rapidly
perceive emotional cues no longer exists (Adolphs, Tranel, Damasio, &
Damasio, 2002; Calder et al., 1996). As with most research in this area,
very little work has been done with children; the few studies that do exist
suggest that amygdalar processing of emotions does not appear identical
from childhood to adulthood (Thomas, Drevets, Whalen, et al., 2001).
Therefore, important questions remain about what kind of maturational
and learning experiences contribute to adult organization of these systems
that are crucial for emotion processing.

Experience with faces and other social cues may play a role in the
development of the neural circuits underlying emotion perception. In primates, although fundamental properties of the inferior temporal cortex
appears very similar to adults', this area undergoes a protracted period of
postnatal development that allows visual experience to influence functioning of this brain region (Rodman, 1994). For example, in one study, children 5–11 years old did show activation to faces in the ventral processing
stream that was similar to adults (Gathers, Bhatt, Corbly, Farley, &
Joseph, 2004). However, the loci of face-preferential activation for the 5-
to 8-year-old group were not in the traditionally defined fusiform area, as

they were in the 9- to 11-year-olds and adults. The authors suggested that these developmental changes reflect the effects of learning and experience with a variety of facial information on the fine-tuning of visual perception areas. Such developmental findings are consistent with studies of adults that have reported increased fusiform activation when fine-grained discriminations of perceptual stimuli for which the individuals have a high degree of expertise are undertaken (Tarr & Gauthier, 2000). In addition, prior experience with particular classes or types of faces has been shown to bias subsequent perception (Webster, Kaping, Mizokami, & Duhamel, 2004). This biasing of perceptual processes would necessarily lead to changes in the eventual behavioral response of the perceiver.

Summary

To summarize, in psychological terms, perception serves as the entry point for the processing of emotional information. For example, as a child gains experience with a variety of different faces, he or she may become increasingly able to detect subtler changes in facial expressions of emotion. And as these features of facial musculature are tied to significant events in the environment, the changes will be reflected in the functional connections within and between the brain regions important for facial perception. These small changes in the stimulus array may or may not be relevant to any particular social context and thus may subsequently be either selectively attended to or ignored and either used or not used in generating an emotional response. If thresholds for a child's sensory systems are set too high or too low, he or she may miss or overprocess changes in the emotional environment, which could lead to ineffective or maladaptive behavioral responses; examples of these situations are discussed below.

ATTENTION TO EMOTIONAL SIGNALS

Children must learn to attend to the cues that are emotionally significant while filtering out irrelevant or redundant information. In an interpersonal context there are myriad potential emotional cues available to the child, including interoceptive (e.g., subjective feeling states: distress, pain, comfort, anxiety, pleasure) and contextual (e.g., social signals being expressed by others, familiarity/novelty of settings or people) information. To successfully use these cues, children rely on attentional processes that allow them to rapidly orient to, and notice, salient stimuli, filter or ignore irrelevant stimuli, shift their attention between multiple sources of information, and sustain attention over time. Because some features of the environment are attended to more than others, attentional processes will influence which emotional signals from the environment are likely to influence children's memories and behaviors (Egeth & Yantis, 1997; Posner, 1994).

What a child attends to at any given time will be based on behavioral or internal goals as well as the environmental context. Humans appear to be particularly biased to attend to information relevant to primary motivational systems, as evidenced by increased visual cortex activity to highly emotionally arousing stimuli compared to neutral and less emotionally arousing stimuli (Bradley, Sabatinelli, Lang, Fitzsimmons, King, & Desai, 2003). Over the course of development children are confronted with innumerable opportunities to attach significance to different emotional cues. For this reason, the attentional system must be selectively tuned to the most biologically relevant stimuli, while, at the same time, inhibiting attention to less significant information. For example, between the ages of 7 and 11 years, children begin to attend to inner facial features (i.e., eyes, nose, and mouth) more than external features of the face and head (Want, Pascalis, Coleman, & Blades, 2003). Furthermore, the type and quality of emotional input to which the child is exposed changes how attention is allocated and controlled. Recent electrophysiological studies of severely abused children revealed that auditory anger cues from their own mothers engaged more attentional resources in these children relative to controls (Shackman & Pollak, 2005), highlighting the salient nature of these cues for this group of children. However, questions remain about whether and how the type and amount of emotional experience children receive throughout development serve to organize the neural systems that subserve the processing of, and attention to, emotional cues.

In terms of behavioral regulation, attentional processes are key adaptive mechanisms by virtue of the fact that emotion systems draw our attention to important features or changes in the environment while also allowing us to control or regulate our responses to these changes (Posner & Rothbart, 1998). Perhaps the most extensive research within the area of affective neuroscience has been directed at examining the brain systems linking attention, emotion, and behavior. Regions of the parietal and frontal lobes mediate attentional control (for review, see Goldberg, Bisley, Powell, Gottlieb, & Kusunoki, 2002). But adults recruit more prefrontal and parietal resources than children when switching attention between stimuli, suggesting that cortical involvement in attention increases with age (Casey et al., 2004). More specifically, the parietal cortex represents a general-purpose mechanism for directing visual attention that is reflected in behaviors such as orienting toward some stimuli while ignoring others (Mirsky, 1996; Wojciulik & Kanwisher, 1999; Yamasaki, LaBar, & McCarthy, 2002). Other cortical areas within the prefrontal cortex (PFC), including the left dorsolateral and medial regions of the PFC, allow children to maintain attentional focus (Compton et al., 2003). Attention to emotionally salient cues is enhanced via the extensive projections from the amygdala to the occipital cortex, described above (Amaral, Price, Pitkanen, & Carmichael, 1992).

As in the perceptual studies described above, modulation of attention to emotional cues is abolished by amygdalar damage (Vuilleumier, Richardson, Armony, Driver, & Dolan, 2004). More recently, a region of the brain collectively referred to as the anterior cingulate cortex (ACC) has been implicated in the processing of emotion information (Fichtenholtz et al., 2004). Interestingly, activation of the ACC has also been observed when subjects are attending to their own internal emotional responses (Lane, Fink, Chau, & Dolan, 1997), further supporting and broadening the role of the ACC in mediating attention to various types of emotion signals. Thus, the development of ACC-mediated networks likely contributes to children's ability to attend to emotionally salient information, although the specifics of these networks and their links to emotional behavior are not yet fully understood.

The frontal lobes, ACC, and areas of the parietal cortex undergo prolonged periods of postnatal development that extend into late childhood or puberty (Stuss, 1992; Yakovlev & Lecours, 1967; see also Lenroot & Giedd, Chapter 3, this volume). Therefore, it is likely that neural attentional mechanisms involved in emotion information processing continue to be fine-tuned throughout early childhood (Klingberg, Forssberg, & Westerberg, 2002). In fact, across development, children's attentional control improves, which leads to improved efficiency on tasks that require irrelevant information to be ignored while relevant information is being processed (Rueda et al., 2004; see Enns, 1990, for review). As expected, better behavioral performance on attention tasks is related to changes in activation in these brain regions across development (Casey et al., 1997, 2004).

There are many aspects of brain development that change in midchildhood, all of which may influence children's behavior. Dopamine (DA) is a neurotransmitter that acts as a powerful regulator of many aspects of cognitive functioning (Nieoullon, 2002). For example, DA motivates behavioral responses to both aversive and positive emotional events (Berridge & Robinson, 1998; Redgrave, Prescott, & Gurney, 1999; Salamone, Cousins, & Snyder, 1997). Key emotion processing areas, such as the frontal and midbrain networks involved in attention, are regulated, in part, by DA systems (King, Tenney, Rossi, Colamussi, & Burdick, 2003; Pruessner, Champagne, Meaney, & Dagher, 2004; Stanford & Santi, 1998). Accordingly, behavioral deficits, such as difficulty focusing attention and increased distractibility, have been related to alterations in DA transmission (Nieoullon, 2002).

Brain systems linked to emotional responses also influence attentional abilities. For example, perceived stress leads to impaired selective attention (Bernstein-Bercovitz, 2003), and degradations in attentional functioning are associated with high levels of stress reactivity in the hypothalamic–pituitary–adrenal axis (HPA) system (Molle, Albrecht, Marshall, Fehm, & Born, 1997; Skosnik, Chatterton, Swisher, & Park, 2000). In adults, high levels of the stress hormone cortisol are negatively related to memory for angry and happy facial expressions (Van Honk et al., 2003). Taken together, these studies suggest that if emotional arousal is too high in a given context, children's utilization of emotional cues may be undermined. In these situations children's behavioral responses could be ineffective because they are not able to filter irrelevant cues, attend to relevant cues, or focus on strategic regulatory strategies.

What a child attends to will influence the types of associations, cognitions, and memories activated, influence the ongoing perception of emotional information, and direct the child's overt behavioral response. For example, a child who selectively attends to his or her mother's angry facial expression may call forth memories of when the mother has been angry in the past, perhaps leading to both a withdrawal response and a subsequent bias to perceive and selectively attend to other available cues indicating anger (e.g., mother's angry tone of voice). Experiencing overwhelming emotional arousal in response to his or her mother's anger, as appears to be the case in children who have experienced physical abuse, could lead to the child missing other important cues (e.g., anger was actually directed at someone else), resulting in an inappropriate behavioral response. In this way, past experiences as well as current emotional states are likely to influence attention to emotion information. Repeated exposure to particular types of emotion eliciting events may strengthen particular connections within the parietal and frontal attention networks, thus creating a more general attentional bias for particular types of emotion cues.

ASSOCIATIVE LEARNING, MEMORY, AND EMOTION

The information to which the child has attended creates an accumulation of stored associations and memories that imparts meaning and motivates behavior. Stored associations may be simple stimulus–response relationships in which the child learns to associate specific emotion-related cues with certain outcomes. Associations may also be more elaborated, whereby the child learns relationships between emotional signals and general rules or categories that guide his or her behavior in novel situations (Call, 2001). Essentially, these associations become the background knowledge and beliefs that the child holds about his or her emotional world. This knowledge is important for navigating the complex emotional world of humans and nonhuman primates. With increasing age, cognitive capacities, and social experiences, children develop more sophisticated and detailed associations, including knowledge about the emotional or motivational significance of particular cues, and the regularity of certain emotions and outcomes, and emotional traits of familiar people, and they become able to predict emotions in certain contexts. In addition, this background of stored associations and memories about past emotional events allows children to rapidly decode and use emotional cues in novel situations.

Associative learning depends on the child's ability to detect regularities in, predictiveness of, and temporal contiguity between, occurrences of emotional cues and the events they signal. In humans, the nature of the infant–caregiver relationship often involves highly repetitive, predictable, and contingent social interactions; indeed, the infant–caregiver patterns of interactions are probably more predictable than any other sequence (Lamb, 1981). Perhaps as a result, infants as young as 3 months demonstrate the ability to understand social contingencies (Bigelow & DeCoste, 2003). Neural circuitry in the amygdala, ventromedial frontal cortex, and medial thalamic nucleus (MD) appear to be important for associative learning and for utilization of associative memory stores in guiding emotional behavior. Nonhuman animal studies suggest that the MD, amygdala, and orbitofrontal cortex may function together to aid in assigning emotional significance to stimuli—a key aspect of learning about emotions (Gaffan & Murray, 1990).

The Amygdala

Research on the biological basis of emotional behavior has largely focused on the role of the amygdala because of clinical evidence linking this region with emotion perception and learning (see Aggleton & Young, 2000, for review). Early reports of amygdalar lesions in monkeys described profound emotional changes, including a complete lack of awareness of the emotional significance of stimuli (Kluver & Bucy, 1939). Similarly, human lesion studies have consistently found deficits in the recognition of facial expressions of emotion following bilateral amygdalar damage (Adolphs, Baron-Cohen, Tranel, 2002; Adolphs et al., 1999; Broks et al., 1998; Calder et al., 1996). The amygdala also appears crucial for making social attributions: Patients with bilateral amygdalar damage tend to be unusually friendly toward others and give favorable ratings to faces that controls judged to be extremely untrustworthy or unapproachable (Adolphs, Tranel, & Damasio, 1998).

In terms of learning and emotional skill development, the amygdala plays a critical role in stimulus-reinforcement conditioning, the process whereby neutral cues acquire positive and negative incentive status and emotional meaning (Aggleton & Young, 2000; Bechara et al., 1995; Emery & Amaral, 2000; Gottfried, O'Doherty, & Dolan, 2003; LeDoux, 1996). Complete amygdalar lesions cause a decline in affiliative behavior, social communication, and emotional responses to other animals—purportedly because, without amygdalar processing, the animals are unable to associate complex stimuli with positive or negative emotional meaning and therefore cannot use emotional cues to guide behavior (Emery & Amaral, 2000; Kling & Brothers, 1992). For example, individuals with large lesions to the amygdala show poorer performance on an associative learning task involving facial expressions of emotion than individuals with smaller lesions or control subjects (Boucsein, Weniger, Mursch, Steinhoff, & Irle, 2001). Both adult and infant monkeys with amygdalar lesions show a lack of social inhibition and wariness of new conspecifics, indicating a failure to perceive potential threat in the social environment (Bauman, Lavenex, Mason, Capitanio, & Amaral, 2004; Emery et al., 2001). In one of the few studies to investigate amygdalar functioning in children, Baird and colleagues (1999) demonstrated amygdalar activation to fearful faces in 12- to 17-year-olds. Results of another study suggested that children also show greater amygdalar activation to neutral faces when compared to adults (Thomas, Drevets, Whalen, et al., 2001). These studies are suggestive of a developmental progression in the ability to decode and understand neutral faces, but they also highlight the need for more research in this area on younger children and on children with emotion regulation difficulties. Indeed, lesion data indicate that this brain region is important developmentally for the acquisition of emotion expression recognition but may play less of a role once this emotion processing ability has been established (Adolphs, Damasio, Tranel, & Damasio, 1996).

How might the amygdala play a role in emotional development? Addressing this question requires some extrapolation from studies of mature nonhuman animals. In primates, the amygdala projects directly to the MD, which, in turn, projects to the ventromedial PFC. Significant increases in myelination over the first 2 years of development in humans appear to strengthen both cortical and subcortical pathways and lead to improved efficiency of the connections between the amygdala and cerebral cortex (Herschkowitz, 2000). This amygdala–MD–ventromedial PFC circuit is often discussed as the main circuitry involved in emotional learning and memory-related processes (Aggleton & Mishkin, 1984; Sarter & Markowitsch, 1983). Convergent evidence about the importance of this neural circuit includes observations that monkeys with lesions of the MD demonstrate impaired object–reward association memory (Gaffan & Parker, 2000) and that rats with lesions of this area have impaired contextual fear conditioning (Li, Inoue, Nakagawa, & Koyama, 2004). Recordings of neuronal activity within the MD in rats also indicate that the MD is responsive to auditory and visual stimuli predictive of reward (Oyoshi, Nishijo, Asakura, Takamura, & Ono, 1996). In addition, neurons in this region change their response patterns during extinction and relearning trials, which suggests that the MD is critical for learning the emotional significance of stimuli in the environment.

The Frontal Lobe

The other brain region most frequently studied by emotion researchers is the frontal lobe. The circuitry in this region is linked to learning of associations because of its role in the formation of mental representations related to expectancies for reward and punishment (Dawson, Hessl, & Frey, 1994). The ventromedial (VM) cortex, which includes the orbitofrontal cortex (OFC), is critical for associating incoming stimuli with existing response-reinforcement contingencies and their motivational significance (Adolphs, 2002; Bechara, Damasio, & Damasio, 2000). This brain region is also partially responsible for holding the representations of behavioral reinforcement contingencies in working memory as motor strategies are selected over time (Damasio, 1999; Goldman-Rakic, 1987; O'Doherty, Kringelbach, Rolls, Hornak, & Andrews, 2001). Therefore, the maturation of this neural system is likely to be important for behavioral regulation, allowing the child to associate certain behaviors with reward and to update behavioral repertoires as interpersonal contexts and emotional signals become more complex and nuanced. We can speculate that this system also allows children to learn that some emotional behaviors are acceptable in some contexts, whereas others are not.

Earlier we highlighted the role of the dopamine system in attentional functioning; this neurotransmitter system appears to facilitate associative learning as well. Dopamine-synthesizing neurons within the ventral tegmental area (VTA) and neuronal connections between the VTA and other limbic and cortical areas modulate the functioning of the prefrontal cortex, limbic cortex, and parietal cortex (Nieoullon, 2002; Stevenson & Gratton, 2003). These activities correspond to, or are associated with, psychological processes such as executive functions, inhibition, learning, memory, and attention. For example, in the rat, pairing of a neutral stimulus with a stimulus predictive of reward consistently led to increases in DA in the nucleus accumbens (Datla, Ahier, Young, Gray, & Joseph, 2002). These increases in DA were specifically associated with *new* associative learning, rather than in the behavioral expression of previously acquired associative contingencies. This circuitry relies upon corticolimbic afferents from such areas as the amygdala, hippocampus, and prefrontal cortex, all of which carry contextual information predictive of reward. These afferents activate DA neurons in the VTA, which subsequently release DA into the nucleus accumbens shell, thereby facilitating reward motivation and approach to rewarding objects (Depue & Morrone-Strupinsky, 2005).

In a previous generation of emotion research, many of these processes were referred to under the psychological rubric of "attribution." But one benefit of increased neuroscience-based approaches in emotion research has been a finer conceptualization and examination of behavioral constructs. Adaptive emotional behavior does involve perception of, and attention to, relevant information. But at some point, signals from the environment become elaborated and take on motivational meaning or significance. For example, a happy facial expression, although recognized by young infants, may not take on meaning (e.g., approach) until the child has been exposed to repeated pairings of happy facial expressions and positive outcomes following approach behaviors. A lack of such associative learning experiences (as occurs with neglected infants, who experience fewer pairings of emotional expressions and reliable or predicted outcomes) may lead to an insufficiency of stored associations and subsequent difficulties in interpreting and understanding emotion cues (Wismer Fries & Pollak, 2004). Uncovering when and how these processes occur awaits future empirical research.

BEHAVIORL RESPONSES

Internal emotional processes become visible when children generate behavioral responses. Children's responses to emotional cues are most often discussed in terms of executive function processes such as inhibitory control (see Bell, Wolfe, & Adkins, Chapter 9, this volume). Memory processes also influence behavioral choices as the child relies on his or her knowledge about the probability of success or failure of particular response options, based on his or her previous experiences. Over the course of development, features of children's behavioral responses will change and come to include an increasingly flexible repertoire of response options, increased skill at adapting quickly to changing contingencies, and increasing abilities to inhibit prepotent responses if alternative responses are more appropriate.

As an example, aggressive children are relatively inflexible in their ability to access a response, and they have a difficult time changing to a new response if the initial one is not successful (Rubin, Bream, & Rose-Krasnor, 1991). Additionally, rates of aggressive behavior are negatively associated with the number of responses generated (Shure & Spivack, 1980), suggesting that aggressive children may rely too heavily on their dominant (and often maladaptive) responses in any particular social situation rather than accessing less salient (but perhaps more prosocial) response options. This pattern may be especially true for children prone to proactive aggression (Crick & Dodge, 1996). The choice to enact a particular response may be based on a variety of factors, including anticipated interpersonal, intrapersonal, and/or instrumental outcomes (Dodge, 1993). These kinds of behavioral regulation issues seem to us to be closely linked to the discussion of contingency, reward, and reversal learning of emotional cues discussed above.

The Frontal Lobe Once Again

Several regions of the frontal cortex appear to be involved in organizing these kinds of behaviors (Bechara, Damasio, Damasio, & Anderson, 1994; Eslinger, Flaherty-Craig, & Benton, 2004). In both humans and nonhuman primates, the orbital region of the frontal cortex is linked to regulation of interpersonal relationships, social cooperativity, moral behavior, and social aggression (Damasio, 1994; Davidson, Putnam, & Larson, 2000; Machado & Bachevalier, 2006). In terms of psychological processes, the circuitry in these regions appears to facilitate the making of judgments based on emotional cues and flexibly representing the meaning of those signals (Machado & Bachevalier, 2006). Clinical evidence indicates that humans who suffer damage to the VM area of the frontal cortex show inappropriate social behavior, diminished capacity to respond to punishment, and lack of empathy; yet these patients do not show impairments in general cognitive abilities (Damasio, 1994; Rolls, Hornak, Wade, McGrath, 1994). Individuals with damage to either VM or orbital areas show high levels of impulsive behaviors that undermine interpersonal social relations, such as inappropriate social behavior, aggression, irritability, and uncooperativeness (Berlin, Rolls, & Kischka, 2004). These findings suggest that in the absence of a mature, intact PFC it is difficult for humans and nonhuman primates to plan, inhibit responses, and flexibly change their behaviors (Kolb, 1990).

In humans, the frontal cortex is a late developing structure, not fully mature until puberty or later (Gogtay at al., 2004; Huttenlocher, 1990; see also Lenroot & Giedd, Chapter 3, this volume). The lengthy developmental time course of the frontal cortex is likely related to the emotional behaviors of children. Because of the lack of a fully mature frontal cortex, young children typically have difficulty regulating their behaviors appropriately, inhibiting inappropriate behaviors, and successfully reacting to many changes in the environment (which parents will recognize as the experience of "tantrums" that occur when environmental changes trigger unregulated emotional responses). These emotional skills develop over the course of the first several years of life. In children, individual differences in frontal cortex maturation are associated with improved performance on tasks known to recruit frontal lobe activation (Fox & Bell, 1990), as well as improvements in the regulation of emotional behavior throughout childhood (Dawson, 1994). For example, children learn that, at times, they must inhibit a prepotent response or reaction, especially if their predominant response is not suitable or appropriate for the given situation. And competent emotional functioning also requires dynamic planning and response selection—as children begin to understand what another person is communicating to them, they make rapid decisions about what to say and how to respond, and they update their course of behavior (Wood & Grafman, 2003). In addition, as the orbital area of the frontal cortex develops, children become better able to activate and hold representations of behavioral reinforcement contingencies in working memory (Berlin et al., 2004; Damasio, 1999). This retention makes it likely that children will be able to use their past successful and unsuccessful social experiences to guide their present emotional responses.

Which mechanisms within the PFC appear to support the emergence of competent emotional behaviors? Several lines of research suggest that mesolimbic DA pathways are critical for emotion regulation (Murphy, Arnsten, Goldman-Rakic, & Roth, 1996; Sawaguchi & Goldman-Rakic, 1991). In addition, the DA system appears to be critical for linking the PFC to other networks tied to emotional behavior regulation, such as the amygdala, hippocampus, and nucleus accumbens (NAC; Yang & Mogenson, 1984). Typically, the circuitry within the medial PFC allows an individual to make goal-directed plans, but various motor responses appear to be selected based on input from the NAC. The information processed in the NAC, in turn, originates from both the hippocampus and amygdala, where contextual information and emotional associations become integrated (Grace, 2000; Heidbreder et al., 2000). Therefore, this connection between the NAC and hippocampal–amygdalar complex creates a neural network whereby associations and memories activated by attended emotion cues are able to directly influence the enactment of a motor response. Over development, it appears that children strengthen the connectivity among these regions (see Casey, Tottenham, Liston, & Durston, 2005, for review).

Individual Differences in Emotional Reactivity

To this point, we have described the developing emotion processing system as if only the child's early perceptual and attentional processing of emotional information would culminate in a behavioral response. But ask any parent who cares for more than one child and it becomes immediately apparent that individual differences in children's emotional reactivity will modulate these early processes and affect children's behavioral responses as well. Although beyond the scope of this chapter, a large body of research has explored the role of individual differences in temperamental characteristics (such as inhibited or uninhibited temperaments) in emotional behavior, social functioning, and the development of psychological problems (Kagan, 1997; see Goldsmith, Lemery, Aksan, & Buss, 2000, for review; see also Kagan & Snidman, Chapter 8, this volume). Relatedly, it appears that the left and right hemispheres may be differentially involved in the mediation of approach and withdrawal emotions and behavioral responses, respectively (Davidson, 2000). Individual differences in relative asymmetry of left and right prefrontal regions involved in this motivational system may have important implications in further understanding children's unique patterns of behavioral responding (Davidson & Rickman, 1999).

Development of Socioemotional Regulatory Systems

The ability to appropriately match a behavioral response to a given interpersonal context is the hallmark of healthy emotional functioning. Socially competent children are emotionally responsive yet able to modulate their emotional reactions as necessary. Either underregulation or overregulation of emotion can lead to behavioral difficulties (Cole, Zahn-Waxler, Fox, Usher, & Welsh , 1996; Eisenberg & Fabes, 1992). For example, low regulation of anger is predictive of high levels of externalizing problem behavior in elementary school children (Rydell, Berlin, & Bohlin, 2003). On the other hand, children with well developed emotion regulation abilities are able to act in more prosocial ways with others (Kalpidou, Power, Cherry, & Gottfried, 2004). For instance, in one study of children's behavioral responses to a crying infant, children who demonstrated better emotion regulatory skills were able to respond in a comforting manner (Fabes, Eisenberg, Karbon, Troyer, & Switzer, 1994).

Two different regulatory systems appear to develop early and guide children's responses to emotional situations. One system of neural circuitry becomes activated in response to fear and leads to improved efficiency of connections between the amygdala and cerebral cortex and the amygdala and hippocampus toward the latter part of the first year of life (Caldji, Diorio, & Anisman, 2004; Herschkowitz, 2000; Kalynchuk & Meaney, 2003). Such a *fear system* might protect the infant from the environment, motivate proximity to caregivers to deal with stress, or generate cries that alert the caregiver to perceived threat over the course of development (LeBar & LeDoux, 2003). However, exaggerated responses to fearful stimuli during childhood may play a role in the development of anxiety disorders (Thomas, Drevets, Dahl, et al., 2001). This fear system becomes coordinated with an *affiliation system* that motivates social contact, including shared affect between infant and caregiver. For example, the neuropeptide oxytocin (OT), produced in the hypothalamus and released centrally and peripherally into the bloodstream via axon terminals in the posterior pituitary (Kendrick, Keverne, Baldwin, & Sharman, 1986), appears to be part of the neural system of reward circuitry that includes the NAC (Lovic & Fleming, 2004). In the prairie vole, a monogamous rodent, higher levels of OT are associated with decreases in stress hormones and increases in positive emotional interactions and attachment behaviors (Witt, Carter, & Walton, 1990). Multiple systems (including oxytocin, dopamine, estradiol, arginine, vasopressin, serotonin, and progesterone) are implicated in feedback loops involving reward circuitry and the regulation of positive emotional responses (Insel & Fernald, 2004).

Summary

In brief, the overt emotional behaviors that are most easily observed in children are an end product of interactions among multiple neural systems. Remarkably, these neural systems become so well integrated over the course of development that parsing emotion processing down to its constituent parts is not only difficult but can appear, and may be at some level, arbitrary. Nevertheless, it is helpful to remember that underlying the overt manifestation of emotion are many component processes. At the same time, while emotional responses are being generated, new perceptions, associations, and feeling states are being processed by the brain in an iterative cycle.

EMOTIONAL DEVELOPMENT AND CHILDREN AT RISK

Work from our laboratory has been examining the ways in which children's emotional experiences may affect the development of the neural systems involved in emotion processing. These studies suggest that the brain mechanisms that children use to perceive and understand emotions are responsive to the kinds of experiences to which children are exposed. This responsivity may account for why early stressful environments are associated with so many behavioral problems in childhood and adulthood (Pollak, 2004). For example, physically abused preschool-age children perceived angry faces as highly salient relative to faces with other emotions (Pollak, Cicchetti, Hornung, & Reed, 2000), displayed broader perceptual category boundaries for perceiving anger than nonabused children (Pollak & Kistler, 2002), and required less visual information than nonabused children to detect the presence of angry facial expressions (Pollak & Sinha, 2002). Event-related potential (ERP) studies reveal that attention to anger distinguishes physically abused children's neural processing of faces (Pollak, Cicchetti, Klorman, & Brumaghim, 1997; Pollak, Klorman, Thatcher, & Cicchetti, 2001; Pollak & Tolley-Schell, 2003) and voices (Shackman & Pollak, 2005). These perceptual processes influence children's abilities to regulate their arousal and attention (Pollak, Vardi, Bechner, & Curtin, 2005; Wismer Fries, Shirtcliff, & Pollak, 2005) and to utilize contextual cues to understand emotional situations (Wismer Fries & Pollak, 2004).

The issue of greatest concern is the extent to which children develop the ability to successfully regulate their emotion-related processes. Importantly, a child's early experiences appear to alter the development of the HPA axis (e.g., Shea, Walsh, MacMillan, & Steiner, 2004). Behaviorally, such changes are indexed as an individual's diminished capacity to maintain homeostasis if challenged by adverse events. Both the level of emotion (i.e., how intensely emotions are aroused) and the individual's proficiency in regulating emotion will have implications for attentional, associative, and behavioral processes related to the emotion. An individual with consistently low levels of emotional arousal and a high threshold for reactivity may demonstrate adequate social functioning despite possessing only meager regulation skills. Conversely, an individual predisposed to high reactivity, and thus high levels of emotional arousal, may require exceptional regulatory skills to function equally well.

Education and Intervention

Emotional development is important for children's social development but also serves as a foundation for emerging cognitive competence and academic achievement. For example, early psychosocial factors during the first 3 years of life significantly predict academic achievement in elementary school, even after controlling for IQ and prior achievement (Teo, Carlson, Mathieu, & Egeland, 1996). Additionally, social and emotional adjustment during early and middle childhood are predictive of later high school adjustment (defined as the degree to which the adolescent successfully progresses toward graduation; Carlson et al., 1999). And longitudinal studies of children at risk suggest that delays in emotional development may interfere with young children's formation of close relationships with their teachers, which in turn can result in poor school achievement (Egeland, 1991). As discussed above, children's perception and understanding of emotional cues trigger neural and hormonal responses that allow them to relate effectively to teachers, feel comfortable and confident so that school is enjoyable, and learn from peers—factors clearly important to educational success. On the other hand, research also suggests that increases in stress reactivity and subsequent elevations in stress hormone levels, such as cortisol, actually impair cognitive performance, including memory and learning abilities (de Quervain et al., 2003; Newcomer et al., 1999).

In addition to the idea that the development of emotional competence can foster academic success, it is important to recognize that school settings are ideal situations in which to foster the development of socioemotional skills. Some school-based primary prevention programs have been developed to address problem behaviors with the goal of changing maladaptive cognitions (Crick & Dodge, 1994; Shure & Spivack, 1982), but few have specifically taken into account the role of emotion in creating behavior problems. Reduced behavior problems and more prosocial behaviors in a school setting are likely to lead to better academic achievement. In fact, children who exhibit prosocial behavior and not antisocial behavior tend to have higher academic achievement (Elias et al., 1997), perhaps because the same social cognitions and emotions play a role in both social and academic competence (Bear, Manning, & Izard, 2003). Emotion knowledge (i.e., ability to recognize emotions and label emotion expressions) during the preschool years contributes significantly to academic competence (i.e., skills in reading, skills in arithmetic, motivation to succeed academically) at age 9, and emotion knowledge serves as a mediator between verbal ability and academic competence (Izard et al., 2001). This relationship between emotional skills and academic success continues to be important even into young adulthood; social skills are a significant predictor of grade-point average over the first 2 years of college (Strahan, 2003). For these reasons, future research on the neural mechanisms underlying emotional development may foster targeted intervention programs for children at risk. For example, one promising intervention for children in foster care placements has been developed to target the biopsychosocial sequelae of child maltreatment (Fisher, Gunnar, Chamberlain, & Reid, 2000). Pilot data from this intervention program found evidence for enhanced emotional functioning in terms of both increases in prosocial behavior and improvements in physiological measures related to emotion regulation.

Emotion-related skills such as the ability to recognize emotional signals and match emotion outcomes to contextual cues are requisites for competent social interactions (Cassidy, Parke, Butkovsky, & Braungart, 1992; Denham, 1986; Denham, McKinley, Couchoud, & Holt, 1990; Garner, Carlson Jones, & Miner, 1994) and predict both prosocial behaviors and positive peer relationships (Izard et al., 2001). Not surprisingly, children who are adept at processing emotional stimuli and understanding the causes of emotions are also better at regulating their own emotional arousal (Schultz, Izard, Ackerman, & Youngstrom, 2001). Children who develop within emotionally impoverished environments may have difficulties as they confront increasingly challenging and complex social interactions. Clearly, more research is required to better understand the affective mechanisms influenced by early experience and to generate effective interventions that support and promote optimal development for children who are at risk for socioemotional difficulties.

CONCLUSION

In this chapter we have outlined numerous mechanisms of emotional behavior that are informed by, and consistent with, research findings drawn from behavioral, psychological, and neurobiological approaches. The framework developed is meant to serve as a heuristic, a way to begin to bridge various bodies of literature relevant to the emergence of emotional behavior in children. To achieve this goal, we organized the chapter in terms of a sequential process of key brain systems subserving emotion processing. At the same time, we have emphasized that the brain appears to work in a parallel fashion. The complexity and interconnectivity of brain systems suggest that multiple neural systems contribute to multiple aspects of processing and feedback circuitry. We expect that future research will elaborate on the processes involved in the development of emotion processing and specify more precisely the critical neurobiological systems affected by normal and atypical experience.

An integrated view of affect regulation and brain function, even if rudimentary and incomplete, has enormous potential for improving our understanding of emotional development. We concur with Mayberg (2002), who has argued that although individual regions of brain activation may be interesting, an understanding of emotion processing will require understanding interactive loops of brain activity. How is it that sensory, motor, cognitive, and affective systems become coordinated? The goal of such research endeavors must be to define networks of connectivity linked to complex affective behaviors. In this chapter we have attempted to sketch the characteristics of these networks based on extant studies. However, most research investigating the neural correlates of emotion processing has been carried out with adults or nonhuman animals, some of which have emotional lives that may be quite different from humans. Moreover, given that the brain continues to develop at least into young adulthood, it is possible that the brain circuits required for carrying out processing of emotion information that we study in adults are not the same as those necessary for acquiring emotional skills during childhood. In this regard, we hope and expect to see more biologically informed emotion research that actually involves human children over the next decade.

ACKNOWLEDGMENTS

Seth D. Pollak was supported by grants from the National Institute of Mental Health (Nos. R01 MH068858 and R01 MH61285) and a core grant from the National Institute of Child Health and Human Development (No. P30 HD03352). Alison B. Wismer Fries was supported by a National Institutes of Health Training Program in Emotion Research (No. T32 MH18931), the University of Wisconsin Graduate School, and a Hoffman Memorial Distinguished Fellowship from the Waisman Center. Seth Pollak is also very grateful to the Montreal Neurological Institute and McGill University for hosting him during a sabbatical leave that facilitated completion of the present work. We extend our thanks to Jamie Hanson for his help with the preparation of this chapter.

REFERENCES

Adolphs, R. (2002). Recognizing emotion from facial expressions: Psychological and neurological mechanisms. *Behavioral and Cognitive Neuroscience Reviews, 1*, 21–61.

Adolphs, R., Baron-Cohen, S., & Tranel, D. (2002). Impaired recognition of social emotions following amygdala damage. *Journal of Cognitive Neuroscience, 14*, 1264–1274.

Adolphs, R., Damasio, H., Tranel, D., & Damasio, A. R. (1996). Cortical systems for the recognition of emotion in facial expressions. *Journal of Neuroscience, 16*, 7678–7687.

Adolphs, R., Tranel, D., & Damasio, A. R. (1998). The human amygdala in social judgment. *Nature, 393*, 470–474.

Adolphs, R., Tranel, D., Damasio, H., & Damasio, A. R. (2002). Impaired recognition of emotion in facial expressions following bilateral damage to the human amygdale. *Nature, 372*, 669–672.

Adolphs, R., Tranel, D., Hamann, S., Young, A., Calder, A., Anderson, A., et al. (1999). Recognition of facial emotion in nine individuals with bilateral amygdala damage. *Neuropsychologia, 37,* 1111–1117.

Aggleton, J. P., & Mishkin, M. (1984). Projections of the amygdala to the thalamus in the cynomolgus monkey. *Journal of Comparative Neurology, 222,* 56–68.

Aggleton, J. P., & Young, A. W. (2000). The enigma of the amygdala: On its contribution to human emotion. In R. D. Lane & L. Nadel (Eds.), *Cognitive neuroscience of emotion* (pp. 106–128). London: Oxford University Press.

Amaral, D. G., Price, D. L., Pitkanen, A., & Carmichael, S. T. (1992). In J. P. Aggleton (Ed.), *The amygdala* (pp. 1–66). New York: Wiley–Liss.

Anderson, A. K., & Phelps, E. A. (2001). Lesions of the human amygdala impair enhanced perception of emotionally salient events. *Nature, 411,* 305–309.

Armony, J. L., & Dolan, R. J. (2002). Modulation of spatial attention by fear-conditioned stimuli: An event-related fMRI study. *Neuropsychologia, 40,* 807–826.

Baird, A. A., Gruber, S. A., Fein, D. A., Maas, L. C., Steingard, R. J., Renshaw, P. E., et al. (1999). Functional magnetic resonance imaging of facial affect recognition in children and adolescents. *Journal of the American Academy of Child and Adolescent Psychiatry, 38,* 195–199.

Bauman, M. D., Lavenex, P., Mason, W. A., Capitanio, J. P., & Amaral, D. G. (2004). The development of social behavior following neonatal amygdala lesions in rhesus monkeys. *Journal of Cognitive Neuroscience, 16,* 1388–1411.

Bear, G. G., Manning, M. A., & Izard, C. E. (2003). Responsible behavior: The importance of social cognition and emotion. *School Psychology Quarterly, 18,* 140–157.

Bechara, A., Damasio, H., & Damasio, A. R. (2000). Emotion, decision making and the orbitofrontal cortex. *Cerebral Cortex, 10,* 295–307.

Bechara, A., Damasio, A. R., Damasio, H., & Anderson, S. W. (1994). Insensitivity to future consequences following damage to human prefrontal cortex. *Cognition, 50,* 7–15.

Bechara, A., Tranel, D., Damasio, H., Adolphs, R., Rockland, C., & Damasio, A. R. (1995). Double dissociation of conditioning and declarative knowledge relative to the amygdala and hippocampus in humans. *Science, 269,* 1115–1118.

Belin, P., Zatorre, R. J., Lafaille, P., Ahad, P., & Pike, B. (2000). Voice-selective areas in human auditory cortex. *Nature, 403,* 309–312.

Berlin, H. A., Rolls, E. T., & Kischka, U. (2004). Impulsivity, time perception, emotion and reinforcement sensitivity in patients with orbitofrontal cortex lesions. *Brain, 127,* 1108–1126.

Bernstein-Bercovitz, H. (2003). Does stress enhance or impair selective attention? The effects of stress and perceptual load on negative priming. *Anxiety, Stress and Coping: An International Journal, 16,* 345–357.

Berridge, K. C., & Robinson, T. E. (1998). What is the role of dopamine in reward: Hedonic impact, reward learning, or incentive salience? *Brain Research Reviews, 28,* 309–369.

Bigelow, A. E., & DeCoste, C. (2003). Sensitivity to social contingency from mothers and strangers in 2-, 4-, and 6-month-old infants. *Infancy, 4,* 111–140.

Boucsein, K., Weniger, G., Mursch, K., Steinhoff, B. J., & Irle, E. (2001). Amygdala lesion in temporal lobe epilepsy subjects impairs associative learning of emotional facial expressions. *Neuropsychologia, 39*, 231–236.

Bradley, M. M., Sabatinelli, D., Lang, P. J., Fitzsimmons, J. R., King, W., & Desai, P. (2003). Activation of the visual cortex in motivated attention. *Behavioral Neuroscience, 117*, 369–380.

Broks, P., Young, A. W., Maratos, E. J., Coffey, P. J., Calder, A. J., Isaac, C. L., et al. (1998). Face processing impairments after encephalitis: Amygdala damage and recognition of fear. *Neuropsychologia, 36*, 59–70.

Calder, A. J., Young, A. W., Rowland, D., Perrett, D. I., Hodges, J. R., & Etcoff, N. L. (1996). Facial emotion recognition after bilateral amygdala damage: Differentially severe impairment of fear. *Cognitive Neuropsychology, 13*, 699–745.

Caldji, C., Diorio, J., & Anisman, H. (2004). Maternal behavior regulates benzo-diazepine/GABA-sub(A) receptor subunit expression in brain regions associated with fear in BALB/c and C57BL/6 mice. *Neuropsychopharmacology, 29*(7), 1344–1352.

Call, J. (2001). Chimpanzee social cognition. *Trends in Cognitive Sciences, 5*, 388–393.

Carlson, E. A., Sroufe, L. A., Collins, W. A., Jimerson, S., Weinfield, N., Henninghausen, K., et al. (1999). Early environmental support and elementary school adjustment as predictors of school adjustment in middle adolescence. *Journal of Adolescent Research, 14*, 72–94.

Casey, B. J., Davidson, M. C., Hara, Y., Thomas, K. M., Martinez, A., Galvan, A., et al. (2004). Early development of subcortical regions involved in non-cued attention switching. *Developmental Science, 7*, 534–542.

Casey, B. J., Tottenham, N., Liston, C., & Durston, S. (2005). Imaging the developing brain: What have we learned about cognitive development? *Trends in Cognitive Sciences, 9*, 104–110.

Casey, B. J., Trainor, R., Giedd, J., Vauss, Y., Vaituzis, C. K., Hamburger, S., et al. (1997). The role of the anterior cingulate in automatic and controlled processes: A developmental neuroanatomical study. *Developmental Psychobiology, 30*, 61–69.

Cassidy, J., Parke, R. D., Butkovsky, L., & Braungart, J. M. (1992). Family–peer connections: The roles of emotional expressiveness within the family and children's understanding of emotions. *Child Development, 63*, 603–618.

Cole, P. M., Zahn-Waxler, C., Fox, N. A., Usher, B. A., & Welsh, J. D. (1996). Individual differences in emotion regulation and behavior problems in preschool children. *Journal of Abnormal Psychology, 105*, 518–529.

Compton, R. J., Banich, M., Mohanty, A., Milham, M. P., Herrington, J., Miller, G. A., et al. (2003). Paying attention to emotion: An fMRI investigation of cognitive and emotional Stroop tasks. *Cognitive, Affective, and Behavioral Neuroscience, 3*, 81–96.

Crick, N. R., & Dodge, K. A. (1994). A review and reformulation of social information processing mechanisms in children's social adjustment. *Psychological Bulletin, 115*, 74–101.

Crick, N. R., & Dodge, K. A. (1996). Social information-processing mechanisms on reactive and proactive aggression. *Child Development, 67,* 993–1002.

Damasio, A. R. (1994). *Descartes' error.* New York: Putnam.

Damasio, A. R. (1999). *The feeling of what happens: Body and emotion in the making of consciousness.* New York: Harcourt.

Datla, K. P., Ahier, R. G., Young, A. M., Gray, J. A., & Joseph, M. H. (2002). Conditioned appetitive stimulus increases extracellular dopamine in the nucleus accumbens of the rat. *European Journal of Neuroscience, 16,* 1987–1993.

Davidson, R. J. (2000). The functional neuroanatomy of affective style. In R. D. Lane & L. Nadel (Eds.), *Cognitive neuroscience of emotion* (pp. 371–388). New York: Oxford University Press.

Davidson, R. J., Putnam, K. M., & Larson, C. L. (2000). Dysfunction in the neural circuitry of emotion regulation: A possible prelude to violence. *Science, 289,* 591–594.

Davidson, R. J., & Rickman, M. (1999). Behavioral inhibition and the emotional circuitry of the brain: Stability and plasticity during the early childhood years. In L. A. Schmidt & J. Schulkin (Eds.), *Extreme fear, shyness, and social phobia: Origins, biological mechanisms, and clinical outcomes* (pp. 67–87). New York: Oxford University Press.

Dawson, G. (1994). Development of emotional expression and emotion regulation in infancy: Contributions of the frontal lobe. In G. Dawson & K. W. Fischer (Eds.), *Human behavior and the developing brain* (pp. 346–379). New York: Guilford Press.

Dawson, G., Hessl, D., & Frey, K. (1994). Social influences on early developing biological and behavioral systems related to risk for affective disorder. *Development and Psychopathology, 6,* 759–779.

Denham, S. A. (1986). Social cognition, prosocial behavior, and emotion in preschoolers: Contextual validation. *Child Development, 57,* 194–201.

Denham, S. A., McKinley, M., Couchoud, E. A., & Holt, R. (1990). Emotional and behavioral predictors of preschool peer ratings. *Child Development, 61,* 1145–1152.

Depue, R. A., & Morrone-Strupinsky, J. V. (2005). A neurobehavioral model of affiliative bonding: Implications for conceptualizing a human trait of affiliation. *Behavioral and Brain Sciences, 28,* 313–350.

De Quervain, D. J., Henke, K., Aerni, A., Treyer, V., McGaugh, J. L., Berthold, T., et al. (2003). Glucocorticoid-induced impairment of declarative memory retrieval is associated with reduced blood flow in the medial temporal lobe. *European Journal of Neuroscience, 17,* 1296–1301.

De Renzi, E. (1997). Prosopagnosia. In T. E. Feinberg & M. J. Farah (Eds.), *Behavioral neurology and neuropsychology* (pp. 245–255). New York: McGraw-Hill.

Dodge, K. A. (1993). Social cognitive mechanisms in the development of conduct disorder and depression. *Annual Review of Psychology, 44,* 559–584.

Egeland, B. (1991). A longitudinal study of high risk families: Issues and findings. In R. H. Starr, Jr. & D. A. Wolfe (Eds.), *The effects of child abuse and neglect: Issues and research* (pp. 33–56). New York: Guilford Press.

Egeth, H. E., & Yantis, S. (1997). Visual attention: Control, representation, and time course. *Annual Review of Psychology, 48,* 269–297.

Eisenberg, N., & Fabes, R. A. (1992). Emotion, regulation, and the development of social competence. In M. S. Clark (Ed.), *Emotion and social behavior* (pp. 119–150). Thousand Oaks, CA: Sage.

Elias, M. J., Zins, J. E., Weissberg, R. P., Frey, K. S., Greenberg, M. T., Haynes, N. M., et al. (1997). *Promoting social and emotional learning: Guidelines for educators.* Alexandria, VA: Association for Supervision and Curriculum Development.

Emery, N. J., & Amaral, D. (2000). The role of the amygdala in primate social cognition. In R. D. Lane & L. Nadel (Eds.), *Cognitive neuroscience of emotion* (pp. 156–191). London: Oxford University Press.

Emery, N. J., Capitanio, J. P., Mason, W. A., Machado, C. J., Mendoza, S. P., & Amaral, D. G. (2001). The effects of bilateral lesions of the amygdala on dyadic social interactions in rhesus monkeys (*Macaca mulatta*). *Behavioral Neuroscience, 115,* 515–544.

Enns, J. T. (1990). Relations between components of visual attention. In J. T. Enns (Ed.), *The development of attention: Research and theory* (pp. 139–158). Amsterdam: Elsevier Science.

Eslinger, P. J., Flaherty-Craig, C. V., & Benton, A. L. (2004). Developmental outcomes after early prefrontal cortex damage. *Brain and Cognition, 55,* 84–103.

Fichtenholtz, H. M., Dean, H. L., Dillon, D. G., Yamasaki, H., McCarthy, G., & LaBar, K. S. (2004). Emotion–attention network interactions during a visual oddball task. *Cognitive Brain Research, 20,* 67–89.

Field, T. M., Woodson, R., Greenberg, R., & Cohen, D. (1982). Discrimination and imitation of facial expressions by neonates. *Science, 218,* 179–181.

Fisher, P. A., Gunnar, M. R., Chamberlain, P., & Reid, J. B. (2000). Preventive intervention for maltreated preschool children: Impact on children's behavior, neuroendocrine activity and foster parent functioning. *Journal of the American Academy of Child and Adolescent Psychiatry, 39,* 1356–1364.

Fox, N. A., & Bell, M. A. (1990). Electrophysiological indices of frontal lobe development: Relations to cognitive and affective behavior in human infants over the first year of life. *Annals of the New York Academy of Sciences, 608,* 677–704.

Gaffan, D., & Murray, E. A. (1990). Amygdalar interaction with the mediodorsal nucleus of the thalamus and the ventromedial prefrontal cortex in stimulus–reward associative learning in the monkey. *Journal of Neuroscience, 10,* 3479–3493.

Gaffan, D., & Parker, A. (2000). Mediodorsal thalamic function in scene memory in rhesus monkeys. *Brain, 123,* 816–827.

Ganis, G., Thompson, W. L., & Kosslyn, S. M. (2004). Brain areas underlying visual mental imagery and visual perception: An fMRI study. *Cognitive Brain Research, 20,* 226–241.

Garner, P. W., Carlson Jones, D., & Miner, J. L. (1994). Social competence among low income preschoolers: Emotion socialization practices and social cognitive correlates. *Child Development, 65,* 622–637.

Gathers, A. D., Bhatt, R., Corbly, C. R., Farley, A. B., & Joseph, J. E. (2004). Developmental shifts in cortical loci for face and object recognition. *Neuro-Report, 15*, 1549–1553.

Gogtay, N., Giedd, J. N., Lusk, L., Hayashi, K. M., Greenstein, D., Vaituzis, A. C., et al. (2004). Dynamic mapping of human cortical development during childhood through early adulthood. *Proceedings of the National Academy of Sciences, 101*, 8174–8179.

Goldberg, M. E., Bisley, J., Powell, K. D., Gottlieb, J., & Kusunoki, M. (2002). The role of the lateral intraparietal area of the monkey in the generation of saccades and visuospatial attention. *Annals of the New York Academy of Sciences, 956*, 205–215.

Goldman-Rakic, P. S. (1987). Circuit basis of a cognitive function in non-human primates. In S. M. Stahl & S. D. Iversen (Eds.), *Cognitive neurochemistry* (pp. 90–110). London: Oxford University Press.

Goldsmith, H. H., Lemery, K. S., Aksan, N., & Buss, K. A. (2000). Temperamental substrates of personality. In V. J. Molfese & D. L. Molfese (Eds.), *Temperament and personality development across the life span* (pp. 1–32). Mahwah, NJ: Erlbaum.

Gottfried, J. A., O'Doherty, J., & Dolan, R. J. (2003). Encoding predictive reward value in human amygdala and orbitofrontal cortex. *Science, 301*, 1104–1107.

Grace, A. A. (2000). Gating of information flow within the limbic system and the pathophysiology of schizophrenia. *Brain Research Review, 31*, 330–341.

Heidbreder, C. A., Weiss, I. C., Domeney, A. M., Pryce, C., Homberg, J., Hedou, G., et al. (2000). Behavioral, neurochemical and endocrinological characterization of the early social isolation syndrome. *Neuroscience, 100*, 749–768.

Herschkowitz, N. (2000). Neurobiological bases of behavioural development in infancy. *Brain and Development, 22*, 411–416.

Hoffman, E. A., & Haxby, J. V. (2000). Distinct representations of eye gaze and identity in the distributed human neural system for face perception. *Nature Neuroscience, 3*, 80–84.

Huttenlocher, P. R. (1990). Morphometric study of human cerebral cortex development. *Neuropsychologia, 28*, 517–527.

Insel, T. R., & Fernald, R. D. (2004). How the brain processes social information: Searching for the social brain. *Annual Review of Neuroscience, 27*, 697–722.

Izard, C., Fine, S., Schultz, D., Mostow, A., Ackerman, B., & Youngstrom, E. (2001). Emotion knowledge as a predictor of social behavior and academic competence in children at risk. *Psychological Science, 12*, 18–23.

Johnson, M. H., Dziurawiec, S., Bartrip, J., & Morton, J. (1992). The effects of movement of internal features on infants' preferences for face-like stimuli. *Infant Behavior and Development, 15*, 129–136.

Kagan, J. (1997). Temperament and the reactions to unfamiliarity. *Child Development, 68*, 139–143.

Kalpidou, M. D., Power, T. G., Cherry, K. E., & Gottfried, N. W. (2004). Regulation of emotion and behavior among 3- and 5-year-olds. *Journal of General Psychology, 131*, 159–178.

Kalynchuk, L. E., & Meaney, M. J. (2003). Amygdala kindling increases fear responses and decreases glucocorticoid receptor mRNA expression in hippo-campal regions. *Progress in Neuro-Psychopharmacology and Biological Psychiatry, 27,* 1225–1234.

Kanwisher, N., McDermott, J., & Chun, M. M. (1997). The fusiform face area: A module in human extrastriate cortex specialized for face perception. *Journal of Neuroscience, 17,* 4302–4311.

Kawasaki, H., Adolphs, R., Kaufman, O., Damasio, H., Damasio, A. R., Granner, M., et al. (2001). Single-neuron responses to emotional visual stimuli recorded in the human ventral prefrontal cortex. *Nature Neuroscience, 4,* 15–16.

Kendrick, K. M., Keverne, E. B., Baldwin, B. A., & Sharman, D. F. (1986). Cerebrospinal fluid levels of acetylcholinesterase, monoamines and oxytocin during labor, parturition, vaginocervical stimulation, lamb separation and suckling in sheep. *Neuroendocrinology, 44,* 149–156.

Kesler, M. L., Andersen, A. H., Smith, C. D., Avison, M. J., Davis, C. E., Kryscio, R. J., et al. (2001). Neural substrates of facial emotion processing using fMRI. *Cognitive Brain Research, 11,* 213–226.

King, J. A., Tenney, J., Rossi, V., Colamussi, L., & Burdick, S. (2003). Neural substrates underlying impulsivity. *Annals of the New York Academy of Sciences, 1008,* 160–169.

Kling, A. S., & Brothers, L. A. (1992). The amygdala and social behavior. In J. P. Aggleton (Ed.), *Amygdala: Neurobiological aspects of emotion, memory, and mental dysfunction* (pp. 353–377). New York: Wiley–Liss.

Klingberg, T., Forssberg, H., & Westerberg, H. (2002). Increased brain activity in frontal and parietal cortex underlies the development of visuospatial working memory capacity during childhood. *Journal of Cognitive Neuroscience, 14,* 1–10.

Kluver, H., & Bucy, P. C. (1939). Preliminary analysis of functions of the temporal lobes in monkeys. *Archives of Neurology and Psychiatry, 42,* 979–997.

Kolb, B. (1990). Prefrontal cortex. In B. Kolb & R. C. Tees (Eds.), *Cerebral cortex of the rat* (pp. 437–458). Cambridge, MA: MIT Press.

Lamb, M. E. (1981). The development of social expectations in the first year of life. In M. E. Lamb & L. R. Sherrod (Eds.), *Infant social cognition: Empirical and theoretical considerations* (pp. 155–175). Hillsdale, NJ: Erlbaum.

Lane, R. D., Fink, G. R., Chau, P. M. L., & Dolan, R. J. (1997). Neural activation during selective attention to subjective emotional responses. *NeuroReport, 8,* 3969–3972.

LeBar, K. S., & LeDoux, J. E. (2003). Fear conditioning in relation to affective neuroanatomy. In R. J. Davidson & K. R. Scherer (Eds.), *Handbook of affective sciences* (pp. 52–65). London: Oxford University Press.

LeDoux, J. E. (1992). Emotion and the amygdala. In J. P. Aggleton (Ed.), *The amygdala: Neurobiological aspects of emotion, memory, and mental dysfunction* (pp. 339–351). New York: Wiley–Liss.

LeDoux, J. E. (1996). *The emotional brain: The mysterious underpinnings of emotional life.* New York: Simon & Schuster.

Li, X. B., Inoue, T., Nakagawa, S., & Koyama, T. (2004). Effect of mediodorsal thalamic nucleus lesion on contextual fear conditioning in rats. *Brain Research, 1008*, 261–272.

Lovic, V., & Fleming, A. S. (2004). Artificially-reared female rats show reduced prepulse inhibition and deficits in the attentional set shifting task-reversal of effects with maternal-like licking stimulation. *Behavioural Brain Research, 148*, 209–219.

Machado, C. J., & Bachevalier, J. (2006). The impact of amygdala, orbital frontal cortex, or hippocampal formation on established social relationships in rhesus monkeys (*Macaca mulatta*). *Behavioral Neuroscience, 120*, 761–786.

Mayberg, H. (2002). Mapping mood: An evolving emphasis on frontal–limbic interactions. In D. T. Stuss & R. T. Knight (Eds.), *Principles of frontal lobe function* (pp. 376–391). London: Oxford University Press.

Mirsky, A. F. (1996). Disorders of attention: A neuropsychological perspective. In G. R. Lyon & N. A. Krasnegor (Eds.), *Attention, memory, and executive function* (pp. 71–95). Baltimore: Brookes.

Molle, M., Albrecht, C., Marshall, L., Fehm, H. L., & Born, J. (1997). Adrenocorticotropin widens the focus of attention in humans: A non-linear electroencephalographic analysis. *Psychosomatic Medicine, 59*, 497–502.

Morris, J. S., Friston, K. J., Buchel, C., Frith, C. D., Young, A. W., Calder, A. J., et al. (1998). A neuromodulatory role for the human amygdala in processing emotional facial expressions. *Brain, 121*, 47–57.

Morris, J. S., Scott, S. K., & Dolan, R. J. (1999). Saying it with feeling: Neural responses to emotional vocalizations. *Neuropsychologia, 37*, 1155–1163.

Murphy, B. L., Arnsten, A. F., Goldman-Rakic, P. S., & Roth, R. H. (1996). Increased dopamine turnover in the prefrontal cortex impairs spatial working memory performance in rats and monkeys. *Proceedings of the National Academy of Sciences, 93*, 1325–1329.

Newcomer, J. W., Selke, G., Melson, A. D., Hershey, T., Craft, S., Richards, K., et al. (1999). Decreased memory performance in healthy humans induced by stress-level cortisol treatment. *Archives of General Psychiatry, 56*, 527–533.

Nieoullon, A. (2002). Dopamine and the regulation of cognition and attention. *Progress in Neurobiology, 67*, 53–83.

O'Doherty, J., Kringelbach, M. L., Rolls, E. T., Hornak, J., & Andrews, C. (2001). Abstract reward and punishment representations in the human orbitofrontal cortex. *Nature Neuroscience, 4*, 95–102.

Oyoshi, T., Nishijo, H., Asakura, T., Takamura, Y., & Ono, T. (1996). Emotional and behavioral correlates of mediodorsal thalamic neurons during associative learning in rats. *Journal of Neuroscience, 16*, 5812–5829.

Phillips, M. L., Young, A. W., Scott, S. K., Calder, A. J., Andrew, C., Giampietro, V., et al. (1998). Neural responses to facial and vocal expressions of fear and disgust. *Proceedings in Biological Science, 265*, 1809–1817.

Pollak, S. D. (2004). Experience-dependent affective learning and risk for psychopathology in children. In J. A. King, C. F. Ferris, & I. I. Lederhendler (Eds.), *Roots of mental illness in children. Annals of the New York Academy of Sciences, 1008*, 102–111.

Pollak, S. D., Cicchetti, D., Hornung, K., & Reed, A. (2000). Recognizing emotion in faces: Developmental effects of child abuse and neglect. *Developmental Psychology, 36,* 679–688.

Pollak, S. D., Cicchetti, D., Klorman, R., & Brumaghim, J. T. (1997). Cognitive brain event-related potentials and emotion processing in maltreated children. *Child Development, 68,* 773–787.

Pollak, S. D., & Kistler, D. J. (2002). Early experience is associated with the development of categorical representations for facial expression of emotion. *Proceedings of the National Academy of Sciences, 99,* 9072–9076.

Pollak, S. D., Klorman, R., Thatcher, J. E., & Cicchetti, D. (2001). P3b reflects maltreated children's reactions to facial displays of emotion. *Psychophysiology, 38,* 267–274.

Pollak, S. D., & Sinha, P. (2002). Effects of early experience on children's recognition of facial displays of emotion. *Developmental Psychology, 38,* 784–791.

Pollak, S. D., & Tolley-Schell, S. A. (2003). Selective attention to facial emotion in physically abused children. *Journal of Abnormal Psychology, 112,* 323–338.

Pollak, S. D., Vardi, S., Bechner, A., & Curtin, J. (2005). Maltreated children's regulation of attention in response to anger. *Child Development, 76,* 968–977.

Posner, M. I. (1994). Attention: The mechanisms of consciousness. *Proceedings of the National Academy of Sciences, 91,* 7398–7403.

Posner, M. I., & Rothbart, M. K. (1998). Attention, self regulation and consciousness. *Philosophical Transactions of the Royal Society B: Biological Sciences, 353,* 1915–1927.

Pourtois, G., de Gelder, B., Bol, A., & Crommelinck, M. (2005). Perception of facial expressions and voices and of their combination in the human brain. *Cortex, 41,* 49–59.

Pruessner, J. C., Champagne, F., Meaney, M. J., & Dagher, A. (2004). Dopamine release in response to a psychological stress in humans and its relationship to early life maternal care: A positron emission tomography study using [^{11}C]raclopride. *Journal of Neuroscience, 24,* 2825–2831.

Puce, A., Allison, T., Bentin, S., Gore, J. C., & McCarthy, G. (1998). Temporal cortex activation in humans viewing eye and mouth movements. *Journal of Neuroscience, 18,* 2188–2199.

Puce, A., & Perrett, D. (2003). Electrophysiology and brain imaging of biological motion. *Philosophical Transactions of the Royal Society B: Biological Sciences, 358,* 435–445.

Redgrave, P., Prescott, T. J., & Gurney, K. (1999). Is the short-latency dopamine response too short to signal reward error? *Trends in Neurosciences, 22,* 146–151.

Rodman, H. R. (1994). Development of inferior temporal cortex in the monkey. *Cerebral Cortex, 4,* 484–498.

Rolls, E. T., Hornak, J., Wade, D., & McGrath, J. (1994). Emotion-related learning in patients with social and emotional changes associated with frontal lobe damage. *Journal of Neurology, Neurosurgery, and Psychiatry, 57,* 1518–1524.

Rubin, K. H., Bream, L. A., & Rose-Krasnor, L. (1991). Social problem solving and aggression in childhood. In D. J. Pepler & K. H. Rubin (Eds.), *Development and treatment of childhood aggression* (pp. 219–248). Hillsdale, NJ: Erlbaum.

Rueda, R., Fan, J., McCandliss, B. D., Halparin, J. D., Gruber, D. B., Lercari, L. P., et al. (2004). Development of attentional networks in childhood. *Neuropsychologia, 42,* 1029–1040.

Rydell, A., Berlin, L., & Bohlin, G. (2003). Emotionality, emotion regulation, and adaptation among 5- to 8-year-old children. *Emotion, 3,* 30–47.

Salamone, J. D., Cousins, M. S., & Snyder, B. J. (1997). Behavioral functions of nucleus accumbens dopamine: Empirical and conceptual problems with the anhedonia hypothesis. *Neuroscience and Biobehavioral Reviews, 21,* 341–359.

Sarter, M., & Markowitsch, H. J. (1983). Reduced resistance to progressive extinction in senescent rats: A neuroanatomical and behavioral study. *Neurobiology of Aging, 4,* 203–215.

Sato, W., Kochiyama, T., Yoshikawa, S., Naito, E., & Matsumura, M. (2004). Enhanced neural activity in response to dynamic facial expressions of emotion: An fMRI study. *Cognitive Brain Research, 20,* 81–91.

Sawaguchi, T., & Goldman-Rakic, P. S. (1991). D1 dopamine receptors in prefrontal cortex: Involvement in working memory. *Science, 251,* 947–950.

Schultz, D., Izard, C., Ackerman, B., & Youngstrom, E. (2001). Emotional knowledge in economically disadvantaged children: Self-regulatory antecedents and relations to social difficulties and withdrawal. *Development and Psychopathology, 13,* 53–67.

Shackman, J. E., & Pollak, S. D. (2005, April). *Regulation of attention to multimodal expressions of emotions in physically abused children: An ERP investigation.* Poster presented at the biennial meeting of the Society for Research on Child Development, Atlanta, GA.

Shea, A., Walsh, C., MacMillan, H., & Steiner, M. (2004). Child maltreatment and HPA axis dysregulation: Relationship to major depressive disorder and post traumatic stress disorder in females. *Psychoneuroendocrinology, 30,* 162–178.

Shure, M. B., & Spivack, G. (1980). Interpersonal problem-solving as a mediator of behavioral adjustment in preschool and kindergarten children. *Journal of Applied Developmental Psychology, 1,* 29–44.

Shure, M. B., & Spivack, G. (1982). Interpersonal problem-solving in young children: A cognitive approach to prevention. *American Journal of Community Psychology, 10,* 341–356.

Skosnik, P. D., Chatterton, R. T., Jr., Swisher, T., & Park, S. (2000). Modulation of attentional inhibition by norepinephrine and cortisol after psychological stress. *International Journal of Psychophysiology, 36,* 59–68.

Stanford, L., & Santi, A. (1998). The dopamine D2 agonist quinpirole disrupts attention to temporal signals without selectively altering the speed of the internal clock. *Psychobiology, 26,* 258–266.

Stevenson, C. W., & Gratton, A. (2003). Basolateral amygdala modulation of the nucleus accumbens dopamine response to stress: Role of the medial prefrontal cortex. *European Journal of Neuroscience, 17,* 1287–1295.

Strahan, E. Y. (2003). The effects of social anxiety and social skills on academic performance. *Personality and Individual Differences, 34,* 347–366.

Stuss, D. T. (1992). Biological and psychological development of executive functions. *Brain and Cognition, 20,* 8–23.

Tarr, M. J., & Gauthier, I. (2000). FFA: A flexible fusiform area for subordinate-level visual processing automatized by expertise. *Nature Neuroscience, 3,* 764–769.

Teo, A., Carlson, E., Mathieu, P. J., & Egeland, B. (1996). A prospective longitudinal study of psychosocial predictors of achievement. *Journal of School Psychology, 34,* 285–306.

Thomas, K. M., Drevets, W. C., Dahl, R. E., Ryan, N. D., Birmaher, B., Eccard, C. H., et al. (2001). Amygdala response to fearful faces in anxious and depressed children. *Archives of General Psychiatry, 58,* 1057–1063.

Thomas, K. M., Drevets, W .C., Whalen, P. J., Eccard, C. H., Dahl, R. E., Ryan, N. D., et al. (2001). Amygdala response to facial expressions in children and adults. *Biological Psychiatry, 49,* 309–316.

Van Honk, J., Kessels, R. P. C., Putnam, P., Jager, G., Koppeschaar, H. P. F., & Postma, A. (2003). Attentionally modulated effects of cortisol and mood on memory for emotional faces in healthy young males. *Psychoneuroendocrinology, 28,* 941–948.

Vuilleumier, P., Armony, J. L., Driver, J., & Dolan, R. J. (2001). Effects of attention and emotion on face processing in the human brain: An event-related fMRI study. *Neuron, 30,* 829–841.

Vuilleumier, P., Armony, J. L., Driver, J., & Dolan, R. J. (2003). Distinct spatial frequency sensitivities for processing faces and emotional expressions. *Nature Neuroscience, 6,* 624–631.

Vuilleumier, P., Richardson, M. P., Armony, J. L., Driver, J., & Dolan, R. J. (2004). Distant influences of amygdala lesion on visual cortical activation during emotional face processing. *Nature Neuroscience, 7,* 1271–1278.

Walker-Andrews, A. S. (1988). Infants' perception of the affordances of expressive behaviors. In C. K. Rovee-Collier (Ed.), *Advances in infancy research* (pp. 173–221). Norwood, NJ: Ablex.

Walker-Andrews, A. S. (1997). Infants' perception of expressive behaviors: Differentiation of multimodal information. *Psychological Bulletin, 121,* 437–456.

Want, S. C., Pascalis, O., Coleman, M., & Blades, M. (2003). Recognizing people from the inner and outer parts of their faces: Developmental data concerning "unfamiliar" faces. *British Journal of Developmental Psychology, 21,* 125–135.

Webster, M. A., Kaping, D., Mizokami, Y., & Duhamel, P. (2004). Adaptation to natural facial categories. *Nature, 428,* 557–561.

Wismer Fries, A. B., & Pollak, S. D. (2004). Emotion understanding in post-institutionalized Eastern European children. *Development and Psychopathology, 16,* 355–369.

Wismer Fries, A. B., Shirtcliff, E., & Pollak, S. D. (2005, April). *Effects of early social deprivation on emotion regulation in children.* Poster presented at the biennial meeting of the Society for Research on Child Development, Atlanta, GA.

Witt, D. M., Carter, C. S., & Walton, D. (1990). Central and peripheral effects of oxytocin administration in prairie voles. *Pharmacology and Biochemical Behavior, 37*, 63–69.

Wojciulik, E., & Kanwisher, N. (1999). The generality of parietal involvement in visual attention. *Neuron, 23*, 747–764.

Wood, J. N., & Grafman, J. (2003). Human prefrontal cortex: Processing and representational perspectives. *Nature Reviews Neuroscience, 4*, 139–147.

Yakovlev, P. I., & Lecours, A. R. (1967). The myelogenetic cycles of regional maturation of the brain. In A. Minkowski (Ed.), *Regional development of the brain in early life* (pp. 3–70). Oxford, UK: Blackwell.

Yamasaki, H., LaBar, K. S., & McCarthy, G. (2002). Dissociable prefrontal brain systems for attention and emotion. *Proceedings of the National Academy of Sciences, 99*, 11447–11451.

Yang, C. R., & Mogenson, G. J. (1984). Electrophysiological responses of neurons in the nucleus accumbens to hippocampal stimulation and the attenuation of the excitatory responses by mesolimbic dopaminergic system. *Brain Research, 324*, 69–84.

CHAPTER 13

Brain Development
and Adolescent Behavior

Linda Patia Spear

Brain development is a lifelong process. Growth and differentiation of the brain proceed at a particularly rapid pace during the prenatal and early postnatal periods, yet the brain continues to develop well into adulthood (Sowell et al., 2003) and to generate modest numbers of new neurons throughout life (Eriksson et al., 1998). Within this framework of a dynamically changing brain throughout the lifespan, the adolescent period has emerged as a time of particularly dramatic ontogenetic change. Alterations occurring in the brain during adolescence include a considerable loss of connections among neurons—a process of pruning that appears to contribute to the transformation of the brain of the child into a more efficient, less energy-demanding brain of an adult (Spear, 2000).

In this review, adolescence is defined as the time of transition from a state of dependence to (relative) independence. During this gradual transition there are marked changes in body appearance associated with periods of rapid growth and the emergence of secondary sexual characteristics, along with sometimes dramatic changes in mood and behavior. Internal transformations include a variety of pubertal and other hormonal changes in addition to the considerable developmental sculpting of the brain. Determining the absolute boundaries of adolescence is difficult, however, with no single event signaling its onset or offset. Adolescence is often considered to subsume the second decade of life (e.g., Petersen, Silbereisen, & Sorensen, 1996), although consensus is lacking. The timing of adolescence is known to vary with environmental conditions and nutritional status (Enright, Levy, Harris, & Lapsley, 1987; Frisch, 1984) as well as gender, with females typically entering adolescence more quickly and males often lagging behind (Savin-Williams & Weisfeld, 1989). Although some researchers have suggested that puberty (i.e., the series of physiological changes leading to sexual maturation) signals the onset of adolescence (e.g., Petersen, 1998), timing of the temporally restricted phase of puberty has been shown to vary notably within the broader adolescent period, occurring relatively late during adolescence in some individuals (e.g., Dubas, 1991).

ADOLESCENCE FROM AN EVOLUTIONARY PERSPECTIVE

To set the stage for reviewing neural and behavioral characteristics of adolescence, the potential adaptive significance of these characteristics is first considered. To the extent that adolescence is defined as the transformation from dependence to independence, by definition developing organisms of all mammalian species go through an adolescent period. During this transition, human adolescents as well as their counterparts in other species exhibit certain common developmental features that include hormonal and physiological alterations associated with puberty, characteristic brain transformations, as well as certain commonalities in adolescent-typical behaviors. Similarities along these dimensions across species seemingly represent highly conserved developmental traits driven by common evolutionary pressures.

The maturing sexuality of adolescence creates a challenge: how to avoid mating with genetically related individuals. Genetic inbreeding is a serious threat to species survival in that it results in greater expression of lethal or otherwise detrimental recessive genes in offspring, a phenomenon known as "inbreeding depression." One strategy to avoid inbreeding is for sexually emergent adolescents to emigrate away from the home territory (Bixler, 1992; Moore, 1992). Indeed, emigration to areas away from genetic relatives is characteristic among adolescents of either or both sexes in virtually all mammalian species (e.g., Keane, 1990), including humans in preindustrial societies (Schlegel & Barry, 1991). Certain common adolescent behaviors (and their underlying neural and hormonal substrates) may have proved adaptive and hence were evolutionarily conserved, in part, because they served to facilitate emigration. Among the conserved behavioral features of adolescence are increases in risk taking and exploration of novel areas, behaviors, and reinforcers, as well as increased affiliation with peers. Changes in social relationships, including greater affinity for peers along with rising parental conflicts, may aid emigration (see Steinberg, 1989), given that the journey often occurs with peers and may be precipitated by increased conflict between parents and offspring (e.g., Caine, 1986). Increases in novelty-seeking and risk-taking behaviors may also facilitate adolescent emigration from the natal group by providing the impetus to enter unknown territories and sample unfamiliar sources of food that may prove necessary for survival (see Spear, 2000, for discussion). The continued emergence of cognitive capacities during adolescence may help emigrants cope with, and adjust to, the challenges associated with detecting and avoiding novel dangers, discerning new food sources, and merging with or establishing a new social group.

According to this approach, then, certain behavioral propensities seen in human adolescents may be highly conserved leftovers from our evolutionary past. Identifying certain adolescent-typical neural, behavioral, and physiological features that are common across a variety of species, however, should not be construed to diminish the uniqueness and complexity of human adolescence. Certainly, no other species demonstrates the full complexity of brain, behavior, and cognitive function seen during human adolescence (or at any other time of life, for that matter). Considering certain conserved neurobehavioral features of human adolescents from an evolutionary perspective also does not imply that these behavioral features are all necessarily adaptive for today's adolescents. Aside from runaways, emigration with peers and without parental support or assistance is rare among adolescents from industrialized nations. Indeed, many young people maintain financial, physical, and psychological dependence on parents until well after the physiological harbingers of adolescence have passed. Yet even in modern societies in which cultural traditions largely protect against inbreeding, highly conserved adolescent behaviors may be retained for relatively long intervals under relaxed selection pressure or because they serve other adaptive functions (e.g., see argument by Wilson & Daly, 1985, regarding the possible adaptive significance of risk taking in terms of increased reproductive fitness in males). Thus, some adolescent behaviors may partly represent remnants of the evolutionary past, despite their potential cost for some adolescents. Adolescence is inherently a risky business, with mortality rates higher during late adolescence than at most other times of the lifespan in virtually all species, including humans (e.g., Crockett & Pope, 1993; Irwin & Millstein, 1992). These elevated mortality rates during the otherwise relatively healthy period of adolescence are attributable largely to misfortunes associated with risk taking (e.g., Muuss & Porton,

1998), including emigration with its inherent dangers (Crockett & Pope, 1993).

ADOLESCENT-TYPICAL BEHAVIORS

Changing Focus of Social Behaviors

Among the prominent behavioral transitions of adolescence are changes in social relationships that emerge as the social sphere of the adolescent begins to shift. During adolescence, emotional distance and conflict between parents and offspring increases (Steinberg, 1987), with such conflict being especially pronounced early in adolescence (Laursen, Coy, & Collins, 1998). In contrast, social interactions with peers take on particular importance, with adolescents spending about fourfold more time interacting with peers than with adults (Csikszentmihalyi, Larson, & Prescott, 1977). Increases in peer-directed social interactions during adolescence are highly conserved and are evident in adolescents of other mammalian species as well (e.g., Douglas, Varlinskaya, & Spear, 2004). Adolescent-associated increases in the value attributed to social interactions with individuals outside the family may have adaptive significance in helping individuals to develop social skills away from the home environment, in guiding choice behaviors, and in allowing opportunities to practice more independent behavior patterns (see Spear, 2000, for a review).

During puberty, adolescents typically exhibit an emerging interest in the opposite sex. Although primates in general, including humans, are "emancipated" from complete dependence on gonadal hormones for sexual activity (Wallen, 2001), there is no doubt that puberty, with its rising gonadal hormone titers, is associated with increases in sexual interest and sex drive (e.g., Smith, Udry, & Morris, 1985; Udry, Talbert, & Morris, 1986). Overall, 17% of seventh and eighth graders and 49% of ninth through twelfth graders report that they have had sex, with one in five sexually active ninth through twelfth graders having a history of pregnancy (Resnick et al., 1997)—rates that would undoubtedly be higher if there were not a period of relative postpubertal infertility (Short, 1976).

Restorative Behaviors: Eating and Sleeping

Adolescence is associated with an increase in food intake that is seen across a wide variety of species (aside from recent cultural trends for dieting in human female adolescents), with adolescents often having the greatest caloric intake relative to their body weight in comparison to any other time period in the lifespan (e.g., Ganji & Betts, 1995; Nance, 1983). Adolescent-

typical increases in food consumption are associated with elevated meta-
bolic activity and contribute to the growth spurt of adolescence, during
which mature size is reached (Post & Kemper, 1993).

In addition to eating more, adolescents sleep less, spending less total
amount of time in sleep (Levy, Gray-Donald, Leech, Zvagulis, & Pless,
1986) and showing a preference for going to bed and waking later
(Carskadon, Vieira, & Acebo, 1993). This phase delay may be biologically
based, in part, and has been suggested to have been of adaptive significance
during evolution (Dahl & Ryan, 1996). Indeed, signs of a similar phase
delay are seen in other species (Alfoldi, Tobler, & Borbely, 1990). Phase
delays and other alterations in sleep during adolescence may partly reflect
developmental changes in the balance between states of sleep and vigilance
or wakefulness, with complex ontogenetic interactions among systems regulating sleep, affect, arousal, and attention (Dahl, 1996). Such phase delays
may have functional significance, with adolescents performing better later
in the day than in the early morning (Hansen, Janssen, Schiff, Zee, &
Dubocovich, 2005). Indeed, early start times for schools have been linked
to sleep deprivation and daytime sleepiness among adolescents (Carskadon,
Wolfson, Acebo, Tzischinsky, & Seifer, 1998; Dexter, Bijwadia, Schilling,
& Applebaugh, 2003; Hansen et al., 2005; but see Eliasson, King, Gould,
& Eliasson, 2002, for contrary data).

Cognitive Alterations and Affect Regulation

Developmental increases in cognitive abilities occur throughout adolescence (e.g., Graber & Petersen, 1991). Among the cognitive competencies
that generally show improvement during adolescence are those considered
within the realm of "executive functions," consisting of several loose clusters of cognitive abilities that include inhibitory control (Williams, Ponesse,
Schachar, Logan, & Tannock, 1999), working memory, abstract reasoning,
decision making, sensitivity to future consequences (e.g., Crone & van der
Molen, 2004), processing of affective stimuli, and regulation of emotions
(Dahl, 2004; Steinberg, 2005). Although improvements are seen along each
of these dimensions across adolescence, the time course of their ontogeny is
not identical and may be related to differential rates of maturation within
various prefrontal cortical (PFC) regions (e.g., dorsolateral PFC, ventromedial PFC, orbitofrontal cortex, and anterior cingulate cortex) particularly critical for their expression (e.g., see Hooper, Luciana, Conklin, &
Yarger, 2004).

Although collectively the maturation of these competencies results in
considerable improvement in judgment from early to mid- and late adolescence (see Steinberg & Cauffman, 1996, for a review), adolescents do not

always exhibit mature decision making during the course of their daily lives (e.g., Steinberg, 2005). That is, whereas adolescents often display excellent decision making capacity under controlled classroom or laboratory situations, less than optimal decision making may emerge in more emotional and arousing contexts, particularly those involving peers. Emotions may play a particularly important role in decision making during adolescence due to immaturity in affect regulation; that is, in the adolescent's ability to regulate affective reactions to achieve adaptive goals (Dahl, 2004). As a result, adaptive decision making evident in low-stress, low-emotional situations in which rational thinking is promoted (so-called "cold cognitions") may be subverted by affective reactions emerging in the "heat" of the moment ("hot cognitions"; see Dahl, 2001, 2004, for reviews and discussion). Although challenging to examine experimentally, one recent study has investigated the impact of peer presence on decision making in adolescents and adults using a computer task designed to index risk taking. Adults performed similarly whether they were tested alone or in the presence of peers who were asked to observe and comment on their performance, whereas adolescents took more risks when performing the task in the presence of peers than when alone (Steinberg, 2005). Thus, one consequence of less than optimal decision making by adolescents in the presence of peers may be an increase in risk taking. Indeed, as discussed below, elevated risk taking is prototypic of adolescence.

Risk Taking and Novelty Seeking

Relative to individuals at other ages, adolescents exhibit a disproportionate amount of risk-taking and reckless behavior (e.g., Trimpop, Kerr, & Kirkcaldy, 1999). Indeed, under certain circumstances, "most youth will . . . engage in moderately risky acts that sometimes, even though relatively rarely, result in accidents and lead to tragic consequences" (Muuss & Porton, 1998, p. 423). Thus, engaging in some degree of risk taking becomes essentially normative during adolescence, with more than 50% of adolescents engaging in drunk driving, sex without contraception, use of illegal drugs, school misconduct, theft or other minor criminal activities, or fighting (Arnett, 1992; Moffitt, 1993). Adverse consequences of risk taking include increased probability of death due to mishap, along with incarceration, AIDS infection, unintended pregnancy, or alcohol or drug dependence (Irwin, 1989). In some high-risk groups, adolescent risk taking may escalate into a deviant lifestyle characterized by continued criminality and other problem behaviors in adulthood (Lerner & Galambos, 1998). Most adolescents, however, exhibit only a transient ontogenetic increase in risk taking and manage to escape the lottery for harm associated with their risk-taking behaviors.

Although clearly hazardous, risk taking during adolescence may confer some benefits. Risk taking may provide the adolescent with opportunities to explore adult behaviors and privileges (Silbereisen & Reitzle, 1992), to master normal developmental tasks (Muuss & Porton, 1998), and to face and conquer challenges (Csikszentmihalyi & Larson, 1978). Risk taking may enhance self-esteem (Silbereisen & Reitzle, 1992; but see also McCarthy & Hoge, 1984), probably at least in part by increasing acceptance by risk-taking peers (Maggs, Almeida, & Galambos, 1995). Indeed, when risk taking was indexed in terms of drug use, Shedler and Block (1990) found adolescents who engaged in moderate amounts of drug use to be more socially competent during both childhood and adolescence than both abstainers and frequent users, leading them to suggest that modest drug experimentation during adolescence may reflect "developmentally appropriate experimentation" (p. 613).

Adolescent risk taking likely has multiple determinants. As discussed earlier, elevated levels of novelty and sensation seeking have been evolutionarily conserved during adolescence, with adolescents of other species also showing higher levels of novelty seeking than adults (e.g., Douglas, Varlinskaya, & Spear, 2003). From an evolutionary perspective, adolescent risk taking has been suggested to aid emigration (see Spear, 2000) and to increase the probability of reproductive success under circumstances in which an opportunistic mating strategy would be favored, such as in individuals having a history of unstable and uncertain resources (Steinberg & Belsky, 1996; see also Wilson & Daly, 1985). In terms of more proximate causes, some individuals may engage in risk taking as a means of reducing dysphoria or coping with stress (Jessor, Donovan, & Costa, 1996; McCord, 1990), whereas others may do so to obtain arousal benefits associated with novel or intense stimuli (Zuckerman, 1992).

Drug Use and Reward Sensitivity

One particularly prevalent risk behavior of adolescence is alcohol and other drug use. For instance, 78% of 12th graders have tried alcohol, 57% have used cigarettes, and 48% have tried marijuana or hashish, with analogous percentages for 8th graders of 47%, 31%, and 19%, respectively. Some of this use reaches high levels, with, for instance, 29% of 12th graders and 12% of 8th graders reporting that they had consumed five or more drinks in a row within the last 2 weeks (Johnston, O'Malley, & Bachman, 2002). Dependence may develop more rapidly in adolescents than adults under some circumstances (Clark, Kirisci, & Tarter, 1998), with adolescents showing relapse rates approximating those of adults, despite the shorter chronicity of adolescent-use patterns (e.g., Brown, 1993). Nevertheless, much of the heavy use of alcohol is "adolescence limited," with rates of use declining after adolescence in many individuals (Bates & Labouvie, 1997).

Multiple factors undoubtedly contribute to the increased propensity of adolescents to use alcohol and other drugs, sometimes excessively. One contributor is likely biological; this perspective is supported by the observation that such use is elevated in adolescents of other species as well, with, for instance, adolescents in a rodent model often drinking two- to three-fold more alcohol relative to their body weights than adults (Doremus, Brunell, Pottayil, & Spear, 2005; Lancaster, Brown, Coker, Elliott, & Wren, 1996). Research in laboratory animals suggests that the propensity for adolescents to drink large amounts of alcohol may be precipitated, in part, by their relative insensitivity to the effects of alcohol that normally serve as cues to limit intake (e.g., sedative, dysphoric effects), when compared with adults (see Spear & Varlinskaya, 2004, for a review). Although comparable studies are rare in humans due to ethical concerns about administering alcohol to youth, there is a study by Behar and associates (1983) that did examine the behavioral and subjective effects of an intoxicating dose of alcohol given to 8- to 15-year-old boys. The investigators were surprised to find little evidence of inebriation in these boys who were presumably undergoing their first experience with alcohol, noting that they "were impressed by how little gross behavioral change occurred in the children . . . after a dose of alcohol which had been intoxicating in an adult population" (p. 407). Whether adolescents might be similarly less sensitive to the rewarding consequences of alcohol, perhaps necessitating greater consumption to obtain euphoric and reinforcing effects, is unclear.

Indeed, there are opposing theoretical perspectives as to whether the elevated propensity of adolescents to seek out drugs, novelty, risks, and other rewarding stimuli is related to an increase or decrease in the rewarding value they attribute to those stimuli (e.g., contrast Chambers, Taylor, & Potenza, 2003, with Spear, 2000). On the one hand, adolescents might avidly seek out such stimuli because they find them especially rewarding (e.g., Chambers et al., 2003), a position that makes intuitive sense. Alternatively, adolescents might be especially prone to seek out drugs and other rewarding stimuli to compensate for an age-related decline in sensitivity of reward circuits (i.e., partial anhedonia; see Spear, 2000). This latter notion is reminiscent of the decline in sensitivity of reward circuits that has been postulated to motivate drug-taking behavior in addicted individuals, with repeated drug use suggested to progressively decrease sensitivity of these circuits, resulting in escalated drug use to compensate for the reward deficiency (Koob & Le Moal, 2001; Volkow, Fowler, & Wang, 2002). Indeed, there are limited data to suggest that adolescents may exhibit some degree of anhedonia. Adolescents report positive situations to be less pleasurable than both younger or older individuals, a "falling from grace" associated with a 50% decline in reports of feeling "very happy" between childhood and early adolescence (Larson & Richards, 1994). Not only do adolescents rate comparable activities as less pleasurable than do adults (Larson & Richards, 1994), they are also less optimistically biased when compared with college students or adults (Millstein, 1993). To the extent that adolescents already show an age-related bias toward partial anhedonia, that anhedonia might escalate more rapidly with repeated drug use in adolescence than in adulthood, perhaps contributing to the more rapid emergence of drug dependence that has been reported in adolescents as compared to adults (e.g., Clark et al., 1998).

PUBERTY, HORMONAL CHANGES, AND ADOLESCENT BEHAVIOR

There has been much interest in determining the triggers for the often dramatic changes observable in the behaviors of adolescents and in their ways of relating to others. Processes associated with puberty have been prime suspects. As discussed above, puberty has clearly been associated with an emerging interest in the opposite sex, leading to sexual activity in a significant number of adolescents and pregnancy in some. In studies comparing adolescents at different stages of pubertal development, puberty has also been associated with a variety of other adolescent-typical behavior patterns, including increased conflicts with, and greater emotional distance from, parents (Steinberg, 1987, 1988); a preference for going to sleep later (Carskadon et al., 1993); and risk-taking behaviors, including a greater probability of smoking, drinking (Harrell, Bangdiwala, Deng, Webb, & Bradley, 1998; Wilson et al., 1994), and use of marijuana (Martin et al., 2002). Not only the state of pubertal maturation but also the timing of that maturation, relative to other adolescents, may influence adolescent behavior. Going through puberty early relative to one's peers is associated with elevated risk taking and other externalizing behaviors in adolescents of both sexes, although other correlates of early versus late pubertal timing may differ between boys and girls (see Steinberg & Belsky, 1996, for a review).

What is it about puberty that might be associated with behavioral change in adolescence? In some circumstances, behavioral conflicts and environmental stressors may hasten pubertal maturation rather than being a consequence of that maturation, with, for instance, greater prepubertal family conflicts predicting earlier puberty (see Steinberg & Belsky, 1996, for a review). Associations of outcome measures with pubertal status are particularly likely to emerge (and appear stronger than associations with chronological age) when sampling across a limited age range in early adolescence, a time when pubertal status varies markedly among individuals (e.g., see Martin et al., 2002). In studies that sample sufficiently across age, pubertal status is typically correlated highly with chronological age (e.g., Booth, Johnson, Granger, Crouter, & McHale, 2003), with both measures perhaps sometimes serving as a proxy for general developmental progression. Yet, puberty per se may contribute to some emerging adolescent behaviors. Puberty is associated with substantial changes in bodily appearance, including the development of secondary sexual characteristics and notable increases in body size. These transformations in appearance may influence adolescents' self-perceptions or the way that others treat them, contributing to the emergence of adolescent-characteristic behaviors.

Puberty is also associated with a multitude of interrelated hormonal changes (see Worthman, 1999, for a review), the so-called "raging hormones" of adolescence often blamed for adolescent peculiarities in behavior and thinking by parents and the mass media. Of particular prominence in these hormonal transitions is the reawakening of the hypothalamus–pituitary–gonadal (HPG) axis. HPG activity is characterized by a cascade of hormone release, beginning with increased release of gonadotrophin releasing hormone (GnRH) in the hypothalamus, which subsequently induces release of follicle stimulating hormone (FSH) and luteinizing hormone (LH) from the pituitary, which in turn precipitates release of gonadal hormones (estrogens in females and testosterone in males; see Worthman, 1999). Levels of these gonadal hormones are high during the pre- and early postnatal period when they exert "organizational" effects on the brain to promote sex-typical differentiation, with levels subsequently suppressed throughout childhood until puberty. Reactivation of the HPG axis at puberty (see Grumbach, 2002) may convey additional long-lasting "organizational" influences on brain structure as well as exerting more contemporaneous "activational" effects on behavioral expression (Arnold & Breedlove, 1985; Romeo, Richardson, & Sisk, 2002). Although humans are unlike many mammalian species in that they do not require gonadal hormones for induction of reproductive behavior, these hormones play a notable role in sexual motivation (Wallen, 2001), and hence their rising titers likely contribute to the emerging interests of adolescents in romance and the opposite sex. Indeed, increased levels of these and other hormones—especially adrenal hormones such as cortisol and dehydroepiandrosterone (DHEA; see Goodyer, Herbert, & Tamplin, 2003)—have been found in some instances to be modestly correlated with sexual activity as well as other behaviors, including aggression and negative affect (see Steinberg & Belsky, 1996, for a review).

Relationships between adolescent behaviors and levels of hormones or pubertal maturation, however, are often surprisingly weak, with only a small part of the variance in behavior generally attributable to gonadal hormone levels or pubertal status. For instance, although one meta-analysis revealed a positive association between testosterone and aggression that emerged most clearly in adolescence, this relationship was weak, at best, and was moderated by age in males (Book, Starzyk, & Quinsey, 2001). When examining contributors to negative affect, gonadal steroids accounted for only about 4% of the variance, in contrast to estimates that 8–18% of the variance is attributable to social context (Brooks-Gunn, Graber, & Paikoff, 1994). The proportion of effects attributable to pubertal maturation per se is often likewise limited, accounting, for instance, for only about 5% of the variance in relationships between adolescents and parents (Steinberg, 1988). In a meta-analysis specifically parsing age and pubertal status contributions to parent–child conflict across adolescence, few changes in such conflict were found to be reliably related to puberty, whereas parent–child conflict was significantly influenced by chronological age, declining from early to mid- and mid- to late adolescence, whereas the negative affect adolescents attributed to that conflict increased from early to mid-adolescence (Laursen et al., 1998).

It is possible that pubertal-associated hormones may exert more of an influence on adolescent behavior than the generally weak associations that have been detected to date would suggest (see Dahl, 2001, 2004). Release of some hormones is variable within or across days (see Worthman, 1999), and the time course between hormonal release and behavioral impact is typically unknown (see Buchanan, Eccles, & Becker, 1992), potentially challenging detection of relationships between hormones and behaviors. Hormonal effects also may be moderated by environmental variables, complicating their detection. For instance, in a study of 6- to 18-year-olds, little direct relationship between testosterone and risk taking was observed, but testosterone-associated risk taking was revealed under circumstances of lower-quality parent–child relationships (Booth et al., 2003). It is also likely that multiple hormones may interact to influence adolescent behavior and affect (Angold, 2003), such that measurement of multiple hormones could reveal associations not evident in studies examining simple linear relationships between hormones and behaviors during adolescence.

NEURAL ALTERATIONS OF ADOLESCENCE

There is increasing recognition that adolescence is associated with considerable reorganization of the brain and that this sculpting of the brain is a likely contributor to adolescent-typical behavioral characteristics. Developmental changes in the brain during adolescence may serve other functions as well. Some of these neural alterations may help to initiate puberty, particularly alterations occurring in hypothalamic regions critical for controlling pituitary release of hormones (e.g., Terasawa & Fernandez, 2001) or in interconnected forebrain regions that may influence those pubertal transformations (e.g., see Moltz, 1975, for an early review). Other brain changes may reflect delayed organizational effects of hormones induced by rising hormone titers at puberty, whereas still other transformations in the adolescent brain are independent of hormonal changes (e.g., Romeo et al., 2002).

Attempting to relate specific neural alterations to behavioral change during ontogeny is often problematic, given the highly interactive nature of the nervous system, with multitudes of input, output, feedback, and modulatory relations that create interconnected functional networks among brain regions. As reviewed below, however, among the brain regions undergoing dramatic transformations during adolescence are mesocortical and mesolimbic regions of the forebrain that form part of the neural circuitry modulating executive functions and affect regulation and that influence the value attributed to motivationally relevant stimuli, including social stimuli, novelty, alcohol, and other drugs. Indeed, given the notable differences between adolescents and adults in functioning in these brain regions, adolescents would be expected to differ from adults in various aspects of their motivated behaviors, as indeed they do. Before illustrating adolescent-related neural alterations in a number of these brain regions, several broader aspects of adolescent brain development are considered.

Synapse Elimination, Metabolic Decline, and Increases in White Matter

Appropriate brain connectivity is determined early in life through the overproduction of synaptic connections among neurons and the elimination of those connections that do not form functional links prior to, or shortly after, birth (e.g., see Rakic, Bourgeois, & Goldman-Rakic, 1994). Synapse elimination is also very prevalent during adolescence, with estimates of loss up to nearly one-half of the average number of synapses per neuron in some cortical regions—a rate of loss calculated to reach the mind-boggling rate of 30,000 synapses terminated per second in the primate cortex during portions of adolescence (Bourgeois, Goldman-Rakic, & Rakic, 1994; Rakic et al., 1994). Substantial synaptic elimination has also been observed in the human neocortex between the ages of 7 and 16 years (Huttenlocher, 1979), although the scarcity of postmortem tissue has not permitted a more detailed description of the time course of this decline. It seems improbable that such delayed synapse elimination would merely reflect belated elimination of synapses that had failed to establish functional connections; it would be highly inefficient to expend the energy to maintain nonfunctional synapses throughout infancy and childhood, postponing their removal until adolescence. Research has shown that synaptic pruning during adolescence is selective, with certain types of synaptic connections particularly vulnerable to pruning. Excitatory (glutaminergic) input is particularly targeted (Rakic et al., 1994), and synaptic pruning is more pronounced in the PFC and other cortical regions than in subcortical areas. Even within the cortex, regional specificity is seen: Synapses connecting different cortical regions (associational circuitry) are pruned less severely than intrinsic circuitry connecting neurons within a cortical region, with these latter connections being particularly critical for expression of reverberating circuits (see Woo, Pucak, Kye, Matus, & Lewis, 1997). Given the apparent specificity of this pruning, it seems likely that the synapse elimination observed in adolescence reflects a fine-tuning of neural connectivity, perhaps to set the stage for a more mature patterning of brain effort and efficiency. Such pruning could also potentially reflect ongoing brain plasticity and a relatively delayed opportunity for the maturing brain to be sculpted by environmental demands during adolescence, a possibility that has yet to be systematically explored. In this regard, it is interesting that work in transgenic mice has shown that the axonal branches of late adolescent mice are extremely dynamic, being frequently retracted or extended on a time scale of minutes, whereas active growth and retraction of axons is rare once full maturity is reached (Gan, Kwon, Feng, Sanes, & Lichtman, 2003).

Synapse elimination in the cortex during adolescence is one of a number of ontogenetic transformations that serve to refine the brain during this time period. There are also prominent developmental increases during adolescence and into adulthood in axon myelination, a process by which membranous extensions of glial cells wrap protective sheaths around axons, speeding information flow along the axons. Because of the high lipid (fat) content of myelin, in unstained brain tissue, myelinated axons collected together in bundles within fiber tracts connecting different brain regions appear white, whereas brain regions with concentrations of neuronal cell bodies appear gray. Thus, with the continued myelination of axons during adolescence, there is an increase in the ratio of white to gray matter (Sowell et al., 1999). In addition to changes in white matter, changes in gray matter are observed in adolescence. Ontogenetic changes in gray matter proportions are regionally specific, with adolescent-typical declines particularly pronounced in frontocortical regions (Rapoport et al., 1999; Sowell et al., 1999), whereas further ontogenetic increases in gray matter volume of the amygdala and hippocampus are seen during adolescence (Giedd, Castellanos, Rajapakse, Vaituzis, & Rapoport, 1997; Yurgelun-Todd, Killgore, & Cintron, 2003; see also Lenroot & Giedd, Chapter 3, this volume).

The reduction in excitatory synaptic input to the cortex, the decline in synaptic connections supporting reverberating cortical circuitry, and the acceleration of information flow provided by myelination of selected axons likely contribute to the refinements in brain effort and efficiency seen during adolescence. There are reports of an ontogenetic decline from childhood into adolescence in the amount of cortical tissue activated during performance on a given task (e.g., Casey, Giedd, & Thomas, 2000) and an increase in the degree to which the left and right hemispheres can process information independently (Merola & Liederman, 1985). Overall brain energy utilization also undergoes a considerable ontogenetic decline, with various indices of the energy needed for brain activity—rates of glucose metabolism, oxygen utilization, and blood flow—at their highest levels early in childhood and waning gradually during adolescence to reach lower, adult-typical levels (e.g., Chugani, 1994).

Cognitive Development and Frontal Brain Regions During Adolescence

Accompanying ontogenetic improvements of cognitive capabilities during adolescence are considerable transformations in forebrain cortical regions, including PFC regions (Casey et al., 2000; Luna et al., 2001; Pine et al., 2002) that are critical for various aspects of "executive functioning" (see Steinberg, 2005) and where (as discussed previously) synaptic pruning is substantial during adolescence. Thus, neural associates of cognitive development may be characterized more by developmental declines in neuronal connectivity than by the formation of new synaptic connections (e.g., see Casey et al, 2000). Whereas this shift might seem counterintuitive at one level, it is not necessarily the case that more synaptic connections are better. Indeed, some forms of mental retardation are characterized by unusually high numbers of synapses (Goldman-Rakic, Isseroff, Schwartz, & Bugbee, 1983).

Studies using functional magnetic resonance imaging (fMRI) have revealed considerable differences during development in which brain areas are activated during particular cognitive tasks. For instance, developmental declines in task-related brain activation in subcortical regions have been reported between adolescence and adulthood, whereas activation of certain specific frontal regions of cortex conversely has been shown to increase (Bunge, Dudukovic, Thomason, Vaidya, & Gabrieli, 2002; Rubia et al., 2000). Differences in regional patterns of brain activation have been evident not only on a task in which performance improved with age (i.e., a delay task) but also on a task in which performance was similar across ages (i.e., a stop task), suggesting that the brains of adolescents and adults may be activated differently even when performing equivalently on a given task (Rubia et al., 2000). A similar conclusion was reached in a study using electrophysiological measures that found that different neural mechanisms were activated in children and adults even though both groups performed equivalently on the sustained attention task; this study also provided evidence for continued maturation of prefrontal regions through late adolescence (Segalowitz & Davies, 2004). Studies using fMRI have also revealed ontogenetic increases in activation of the PFC during performance of a variety of working memory and response inhibition tasks during adolescence (see Paus, 2005, for a review), with adolescents sometimes showing greater PFC activation than both children and adults during task performance (Luna et al., 2001).

Although there has been substantial focus on maturational changes in prefrontal regions and cognitive development, it is clear that multiple regions throughout the brain are associated with improvements in cognitive performance during adolescence, even within realms associated with executive function (e.g., working memory, inhibitory control, or emotional regulation; Luna et al., 2001). To give but one example, consider a region located distally from the forebrain: the cerebellum. Although the functions of the cerebellum had long been thought to be limited largely to control of motor movements, evidence has emerged for cerebellar involvement in cognitive function (Kim, Ugurbil, & Strick, 1994) and for developmental changes in this region during adolescence. Anatomical studies have shown neural connections linking the cerebellum and prefrontal cortex (Middleton & Strick, 2000, 2001), with lesions of the cerebellum inducing impairments in executive functioning and affect regulation in adult humans that are reminiscent of those seen following prefrontal damage (Schmahmann & Sherman, 1998). Such deficits, however, are less evident following cerebellar damage in childhood, with signs of affective and cognitive disruptions emerging more reliably in older than younger individuals with brain damage across the age span from 3 to 16 years (Levisohn, Cronin-Golomb, & Schmahmann, 2000). Consistent with the notion that developmental increases in cerebellar activity may subserve a cognitive role, fMRI studies have shown developmental increases in cerebellar activation through adolescence and into adulthood during performance of an inhibitory task (Luna et al., 2001) and a memory-guided spatial navigation task (Pine et al., 2002). Although activation of a brain region during task performance does not necessarily imply that it is required for task performance (e.g., see Zald, 2003), these data nevertheless support the conclusion that developmental changes in the cerebellum contribute to maturational changes in cognition during adolescence. Evidence for developmental changes in activation of a variety of brain regions during performance of cognitive tasks has led to the suggestion that age-related improvements in cognitive performance through adolescence are associated with changes in widely distributed brain areas that are interconnected within functional networks (see Luna et al., 2001; Pine et al., 2002).

Emotional Regulation, the Adolescent Amygdala, and Other Forebrain Regions

As discussed previously, logical decision making by adolescents sometimes may be less than optimal due to immaturity in the ability of adolescents to regulate their affect under emotional or arousing circumstances (e.g., Dahl, 2004). Although a number of brain regions have been implicated in affect regulation, relating immaturity in emotional regulation to adolescent-typical brain characteristics remains an ongoing and intriguing challenge.

Affect regulation is thought to involve networks of neural regions that include portions of the prefrontal cortex along with a prominent group of subcortical nuclei collectively termed the amygdala. Nuclei of the amygdala are thought to play critical roles not only in the processing of emotional stimuli and attributing affect to those stimuli (Baxter & Murray, 2002; Bechara, Damasio, Damasio & Lee, 1999), but also in establishing reward expectancies (Holland & Gallagher, 2004), mounting defensive responses (Deakin & Graeff, 1991), and modulating social behavior (Amaral et al., 2003). The amygdala has anatomical connections with orbitofrontal and ventromedial portions of the PFC (e.g., see Happaney, Zelazo, & Stuss, 2004, for a review), and these regions appear to be functionally coupled as well. The orbitofrontal cortex and amygdala are both activated when processing emotional (e.g., aversive) stimuli, whereas activity in each region may be uncoupled under other circumstances (Zald, Donndelinger, & Pardo, 1998). Although the exact functions attributed to specific components of the PFC are still a matter of discussion (e.g., contrast Schaefer et al., 2003; Segalowitz & Davies, 2004; with Hooper et al., 2004; Steinberg, 2005) and are likely to overlap under some conditions, orbitofrontal and ventromedial regions are thought to be more critical for emotional regulation than dorsolateral PFC (DLPFC; Bechara, Damasio, & Damasio, 2000). In addition to evidence for substantial maturation in PFC regions during adolescence, as discussed above, there is some evidence suggesting differential maturational rates among PFC regions. For instance, based on age-related differences in performance on several different types of executive function tasks, Hooper and colleagues (2004) concluded that the ventromedial PFC undergoes protracted development throughout adolescence and into adulthood that is at least, if not more, prolonged than that observed for DLPFC. From his review of imaging, anatomical, and neuropsychological studies, Dahl (2001) conversely suggested that ventral portions of the PFC may mature earlier in adolescence than the DLPFC. Thus, although development of prefrontal regions has been suggested to contribute to improvement in affect regulation during adolescence, additional research is needed to identify the nature and characteristics of the ontogenetic differences in maturational rates across prefrontal regions.

Although limited to date, studies conducted in both laboratory animals and humans have also yielded hints of notable ontogenetic changes in the amygdala during adolescence. A study in human adolescents using volumetric MRI observed an increase in amygdala volume with age during adolescence, with greater amygdala volumes associated with better performance on a number of cognitive tasks (Yurgelun-Todd et al., 2003). In work using a rodent model, excitatory (glutaminergic) input from the basolateral nucleus of the amygdala to the prefrontal cortex was observed to continue to be elaborated throughout adolescence (Cunningham, Bhattacharyya, & Benes, 2002). The adolescent amygdala of rodents was also found to be more sensitive to seizures induced by electrical stimulation than that of younger or older animals (Terasawa & Timiras, 1968) and to exhibit less stress-induced activation of immediate early genes (indexed via c-fos expression) than seen in mature animals (Kellogg, Awatramani, & Piekut, 1998). Moreover, it has long been known from animal studies that the amygdala is unusual among forebrain regions in that damage to this region markedly alters the timing of puberty, with some studies reporting that amygdalar lesions produce precocial puberty, whereas others have found a considerable lesion-induced pubertal delay (see Moltz, 1975). The converse nature of these findings is likely related in part to differences in the specific amygdalar regions damaged across studies, given that the amygdala consists of numerous discrete nuclei with diverse and sometimes opposing functional effects (Swanson & Petrovich, 1998).

Recent human imaging studies have revealed evidence for differential amygdalar activation in response to emotional stimuli in human adolescents, relative to their more mature counterparts, although again the ontogenetic nature of those developmental changes has been found to vary across studies. Killgore and colleagues reported that in female adolescents (but not their male counterparts), amount of activation of the left amygdala induced by viewing faces expressing fearful affect decreased during adolescence, whereas activation of the left dorsolateral PFC in response to these stimuli increased during this period (Killgore, Oki, & Yurgelun-Todd, 2001). These data were interpreted to support a developmental model for progressively greater cortical control of emotional behavior during adolescence, with the continued emergence of PFC modulation of emotional processing occurring in the amygdala. In contrast, Thomas and colleagues (2001) reported that adults exhibited more left-amygdalar activation in response to emotional (fearful) faces than children, whereas children conversely showed greater activation of this region in response to neutral than fearful faces—data interpreted to suggest an ontogenetic increase in left-amygdalar activation by emotional stimuli during adolescence. In other studies, adolescents have been found to be similar to adults in the extent of amygdalar activation elicited by fearful faces (Pine et al., 2001), with males, in particular, showing similar patterns of brain activation across the adolescent-to-adult age span but females showing greater discrimination of unambiguous versus ambiguous threat cues as they matured into adulthood (McClure et al., 2004). Lateralization of activation has also been reported to change ontogenetically, with amygdalar activation to fearful faces reported to be bilateral in children and adults but right-lateralized in adolescents (Killgore & Yurgelun-Todd, 2004). Among the factors that could contribute to these widely differing findings across (and even within) laboratories is the rapid habituation to stimuli often seen in the amygdala, making the timing of assessment critical for the outcomes observed. Current fMRI techniques also lack the spatial resolution to localize the focus of activation to specific amygdalar nuclei (see Zald, 2003, for a review and discussion), an issue that is particularly problematic given that different nuclei have separable—and sometimes even opposing—functional effects (e.g., Swanson & Petrovich, 1998). With the higher spatial resolution provided by scanners with higher field strengths, at some future point it may become possible to discriminate specific nuclei of the amygdalar complex, an advance likely to prove crucial for resolving current inconsistencies in this intriguingly complex literature.

Risk Taking, Sensation Seeking, and Drugs: Dopamine Mesocorticolimbic Circuitry

Among the neural systems that undergo marked remodeling during adolescence are dopamine (DA) systems projecting to cortical (e.g., PFC), limbic (e.g., nucleus accumbens, amygdala), and striatal regions of the forebrain. These projection systems that release DA as a neurotransmitter, along with their forebrain targets and receptors, are thought to be critical for directing behavior toward rewarding stimuli and processing stimuli related to rewards that include drugs of abuse as well as natural rewards (e.g., social stimuli, novelty, food), although the precise nature of the relationship between DA activity in these networks and reward remains controversial (e.g., Di Chiara, 1999; Ikemoto & Panksepp, 1999). Given the marked developmental changes seen in these DA forebrain projection systems during adolescence, it would be surprising, indeed, if adolescents did not differ from both younger and more mature individuals in reward-related behaviors. And as previously discussed, they certainly do, with adolescents differing from adults along a number of dimensions, including sensation seeking, drug-taking propensity, and peer-directed social affiliations. When reviewing data in this area, it should be noted that studies examining the ontogeny of DA forebrain projection systems during adolescence have been conducted, by necessity, largely in laboratory animals, and hence caution is necessary when considering the potential implications of these findings for human adolescents.

Developmental changes are seen in DA mesocortical projections, with DA projections to the PFC continuing to be elaborated throughout adolescence (Benes, Taylor, & Cunningham, 2000), as well as in DA subcortical (mesolimbic and striatal) regions, where dramatic declines in the number of DA receptors are observed during adolescence. For instance, a loss of one-third to one-half or more of the D1 and D2 subtypes of the DA receptor are seen in striatum during adolescence, findings reported both in studies using animal models and human autopsy material (Seeman et al., 1987; Tarazi & Baldessarini, 2000; Teicher, Andersen, & Hostetter, 1995). Although the data are mixed, developmental overproduction and subsequent pruning of D1, D2, and D4 receptors has been observed in the nucleus accumbens as well, with levels of these receptors reported to be about one-third higher in early adolescence than in young adulthood (Tarazi & Baldessarini, 2000; Tarazi, Tomasini, & Baldessarini, 1998, 1999; but see also Teicher et al., 1995). In contrast to the early adolescent peak and subsequent decline in DA receptors in these subcortical regions, D1 and D2 receptor pruning is relatively delayed in PFC, with ontogenetic increases reported into early adulthood (Tarazi & Baldessarini, 2000) and ontogenetic declines observed thereafter (Andersen, Thompson, Rutstein, Hostetter, & Teicher, 2000).

Subcortical and mesocortical DA terminal regions also exhibit different ontogenetic patterns in terms of relative rates of DA synthesis and turnover. Early in adolescence, estimates of DA synthesis and turnover in mesolimbic (nucleus accumbens) and striatal regions are lower than later in adolescence (Andersen, Dumont, & Teicher, 1997; Teicher et al., 1993), whereas DA synthesis and turnover estimates in PFC are conversely higher earlier than later in adolescence (Andersen et al., 1997; Boyce, 1996; although, see also Leslie, Robertson, Cutler, & Bennett, 1991). These converse ontogenetic patterns of DA turnover rates in PFC versus mesolimbic and striatal regions are consistent with the reciprocal relationship that often characterizes relative levels of DA activity between these terminal regions in adult animals (Deutch, 1992; Wilkinson, 1997). Together these ontogenetic findings have led to the suggestion that there is a developmental shift in the balance between these regions during adolescence (Andersen, 2003; Spear, 2000), with mesocortical DA influences peaking early in adolescence, followed later by a shift toward greater mesolimbic and striatal DA activity (see Spear, 2000, for a review). Given the greater sensitivity of mesocortical than mesolimbic and striatal DA projections to activation by stressors (e.g., Dunn, 1988), any shift in balance toward greater mesocortical (and lower mesolimbic and striatal) DA predominance early in adolescence would be expected to be exacerbated further by stressors.

A stress-exacerbated ontogenetic shift in DA balance that results in a transient lowering of DA function in mesolimbic brain regions early in adolescence may be of considerable functional significance. Functional insufficiencies in mesolimbic DA reward pathways have been linked to a "reward deficiency syndrome" (Gardner, 1999), with marked hypo-DA states, for instance, postulated to be characteristic of drug addiction (see Volkow et al., 2002). To the extent that mesolimbic DA activity is transiently attenuated during early adolescence, youth may exhibit signs of a partial "reward deficiency syndrome," and as a result may seek out drugs, environmental risks, and novelty in an attempt to behaviorally remediate this reward deficiency (see earlier discussion and Spear, 2000). It should be noted, however, that there are other hypotheses regarding the relationship between mesolimbic DA activity and reward-related processes that conversely predict a positive relationship between mesolimbic DA activity and drug seeking (see Spanagel & Weiss, 1999, for a review), emphasizing the complexity of the relationship between DA activity and reward.

SUMMARY AND FURTHER REFLECTIONS

Adolescents clearly behave the way that they do for a diversity of reasons. Based on rapidly accumulating knowledge of adolescent brain development, one important contributor to adolescent-related behavioral proclivities appears to be the sculpting that is ongoing in their brains. By framing the discussion of adolescence from an evolutionary perspective, this chapter has considered that some adolescent-typical behavioral characteristics and their neural underpinnings may reflect remnants of an evolutionary past, a past in which expression of behaviors that facilitated emigration of sexually maturing adolescents away from the home area may have served an adaptive function to avoid inbreeding. Thus, antecedents of adolescent behaviors may reflect a myriad of sources with distinct functions, some enduring from childhood, others reflecting, in part, remnants of the evolutionary past, some helping the adolescent cope with the immediate demands of this developmental transition, and still others preparing the adolescent for incorporation of adult roles.

During the adolescent sculpting of the brain, the energy-inefficient brain of the child is eventually converted into the leaner, more rapidly communicative and energy-efficient brain of the adult. At the same time that the brain of the developmental past is being massively pruned and sculpted into a brain suitable to meet future demands, the brain of the adolescent must also multitask to support critical adolescent behaviors and facilitate attainment of puberty and other physiological transformations of this age period. Based on the brain regions undergoing marked restructuring during adolescence and the critical roles that these brain regions play in modulating various cognitive and behavioral functions, including executive functioning, affect modulation, social behaviors, and risk taking, it is not surprising that adolescents differ from individuals in other age groups in the expression of these types of cognitive and behavioral functions.

The emerging neuroscience of adolescence may have a number of implications for educators of adolescents. Under even the best of circumstances, the adolescent brain is subject to serious multitasking. Not only are thousands of synaptic connections being lost per second during portions of adolescence, but also childhood activities are being inhibited and adult-typical activities sometimes emulated, along with an increasing focus on social concerns and activities and other rising issues of importance for the adolescent—all of which can provide significant competition for classroom engagement. Individual differences are of particular significance when educating adolescents, with pubertal status adding a notable complicating factor. In a given adolescent group, one may find individuals who have gone through puberty early and hence who are at a different phase of emotional and cognitive interests than others in the group, who will enter puberty later. Sex differences in interests and cognitive style become particularly pronounced postpubertally, with the implications of early versus late pubertal status being notably different for boys and girls. When attempting to engage adolescents in the classroom, individualized strategies based on level of cognitive and emotional development may be of particular value.

The timing of education is also important. There is clear evidence for a phase shift during adolescence, with adolescents going to bed later and rising later than children. This phase shift is largely biological, with adolescents typically unable to fall asleep at earlier times. For the most part, school systems have not considered this adolescent phase shift, with many systems traditionally having earlier (rather than later) start dates for high school than grade school students. By recognizing the shift in biological rhythms during adolescence and delaying high school start times accordingly, classroom experiences can be matched to the times when adolescents are most alert and attentive.

Research has shown that adolescents often demonstrate excellent decision-making abilities under controlled classroom situations (so-called "cold cognitions"), whereas decisions reached outside the classroom may be less than optimal, particularly under circumstances that are relatively emotional and arousing (i.e., "hot cognitions"). To encourage emergence of good decision making in these higher-affect situations, other strategies are needed. One approach may be to support education conducted under "cold cognition" conditions with training involving role playing or other procedures designed to emulate the greater affective load under which "hot cognitions" are typically made. Development of educational efforts that are effective under these circumstances is important, given that poor decision making under stimulating or emotional circumstances is particularly problematic for adolescents.

Indeed, adolescent-typical behavioral proclivities can sometimes be costly for the adolescent and for those around him or her. Despite the robust health typical of adolescence, death rates soar at this age largely because of misfortunes associated with elevated risk-taking behaviors (e.g., Muuss & Porton, 1998), including use of alcohol and other drugs that may further increase the incidence of risky behaviors (e.g., see Windle & Windle, 2005). To the extent that the motivation for risk taking in adolescence is strong with deep evolutionary roots, attempts to reduce adolescent risk taking by education alone likely would be of limited success, a lack of efficacy supported by the evidence gathered to date (see Steinberg, 2005, for a review). Rather than attempting to limit risk-taking behaviors of adolescents completely, a more effective strategy might be to channel risk taking towards less hazardous activities (e.g., wall climbing, white-water rafting, snowboarding) or circumstances (e.g., skateboard parks, climbing walls, supervised wilderness adventures).

Adolescence may be a vulnerable period not only because of the high prevalence of risk taking, but also because of the potential lasting consequences of perturbations to the brain as it is sculpted during this time. For instance, brain regions undergoing particularly marked remodeling during adolescence (e.g., PFC, amygdala, nucleus accumbens) are among those that are most sensitive to alcohol and other drugs of abuse. This fact raises the possibility that exposure to alcohol or other drugs during adolescence may alter ongoing processes of adolescent brain development, with a long-term impact on neurobehavioral function in adulthood. Data providing support for this possibility are beginning to emerge. Young adults who began drinking heavily in adolescence have been found to exhibit cognitive deficits along with significantly altered brain responses during task perfor-

mance (e.g., Tapert & Schweinsburg, 2005). Moreover, the earlier the initiation of alcohol use, the greater the likelihood of later alcohol abuse and
dependence, with lifetime prevalence rates of alcohol dependence at 40%
when individuals begin drinking before 14 years of age, but only 10%
when drinking is delayed until 20 years of age or later (Grant & Dawson,
1997). It is not necessarily the case, however, that early alcohol use is
causal in these situations. It is possible that some neurocognitive deficits
may precede initiation of alcohol use and may serve as risk factors for early
and prolonged use of alcohol, whereas other deficits may be a consequence
of that use (Hill, 2004). Prospective studies should help distinguish between
these possibilities. Meanwhile, studies using a variety of animal models
have begun to provide some evidence that adolescent exposure to alcohol
and other drugs may exert long-term alterations that are often more robust
than those observed with comparable exposure in adulthood (see Smith,
2003, for a review). For instance, adolescent rats exposed to high doses of
alcohol mimicking "binge" alcohol use were found to exhibit more brain
damage in a number of frontal regions than comparison adult rats (Crews,
Braun, Hoplight, Switzer, & Knapp, 2000). In studies using animals genetically bred for high alcohol use, adolescent alcohol exposure increased alcohol self-administration in adulthood as well as increasing craving and the
potential for relapse (McBride, Bell, Rodd, Strother, & Murphy, 2005).

The sculpting of adolescent brain may not only impart age-specific vulnerabilities, but also potentially may provide unique age-specific opportunities. That is, to the extent that the brain is unusually vulnerable to pertur-
bation during adolescence, it seems feasible that some kinds of adolescent
experiences might exert lasting positive consequences. Although this exciting possibility has been little explored, data from studies of environmental
enrichment in laboratory animals provide hints of particularly beneficial
effects from some experiences during adolescence. In these studies, enrichment of the environment was associated with a variety of positive effects on
brain structure and function, with the most dramatic effects noted when
the enrichment period included adolescence. Environmental enrichment is
typically accomplished in studies using a rodent model by rearing animals
in groups in a large cage containing a daily changing variety of different
toys, ladders, platforms, and textures. Neurobehavioral function of animals
in this enriched condition (EC) is then compared with control groups consisting of animals placed in cages without objects and reared either in social
groups (social condition: SC) or alone (isolate condition: IC). Relative to IC
control animals, animals reared in the EC environment through adolescence exhibited an increase in cortical size, along with an approximate
20% increase in number of synapses per neuron in cortical regions, with
data from SC animals generally intermediate between enriched and isolated

animals (see Greenough & Chang, 1988, for a review). Animals raised in enriched environments also exhibited an increase in number of blood capillaries innervating cortical regions, an increase that exceeded the extra demand associated with the increased numbers of synapses (e.g., Greenough & Black, 1992). Although qualitatively similar effects have been observed following comparable lengths of enrichment in mature animals, the magnitude of enrichment effects in adulthood are less than that associated with enrichment periods that subsume adolescence (e.g., see Greenough & Black, 1992; Greenough & Chang, 1988). Whether the enrichment-associated increase in number of synapses reflects retention of synapses that would ordinarily be eliminated during adolescence or the production of new synapses has yet to be determined, and may vary with the timing, type, or magnitude of the environmental experience (see Greenough & Black, 1992).

It is important to note that these enrichment effects are characterized not only by neuroanatomical alterations, but also by functional consequences, with animals that received environmental enrichment during adolescence learning complex tasks (e.g., mazes) more quickly (e.g., Gardner, Boitano, Mancino, & D'Amico, 1975), responding to novelty more adaptively (e.g., Zimmermann, Stauffacher, Langhans, & Wurbel, 2001), being less prone to self-administer amphetamine (Green, Gehrke, & Bardo, 2002), and showing more recovery following prenatal drug exposure (Rema & Ebner, 1999) than control animals raised in nonenriched environments. It remains to be determined how relevant these findings obtained in laboratory animals are in terms of potential beneficial effects of environmental enrichment in human adolescents. It would be exciting indeed if the normal ontogenetic sculpting of the brain during adolescence provides a unique window of opportunity through which enrichment and educational efforts may confer ameliorative or protective influences on the maturing adolescent.

ACKNOWLEDGMENTS

Preparation of this chapter was supported by Grant Nos. R37 AA12525 and R01 DA019071.

REFERENCES

Alfoldi, P., Tobler, I., & Borbely, A. A. (1990). Sleep regulation in rats during early development. *American Journal of Physiology, 258*, R634–R644.
Amaral, D. G., Capitanio, J. P., Jourdain, M., Mason, W. A., Mendoza, S. P., &

Prather, M. (2003). The amygdala: Is it an essential component of the neural network for social cognition? *Neuropsychologia, 41*(2), 235–240.

Andersen, S. L. (2003). Trajectories of brain development: Point of vulnerability or window of opportunity? *Neuroscience and Biobehavioral Reviews, 27*(1–2), 3–18.

Andersen, S. L., Dumont, N. L., & Teicher, M. H. (1997). Developmental differences in dopamine synthesis inhibition by (+/–)-7-OH-DPAT. *Naunyn–Schmiedeberg's Archives of Pharmacology, 356*(2), 173–181.

Andersen, S. L., Thompson, A. T., Rutstein, M., Hostetter, J. C., & Teicher, M. H. (2000). Dopamine receptor pruning in prefrontal cortex during the periadolescent period in rats. *Synapse, 37*(2), 167–169.

Angold, A. (2003). Adolescent depression, cortisol and DHEA—editorial. *Psychological Medicine, 33*(4), 573–581.

Arnett, J. (1992). Reckless behavior in adolescence: A developmental perspective. *Developmental Review, 12,* 339–373.

Arnold, A. P., & Breedlove, S. M. (1985). Organizational and activational effects of sex steroids on brain and behavior: A reanalysis. *Hormones and Behavior, 19*(4), 469–498.

Bates, M. E., & Labouvie, E. W. (1997). Adolescent risk factors and the prediction of persistent alcohol and drug use into adulthood. *Alcoholism: Clinical and Experimental Research, 21*(5), 944–950.

Baxter, M. G., & Murray, E. A. (2002). The amygdala and reward. *Nature Reviews Neuroscience, 3*(7), 563–573.

Bechara, A., Damasio, H., & Damasio, A. R. (2000). Emotion, decision making and the orbitofrontal cortex. *Cerebral Cortex, 10*(3), 295–307.

Bechara, A., Damasio, H., Damasio, A. R., & Lee, G. P. (1999). Different contributions of the human amygdala and ventromedial prefrontal cortex to decision-making. *Journal of Neuroscience, 19*(13), 5473–5481.

Behar, D., Berg, C. J., Rapoport, J. L., Nelson, W., Linnoila, M., Cohen, M., et al. (1983). Behavioral and physiological effects of ethanol in high-risk and control children: A pilot study. *Alcoholism: Clinical and Experimental Research, 7*(4), 404–410.

Benes, F. M., Taylor, J. B., & Cunningham, M. C. (2000). Convergence and plasticity of monaminergic systems in the medial prefrontal cortex during the postnatal period: Implications for the development of psychopathology. *Cerebral Cortex, 10*(10), 1014–1027.

Bixler, R. H. (1992). Why littermates don't: The avoidance of inbreeding depression. *Annual Review of Sex Research, 3,* 291–328.

Book, A. S., Starzyk, K. B., & Quinsey, V. L. (2001). The relationship between testosterone and aggression: A meta-analysis. *Aggression and Violent Behavior, 6*(6), 579–599.

Booth, A., Johnson, D. R., Granger, D. A., Crouter, A. C., & McHale, S. (2003). Testosterone and child and adolescent adjustment: The moderating role of parent–child relationships. *Developmental Psychology, 39*(1), 85–98.

Bourgeois, J. P., Goldman-Rakic, P. S., & Rakic, P. (1994). Synaptogenesis in the prefrontal cortex of rhesus monkeys. *Cerebral Cortex, 4*(1), 78–96.

Boyce, W. T. (1996). Biobehavioral reactivity and injuries in children and adolescents. In M. H. Bornstein & J. L. Genevro (Eds.), *Child development and behavioral pediatrics* (pp. 35–58). Mahwah, NJ: Erlbaum.

Brooks-Gunn, J., Graber, J. A., & Paikoff, R. L. (1994). Studying links between hormones and negative affect: Models and measures. *Journal of Research on Adolescence, 4*, 469–486.

Brown, S. A. (1993). Recovery patterns in adolescent substance abuse. In J. S. Baer, G. A. Marlatt, & R. J. McMahon (Eds.), *Addictive behaviors across the life span: Prevention, treatment, and policy issues* (pp. 161–183). Newbury Park, CA: Sage.

Buchanan, C. M., Eccles, J. S., & Becker, J. B. (1992). Are adolescents the victims of raging hormones?: Evidence for activational effects of hormones on moods and behavior at adolescence. *Psychological Bulletin, 111*(1), 62–107.

Bunge, S. A., Dudukovic, N. M., Thomason, M. E., Vaidya, C. J., & Gabrieli, J. D. E. (2002). Immature frontal lobe contributions to cognitive control in children: Evidence from fMRI. *Neuron, 33*, 301–311.

Caine, N. G. (1986). Behavior during puberty and adolescence. In G. Mitchell & J. Erwin (Eds.), *Comparative primate biology: Vol. 2A. Behavior, conservation, and ecology* (pp. 327–361). New York: Liss.

Carskadon, M. A., Vieira, C., & Acebo, C. (1993). Association between puberty and delayed phase preference. *Sleep, 16*(3), 258–262.

Carskadon, M. A., Wolfson, A. R., Acebo, C., Tzischinsky, O., & Seifer, R. (1998). Adolescent sleep patterns, circadian timing, and sleepiness at a transition to early school days. *Sleep, 21*(8), 871–881.

Casey, B. J., Giedd, J. N., & Thomas, K. M. (2000). Structural and functional brain development and its relation to cognitive development. *Biological Psychology, 54*, 241–257.

Chambers, R. A., Taylor, J. R., & Potenza, M. N. (2003). Developmental neurocircuitry of motivation in adolescence: A critical period of addiction vulnerability. *American Journal of Psychiatry, 160*, 1041–1052.

Chugani, H. T. (1994). Development of regional brain glucose metabolism in relation to behavior and plasticity. In G. Dawson & K. W. Fischer (Eds.), *Human behavior and the developing brain* (pp. 153–175). New York: Guilford Press.

Clark, D. B., Kirisci, L., & Tarter, R. E. (1998). Adolescent versus adult onset and the development of substance use disorders in males. *Drug and Alcohol Dependence, 49*, 115–121.

Crews, F. T., Braunm, C. J., Hoplight, B., Switzer, R. C., & Knapp, D. J. (2000). Binge ethanol consumption causes differential brain damage in young adolescent rats compared with adult rats. *Alcoholism: Clinical and Experimental Research, 24*, 1712–1723.

Crockett, C. M., & Pope, T. R. (1993). Consequences of sex differences in dispersal for juvenile red howler monkeys. In M. E. Pereira & L. A. Fairbanks (Eds.), *Juvenile primates* (pp. 104–118, 367–415). New York: Oxford University Press.

Crone, E. A., & van der Molen, M. W. (2004). Developmental changes in real life decision making: Performance on a gambling task previously shown to depend on the ventromedial prefrontal cortex. *Developmental Neuropsychology, 25*(3), 251–279.

Csikszentmihalyi, M., & Larson, R. (1978). Intrinsic rewards in school crime. *Crime and Delinquency, 24,* 322–335.

Csikszentmihalyi, M., Larson, R., & Prescott, S. (1977). The ecology of adolescent activity and experience. *Journal of Youth and Adolescence, 6,* 281–294.

Cunningham, M. G., Bhattacharyya, S., & Benes, F. M. (2002). Amygdalo-cortical sprouting continues into early adulthood: Implications for the development of normal and abnormal function during adolescence. *Journal of Comparative Neurology, 453*(2), 116–130.

Dahl, R. E. (1996). The regulation of sleep and arousal: Development and psychopathology. *Development and Psychopathology, 8,* 3–27.

Dahl, R. E. (2001). Affect regulation, brain development, and behavioral/emotional health in adolescence. *CNS Spectrums, 6*(1), 60–72.

Dahl, R. E. (2004). Adolescent brain development: A period of vulnerabilities and opportunities. *Annals of the New York Academy of Sciences, 1021,* 1–23.

Dahl, R. E., & Ryan, N. D. (1996). The psychobiology of adolescent depression. In D. Cicchetti & S. L. Toth (Eds.), *Rochester symposium on developmental psychopathology, adolescence: Opportunities and challenges* (Vol. 7, pp. 197–232). Rochester, NY: University of Rochester Press.

Deakin, J. F. W., & Graeff, F. G. (1991). Critique: 5-HT and mechanisms of defense. *Journal of Psychopharmacology, 5*(4), 305–315.

Deutch, A. Y. (1992). The regulation of subcortical dopamine systems by the prefrontal cortex: Interactions of central dopamine systems and the pathogenesis of schizophrenia. *Journal of Neural Transmission, 36,* 61–89.

Dexter, D., Bijwadia, J., Schilling, D., & Applebaugh, G. (2003). Sleep, sleepiness and school start times: A preliminary study. *Wisconsin Medical Journal, 102*(1), 44–46.

Di Chiara, G. (1999). Drug addiction as dopamine-dependent associative learning disorder. *European Journal of Pharmacology, 375,* 13–30.

Doremus, T. L., Brunell, S. C., Pottayil, R., & Spear, L. P. (2005). Factors influencing elevated ethanol consumption in adolescent relative adult rats. *Alcoholism: Clinical and Experimental Research, 29,* 1796–1808.

Douglas, L. A., Varlinskaya, E. I., & Spear, L. P. (2003). Novel object place conditioning in adolescent and adult male and female rats: Effects of social isolation. *Physiology and Behavior, 80,* 317–325.

Douglas, L. A., Varlinskaya, E. I., & Spear, L. P. (2004). Rewarding properties of social interactions in adolescent and adult male and female rats: Impact of social vs. isolate housing of subjects and partners. *Developmental Psychobiology, 45,* 153–162.

Dubas, J. S. (1991). Cognitive abilities and physical maturation. In R. M. Lerner, A. C. Petersen, & J. Brooks-Gunn (Eds.), *Encyclopedia of adolescence* (Vol. 1, pp. 133–138). New York: Garland.

Dunn, A. J. (1988). Stress-related activation of cerebral dopaminergic systems. *Annals of the New York Academy of Sciences, 537,* 188–205.

Eliasson, A., King, J., Gould, B., & Eliasson, A. (2002). Association of sleep and academic performance. *Sleep and Breathing, 6*(1), 45–48.

Enright, R. D., Levy, V. M., Jr., Harris, D., & Lapsley, D. K. (1987). Do economic conditions influence how theorists view adolescents? *Journal of Youth and Adolescence, 16,* 541–559.

Eriksson, P. S., Perfilieva, E., Bjork-Eriksson, T., Alborn, A.-M., Nordborg, C., Peterson, D. A., et al. (1998). Neurogenesis in the adult human hippocampus. *Nature Medicine, 4*(11), 1313–1317.

Frisch, R. E. (1984). Body fat, puberty and fertility. *Biological Reviews of the Cambridge Philosophical Society, 59*(2), 161–188.

Gan, W. -B., Kwon, E., Feng, G., Sanes, J. R., & Lichtman, J. W. (2003). Synaptic dynamism measured over minutes to months: Age-dependent decline in an autonomic ganglion. *Nature Neuroscience, 6*(9), 956–960.

Ganji, V., & Betts, N. (1995). Fat, cholesterol, fiber and sodium intakes of US population: Evaluation of diets reported in 1987–88 Nationwide Food Consumption Survey. *European Journal of Clinical Nutrition, 49,* 915–920.

Gardner, E. B., Boitano, J. J., Mancino, N. S., & D'Amico, D. P. (1975). Environmental enrichment and deprivation: Effects on learning, memory and exploration. *Physiology and Behavior, 14,* 321–327.

Gardner, E. L. (1999). The neurobiology and genetics of addiction: Implications of the reward deficiency syndrome for therapeutic strategies in chemical dependency. In J. Elster (Ed.), *Addiction: Entries and exits* (pp. 57–119). New York: Sage.

Giedd, J. N., Castellanos, F. X., Rajapakse, J. C., Vaituzis, A. C., & Rapoport, J. L. (1997). Sexual dimorphism of the developing human brain. *Progress in NeuroPsychopharmacology and Biological Psychiatry, 21,* 1185–1201.

Goldman-Rakic, P. S., Isseroff, A., Schwartz, M. L., & Bugbee, N. M. (1983). The neurobiology of cognitive development. In P. H. Mussen (Ed.), *Infancy and developmental psychobiology* (Vol. 2, pp. 281–344). New York: Wiley.

Goodyer, I. M., Herbert, J., & Tamplin, A. (2003). Psychoendocrine antecedents of persistent first-episode major depression in adolescents: A community-based longitudinal enquiry. *Psychological Medicine, 33*(4), 601–610.

Graber, J. A., & Petersen, A. C. (1991). Cognitive changes in adolescence: Biological perspectives. In K. R. Gibson & A. C. Petersen (Eds.), *Brain maturation and cognitive development: Comparative and cross-cultural perspectives* (pp. 253–279). New York: Aldine de Gruyter.

Grant, B. F., & Dawson, D. A. (1997). Age at onset of alcohol use and its association with DSM-IV alcohol abuse and dependence: Results from the National Longitudinal Alcohol Epidemiologic Survey. *Journal of Substance Abuse, 9,* 103–110.

Green, T. A., Gehrke, B. J., & Bardo, M. T. (2002). Environmental enrichment decreases intravenous amphetamine self-administration in rats: Dose–response functions for fixed- and progressive-ratio schedules. *Psychopharmacology, 162,* 373–378.

Greenough, W. T., & Black, J. E. (1992). Induction of brain structure by experience: Substrates for cognitive development. In M. R. Gunnar & C. A. Nelson

(Eds.), *Developmental behavioral neuroscience: The Minnesota symposium on child psychology* (Vol. 24, pp. 155–200). Hillsdale, NJ: Erlbaum.

Greenough, W. T., & Chang, F.-L. F. (1988). Plasticity of synapse structure and pattern in the cerebral cortex. In A. Peters & E. G. Jones (Eds.), *Cerebral cortex: Development and maturation of the cerebral cortex* (pp. 391–440). New York: Plenum Press.

Grumbach, M. M. (2002). The neuroendocrinology of human puberty revisited. *Hormone Research*, 57(Suppl. 2), 2–14.

Hansen, M., Janssen, I., Schiff, A., Zee, P. C., & Dubocovich, M. L. (2005). The impact of school daily schedule on adolescent sleep. *Pediatrics*, 115(6), 1555–1561.

Happaney, K., Zelazo, P. D., & Stuss, D. T. (2004). Development of orbitofrontal function: Current themes and future directions. *Brain and Cognition*, 55(1), 1–10.

Harrell, J. S., Bangdiwala, S. I., Deng, S., Webb, J. P., & Bradley, C. (1998). Smoking initiation in youth. *Journal of Adolescent Health*, 23, 271–279.

Hill, S. Y. (2004). Trajectories of alcohol use and electrophysiological and morphological indices of brain development: Distinguishing causes from consequences. *Annals of the New York Academy of Sciences*, 1021, 245–259.

Holland, P. C., & Gallagher, M. (2004). Amygdala–frontal interactions and reward expectancy. *Neurobiology*, 14, 148–155.

Hooper, C. J., Luciana, M., Conklin, H. M., & Yarger, R. S. (2004). Adolescents' performance on the Iowa gambling task: Implications for the development of decision making and ventromedial prefrontal cortex. *Developmental Psychology*, 40(6), 1148–1158.

Huttenlocher, P. (1979). Synaptic density of human frontal cortex: Developmental changes and effects of aging. *Brain Research*, 163, 195–205.

Ikemoto, S., & Panksepp, J. (1999). The role of nucleus accumbens dopamine in motivated behavior: A unifying interpretation with special reference to reward-seeking. *Brain Research Reviews*, 31(1), 6–41.

Irwin, C. E., Jr. (1989). Risk taking behaviors in the adolescent patient: Are they impulsive? *Pediatric Annals*, 18, 122–133.

Irwin, C. E., Jr., & Millstein, S. G. (1992). Correlates and predictors of risk-taking behavior during adolescence. In L. P. Lipsitt & L. L. Mitnick (Eds.), *Self-regulatory behavior and risk taking: Causes and consequences* (pp. 3–21). Norwood, NJ: Ablex.

Jessor, R., Donovan, J. E., & Costa, F. (1996). Personality, perceived life chances, and adolescent behavior. In K. Hurrelmann & S. F. Hamilton (Eds.), *Social problems and social contexts in adolescence* (pp. 219–233). New York: Aldine de Gruyter.

Johnston, L. D., O'Malley, P. M., & Bachman, J. G. (2002). *Monitoring the future: National survey results on drug use, 1975–2001: Vol. I. Secondary school students* (NIH Publication No. 02-5106). Bethesda, MD: National Institute on Drug Abuse.

Keane, B. (1990). Dispersal and inbreeding avoidance in the white-footed mouse, *Peromyscus leucopus*. *Animal Behaviour*, 40, 143–152.

Kellogg, C. K., Awatramani, G. B., & Piekut, D. T. (1998). Adolescent development alters stressor-induced Fos immunoreactivity in rat brain. *Neuroscience*, 83(3), 681–689.

Killgore, W. D. S., Oki, M., & Yurgelun-Todd, D. A. (2001). Sex-specific developmental changes in amygdala responses to affective faces. *NeuroReport*, 12(2), 427–433.

Killgore, W. D. S., & Yurgelun-Todd, D. A. (2004). Sex-related developmental differences in the lateralized activation of the prefrontal cortex and amygdala during perception of facial affect. *Perceptual and Motor Skills*, 99(2), 371–391.

Kim, S. -G., Ugurbil, K., & Strick, P. L. (1994). Activation of a cerebellar output nucleus during cognitive processing. *Science*, 265, 949–951.

Koob, G. F., & Le Moal, M. (2001). Drug addiction, dysregulation of reward, and allostasis. *Neuropsychopharmacology*, 24, 97–129.

Lancaster, F. E., Brown, T. D., Coker, K. L., Elliott, J. A., & Wren, S. B. (1996). Sex differences in alcohol preference and drinking patterns emerge during the early postpubertal period in Sprague–Dawley rats. *Alcoholism: Clinical and Experimental Research*, 20(6), 1043–1049.

Larson, R., & Richards, M. H. (1994). *Divergent realities: The emotional lives of mothers, fathers, and adolescents*. New York: Basic Books.

Laursen, B., Coy, K. C., & Collins, W. A. (1998). Reconsidering changes in parent–child conflict across adolescence: A meta-analysis. *Child Development*, 69(3), 817–832.

Lerner, R. M., & Galambos, N. L. (1998). Adolescent development: Challenges and opportunities for research, programs, and policies. *Annual Review of Psychology*, 49, 413–446.

Leslie, C. A., Robertson, M. W., Cutler, A. J., & Bennett, J. P., Jr. (1991). Postnatal development of D_1 dopamine receptors in the medial prefrontal cortex, striatum and nucleus accumbens of normal and neonatal 6-hydroxydopamine treated rats: A quantitative autoradiographic analysis. *Developmental Brain Research*, 62(1), 109–114.

Levisohn, L., Cronin-Golomb, A., & Schmahmann, J. D. (2000). Neuropsychological consequences of cerebellar tumour resection in children: Cerebellar cognitive affective syndrome in a paediatric population. *Brain*, 123, 1041–1050.

Levy, D., Gray-Donald, K., Leech, J., Zvagulis, I., & Pless, I. B. (1986). Sleep patterns and problems in adolescents. *Journal of Adolescent Health Care*, 7, 386–389.

Luna, B., Thulborn, K. R., Munoz, D. P., Merriam, E. P., Garver, K. E., Minshew, N. J., et al. (2001). Maturation of widely distributed brain function subserves cognitive development. *NeuroImage*, 13(5), 786–793.

Maggs, J. L., Almeida, D. M., & Galambos, N. L. (1995). Risky business: The paradoxical meaning of problem behavior for young adolescents. *Journal of Early Adolescence*, 15, 344–362.

Martin, C. A., Kelly, T. H., Rayens, M. K., Brogli, B. R., Brenzel, A., Smith, W. J., et al. (2002). Sensation seeking, puberty, and nicotine, alcohol, and marijuana use in adolescence. *Journal of the American Academy of Child and Adolescent Psychiatry, 41*(12), 1495–1502.

McBride, W. J., Bell, R. L., Rodd, Z. A., Strother, W. N., & Murphy, J. M. (2005). Adolescent alcohol drinking and its long-range consequences: Studies with animal models. In M. Galanter (Ed.), *Recent developments in alcoholism: Vol. 17. Alcohol problems in adolescents and young adults* (pp. 123–142). Hingham, MA: Kluwer.

McCarthy, J. D., & Hoge, D. R. (1984). The dynamics of self-esteem and delinquency. *American Journal of Sociology, 90,* 396–410.

McClure, E. B., Monk, C. S., Nelson, E. E., Zarahn, E., Leibenluft, E., Bilder, R. M., et al. (2004). A developmental examination of gender differences in brain engagement during evaluation of threat. *Biological Psychiatry, 55*(11), 1047–1055.

McCord, J. (1990). Problem behaviors. In S. S. Feldman & G. R. Elliott (Eds.), *At the threshold: The developing adolescent* (pp. 414–430). Cambridge, MA: Harvard University Press.

Merola, J. L., & Liederman, J. (1985). Developmental changes in hemispheric independence. *Child Development, 56,* 1184–1194.

Middleton, F. A., & Strick, P. L. (2000). Basal ganglia and cerebellar loops: Motor and cognitive circuits. *Brain Research Reviews, 31,* 236–250.

Middleton, F. A., & Strick, P. L. (2001). Cerebellar projections to the prefrontal cortex of the primate. *Journal of Neuroscience, 21*(2), 700–712.

Millstein, S. G. (1993). Perceptual, attributional, and affective processes in perceptions of vulnerability through the life span. In N. J. Bell & R. W. Bell (Eds.), *Adolescent risk taking* (pp. 55–65). Newbury Park, CA: Sage.

Moffitt, T. E. (1993). Adolescence-limited and life-course-persistent antisocial behavior: A developmental taxonomy. *Psychological Review, 100,* 674–701.

Moltz, H. (1975). The search for the determinants of puberty in the rat. In B. E. Eleftheriou & R. L. Sprott (Eds.), *Hormonal correlates of behavior: A lifespan view* (pp. 35–154). New York: Plenum Press.

Moore, J. M. (1992). Dispersal, nepotism, and primate social behavior. *International Journal of Primatology, 13,* 361–378.

Muuss, R. E., & Porton, H. D. (1998). *Increasing risk behavior among adolescents.* Boston: McGraw-Hill College.

Nance, D. M. (1983). The developmental and neural determinants of the effects of estrogen on feed behavior in the rat: A theoretical perspective. *Neuroscience and Biobehavioral Reviews, 7*(2), 189–211.

Paus, T. (2005). Mapping brain maturation and cognitive development during adolescence. *Trends in Cognitive Sciences, 9*(2), 60–68.

Petersen, A. C. (1998). Adolescence. In E. A. Blechman & K. D. Brownell (Eds.), *Behavioral medicine and women: A comprehensive handbook* (pp. 45–50). New York: Guilford Press.

Petersen, A. C., Silbereisen, R. K., & Sorensen, S. (1996). Adolescent development: A global perspective. In K. Hurrelmann & S. F. Hamilton (Eds.), *Social problems and social contexts in adolescence* (pp. 3–37). New York: Aldine de Gruyter.

Pine, D. S., Grun, J., Maguire, E. A., Burgess, N., Zarahn, E., Koda, V., et al. (2002). Neurodevelopmental aspects of spatial navigation: A virtual reality fMRI study. *NeuroImage, 15*(2), 396–406.

Pine, D. S., Grun, J., Zarahn, E., Fyer, A., Koda, V., Li, W., et al. (2001). Cortical brain regions engaged by masked emotional faces in adolescents and adults: An fMRI study. *Emotion, 1*(2), 137–147.

Post, G. B., & Kemper, H. C. G. (1993). Nutrient intake and biological maturation during adolescence: The Amsterdam Growth and Health Longitudinal Study. *European Journal of Clinical Nutrition, 47*(6), 400–408.

Rakic, P., Bourgeois, J. -P., & Goldman-Rakic, P. S. (1994). Synaptic development of the cerebral cortex: Implications for learning, memory, and mental illness. In J. van Pelt, M. A. Corner, M. B. M. Uylings, & F. H. Lopes da Silva (Vol. Eds.), *Progress in brain research: Vol. 102. The self-organizing brain: From growth cones to functional networks* (pp. 227–243). Amsterdam: Elsevier.

Rapoport, J. L., Giedd, J. N., Blumenthal, J., Hamburger, S., Jeffries, N., Fernandez, T., et al. (1999). Progressive cortical change during adolescence in childhood-onset schizophrenia. *Archives of General Psychiatry, 56*, 649–654.

Rema, V., & Ebner, F. F. (1999) Effect of enriched environment rearing on impairments in cortical excitability and plasticity after prenatal alcohol exposure. *Journal of Neuroscience, 19*, 10993–11006.

Resnick, M. D., Bearman, P. S., Blum, R. W., Bauman, K. E., Harris, K. M., Jones, J., et al. (1997). Protecting adolescents from harm: Findings from the National Longitudinal Study on Adolescent Health. *Journal of the American Medical Association, 278*(10), 823–832.

Romeo, R. D., Richardson, H. N., & Sisk, C. L. (2002). Puberty and the maturation of the male brain and sexual behavior: Recasting a behavioral potential. *Neuroscience and Biobehavioral Reviews, 26*(3), 381–391.

Rubia, K., Overmeyer, S., Taylor, E., Brammer, M., Williams, S. C. R., Simmons, A., et al. (2000). Functional frontalisation with age: Mapping neurodevelopmental trajectories with fMRI. *Neuroscience and Biobehavioral Reviews, 24*(1), 13–19.

Savin-Williams, R. C., & Weisfeld, G. E. (1989). An ethological perspective on adolescence. In G. R. Adams, R. Montemayor, & T. P. Gullotta (Eds.), *Biology of adolescent behavior and development* (pp. 249–274). Newbury Park, CA: Sage.

Schaefer, A., Collette, F., Philippot, P., Vander-Linden, M., Laureys, S., Delfiore, G., et al. (2003). Neural correlates of "hot" and "cold" emotional processing: A multilevel approach to the functional anatomy of emotion. *NeuroImage, 18*(4), 938–949.

Schlegel, A., & Barry, H., III. (1991). *Adolescence: An anthropological inquiry.* New York: Free Press.

Schmahmann, J. D., & Sherman, J. C. (1998). The cerebellar cognitive affective syndrome. *Brain, 121*, 561–579.

Seeman, P., Bzowej, N. H., Guan, H.-C., Bergeron, C., Becker, L. E., Reynolds, G. P., et al. (1987). Human brain dopamine receptors in children and aging adults. *Synapse, 1*, 399–404.

Segalowitz, S. J., & Davies, P. L. (2004). Charting the maturation of the frontal lobe: An electrophysiological strategy. *Brain and Cognition, 55*(1), 116–133.

Shedler, J., & Block, J. (1990). Adolescent drug use and psychological health: A longitudinal inquiry. *American Psychologist, 45*(5), 612–630.

Short, R. V. (1976). The evolution of human reproduction. *Proceedings of the Royal Society of London Series B, 195*(1118), 3–24.

Silbereisen, R. K., & Reitzle, M. (1992). On the constructive role of problem behavior in adolescence: Further evidence on alcohol use. In L. P. Lipsitt & L. L. Mitnick (Eds.), *Self-regulatory behavior and risk taking: Causes and consequences* (pp. 199–217). Norwood, NJ: Ablex.

Smith, E. A., Udry, J. R., & Morris, N. M. (1985). Pubertal development and friends: A biosocial explanation of adolescent sexual behavior. *Journal of Health and Social Behavior, 26,* 183–192.

Smith, R. F. (2003). Animal models of periadolescent substance abuse. *Neurotoxicology and Teratology, 25,* 291–301.

Sowell, E. R., Peterson, B. S., Thompson, P. M., Welcome, S. E., Henkenius, A. L., & Toga, A. W. (2003). Mapping cortical change across the human life span. *Nature Neuroscience, 6*(3), 309–315.

Sowell, E. R., Thompson, P.M., Holmes, C. J., Bath, R., Jernigan, T. L., & Toga, A. W. (1999). Localizing age-related changes in brain structure between childhood and adolescence using statistical parametric mapping. *NeuroImage, 9*(6), 587–598.

Spanagel, R., & Weiss, F. (1999). The dopamine hypothesis of reward: Past and current status. *Trends in Neuroscience, 22*(11), 521–527.

Spear, L. P. (2000). The adolescent brain and age-related behavioral manifestations. *Neuroscience and Behavioral Physiology, 24*(4), 417–463.

Spear, L. P., & Varlinskaya, E. I. (2004). Adolescence: Alcohol sensitivity, tolerance, and intake. In M. Galanter (Ed.), *Recent developments in alcoholism: Vol. 17. Alcohol problems in adolescents and young adults* (pp. 143–159). Hingham, MA: Kluwer.

Steinberg, L. (1987). Impact of puberty on family relations: Effects of pubertal status and pubertal timing. *Developmental Psychology, 23*(3), 451–460.

Steinberg, L. (1988). Reciprocal relation between parent–child distance and pubertal maturation. *Developmental Psychology, 24*(1), 122–128.

Steinberg, L. (1989). Pubertal maturation and parent–adolescent distance: An evolutionary perspective. In G. R. Adams, R. Montemayor, & T. P. Gullotta (Eds.), *Advances in adolescent behavior and development* (pp. 71–97). Newbury Park, CA: Sage.

Steinberg, L. (2005). Cognitive and affective development in adolescence. *Trends in Cognitive Sciences, 9*(2), 69–74.

Steinberg, L., & Belsky, J. (1996). An evolutionary perspective on psychopathology in adolescence. In D. Cicchetti & S. L. Toth (Eds.), *Adolescence: Opportunities and challenges* (pp. 93–124). Rochester, NY: University of Rochester Press.

Steinberg, L., & Cauffman, E. (1996). Maturity of judgement in adolescence:

Psychosocial factors in adolescent decision making. *Law and Human Behavior, 20*(3), 249–272.

Swanson, L. W., & Petrovich, G. D. (1998). What is the amygdala? *Trends in Neurosciences, 21*(8), 323–331.

Tapert, S. F., & Schweinsburg, A. D. (2005). The human adolescent brain and alcohol use disorders. In M. Galanter (Ed.), *Recent developments in alcoholism: Vol. 17. Alcohol problems in adolescents and young adults* (pp. 177–197). Hingham, MA: Kluwer.

Tarazi, F. I., & Baldessarini, R. J. (2000). Comparative postnatal development of dopamine D_1, D_2, and D_4 receptors in rat forebrain. *International Journal of Developmental Neuroscience, 18*(1), 29–37.

Tarazi, F. I., Tomasini, E. C., & Baldessarini, R. J. (1998). Postnatal development of dopamine D_4-like receptors in rat forebrain regions: Comparison with D_2-like receptors. *Developmental Brain Research, 110,* 227–233.

Tarazi, F. I., Tomasini, E. C., & Baldessarini, R. J. (1999). Postnatal development of dopamine D_1-like receptors in rat cortical and striatolimbic brain regions: An autoradiographic study. *Developmental Neuroscience, 21,* 43–49.

Teicher, M. H., Andersen, S. L., & Hostetter, J. C., Jr. (1995). Evidence for dopamine receptor pruning between adolescence and adulthood in striatum but not nucleus accumbens. *Developmental Brain Research, 89,* 167–172.

Teicher, M. H., Barber, N. I., Gelbard, H. A., Gallitano, A. L., Campbell, A., Marsh, E., et al. (1993). Developmental differences in acute nigrostriatal and mesocorticolimbic system response to haloperidol. *Neuropsychopharmacology, 9*(2), 147–156.

Terasawa, E., & Fernandez, D. L. (2001). Neurobiological mechanisms of the onset of puberty in primates. *Endocrine Reviews, 22*(1), 111–151.

Terasawa, E., & Timiras, P. S. (1968). Electrophysiological study of the limbic system in the rat at onset of puberty. *American Journal of Physiology, 215*(6), 1462–1467.

Thomas, K. M., Drevets, W. C., Whalen, P. J., Eccard, C. H., Dahl, R. E., Ryan, N. D., et al. (2001). Amygdala response to facial expressions in children and adults. *Biological Psychiatry, 49,* 309–316.

Trimpop, R. M., Kerr, J. H., & Kirkcaldy, B. (1999). Comparing personality constructs of risk-taking behavior. *Personality and Individual Differences, 26*(2), 237–254.

Udry, J. R., Talbert, L. M., & Morris, N. M. (1986). Biosocial foundations for adolescent female sexuality. *Demography, 23*(2), 217–230.

Volkow, N. D., Fowler, J. S., & Wang, G.-J. (2002). Role of dopamine in drug reinforcement and addiction in humans: Results from imaging studies. *Behavioural Pharmacology, 13*(5–6), 355–366.

Wallen, K. (2001). Sex and context: Hormones and primate sexual motivation. *Hormones and Behavior, 40,* 339–357.

Wilkinson, L. S. (1997). The nature of interactions involving prefrontal and striatal dopamine systems. *Journal of Psychopharmacology, 11,* 143–150.

Williams, B. R., Ponesse, J. S., Schachar, R. J., Logan, G. D., & Tannock, R.

(1999). Development of inhibitory control across the life span. *Developmental Psychology, 35*(1), 205–213.

Wilson, D. M., Killen, J. D., Hayward, C., Robinson, T. N., Hammer, L. D., Kraemer, H. C., et al. (1994). Timing and rate of sexual maturation and the onset of cigarette and alcohol use among teenage girls. *Archives of Pediatrics and Adolescent Medicine, 148,* 789–795.

Wilson, M., & Daly, M. (1985). Competitiveness, risk taking, and violence: The young male syndrome. *Ethology and Sociobiology, 6,* 59–73.

Windle, M., & Windle, R. C. (2005). Alcohol consumption and its consequences among adolescents and young adults. In M. Galanter (Ed.), *Recent developments in alcoholism: Vol. 17. Alcohol problems in adolescents and young adults* (pp. 67–83). Hingham, MA: Kluwer.

Woo, T.-U., Pucak, M. L., Kye, C. H., Matus, C. V., & Lewis, D. A. (1997). Peripubertal refinement of the intrinsic and associational circuitry in monkey prefrontal cortex. *Neuroscience, 80*(4), 1149–1158.

Worthman, C. M. (1999). Epidemiology of human development. In C. Panter-Brick & C. M. Worthman (Eds.), *Hormones, health, and behavior: A socioecological and lifespan perspective* (pp. 47–104). New York: Cambridge University Press.

Yurgelun-Todd, D. A., Killgore, W. D. S., & Cintron, C. B. (2003). Cognitive correlates of medial temporal lobe development across adolescence: A magnetic resonance imaging study. *Perceptual and Motor Skills, 96,* 3–17.

Zald, D. H. (2003). The human amygdala and the emotional evaluation of sensory stimuli. *Brain Research Reviews, 41*(1), 88–123.

Zald, D. H., Donndelinger, M. J., & Pardo, J. V. (1998). Elucidating dynamic brain interactions with across-subjects correlational analyses of positron emission tomographic data: The functional connectivity of the amygdala and orbitofrontal cortex during olfactory tasks. *Journal of Cerebral Blood Flow and Metabolism, 18,* 896–905.

Zimmermann, A., Stauffacher, M., Langhans, W., & Wurbel, H. (2001). Enrichment-dependent differences in novelty exploration in rats can be explained by habituation. *Behavioural Brain Research, 121,* 11–20.

Zuckerman, M. (1992). Sensation seeking: The balance between risk and reward. In L. P. Lipsitt & L. L. Mitnick (Eds.), *Self-regulatory behavior and risk taking* (pp. 143–152). Norwood, NJ: Ablex.

Index

Page numbers followed by *f* indicate figure, *t* indicate table

397